SKILLS CHECKLISTS TO /

MW00837458

Delmar's
FUNDAMENTAL & ADVANCED
NURSING SKILLS

SECOND EDITION

Prepared by
Kathie Doyle, RN, MS
Nursing Faculty
Excelsior College School of Nursing
Albany, New York

THOMSON

DELMAR LEARNING

Australia   Canada   Mexico   Singapore   Spain   United Kingdom   United States

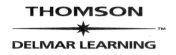

THOMSON

DELMAR LEARNING

Skills Checklist to Accompany
Delmar's Fundamental & Advanced Nursing Skills, 2e
by Gaylene Bouska Altman, RN, PhD, prepared by Kathie Doyle, RN, MS

VP of Healthcare SBU:
William Brottmiller

Editorial Director:
Cathy L. Esperti

Developmental Editor:
Patricia Gaworecki

Marketing Director:
Jennifer McAvey

Channel Manager:
Tamara Caruso

Editorial Assistant:
Patricia M. Osborn

Project Editor:
Jennifer Luck

Art/Design Coordinator:
Robert Plante

Production Coordinator:
Kenneth McGrath

Library of Congress Cataloging-in-Publication Data

ISBN 1-4018-8123-8

International Divisions List

Asia (Including India):
Thomson Learning
60 Albert Street, #15–01
Albert Complex
Singapore 189969
Tel 65 336–6411
Fax 65 336–7411

Australia/New Zealand:
Nelson
102 Dodds Street
South Melbourne
Victoria 3205
Australia
Tel 61 (0)3 9685–4111
Fax 61 (0)3 9685–4199

Latin America:
Thomson Learning
Seneca 53
Colonia Polanco
11560 Mexico, D.F. Mexico
Tel (525) 281–2906
Fax (525) 281–2656

Canada:
Nelson
1120 Birchmount Road
Toronto, Ontario
Canada M1K 5G4
Tel (416) 752–9100
Fax (416) 752–8102

UK/Europe/Middle East/Africa:
Thomson Learning
Berkshire House
1680–173 High Holborn
London WC1V 7AA
United Kingdom
Tel 44 (0)20 497–1422
Fax 44 (0)20 497–1426

Spain (includes Portugal):
Paraninfo
Calle Magallanes 25
28015 Madrid
España
Tel 34 (0)91 446–3350
Fax 34 (0)91 445–6218

Notice to the Reader

Publisher does not warrant or guarantee any of the products described herein or perform any independent analysis in connection with any of the product information contained herein. Publisher does not assume, and expressly disclaims, any obligation to obtain and include information other than that provided to it by the manufacturer.

The reader is expressly warned to consider and adopt all safety precautions that might be indicated by the activities described herein and to avoid all potential hazards. By following the instructions contained herein, the reader willingly assumes all risks in connection with such instructions.

The publisher makes no representations or warranties of any kind, including but not limited to, the warranties of fitness for particular purpose or merchantability, nor are any such representations implied with respect to the material set forth herein, and the publisher takes no responsibility with respect to such material. The publisher shall not be liable for any special, consequential, or exemplary damages resulting, in whole or part, from the reader's use of, or reliance upon, this material.

CONTENTS

Preface   vii

CHAPTER 1 • PHYSICAL ASSESSMENT

1-1   Physical Assessment   1
1-2   Taking a Temperature   15
1-3   Taking a Pulse   23
1-4   Counting Respirations   27
1-5   Taking Blood Pressure   29
1-6   Weighing a Client, Mobile and Immobile 33
1-7   Measuring Intake and Output   37
1-8   Breast Self-Examination   41
1-9   Male Genitalia, Hernia, and
      Rectal Examination   45
1-10 Collecting a Clean Catch, Midstream
      Urine Specimen   49
1-11 Testing Urine for Specific Gravity, Ketones,
      Glucose, and Occult Blood   53
1-12 Performing a Skin Puncture   57
1-13 Measuring Blood Glucose Levels   61
1-14 Collecting Nose, Throat, and Sputum
      Specimens   65
1-15 Testing for Occult Blood with a
      Hemoccult Slide   71

CHAPTER 2 • SAFETY AND INFECTION CONTROL

2-1   Proper Body Mechanics, Safe Lifting,
      and Transferring   75
2-2   Assisting with Ambulation and
      Safe Falling   79

2-3   Applying Restraints   83
2-4   Handwashing   87
2-5   Donning and Removing Clean
      and Contaminated Gloves, Cap,
      and Mask   89
2-6   Removing Contaminated Items   93
2-7   Applying Sterile Gloves via the
      Open Method   97
2-8   Surgical Scrub   99
2-9   Applying Sterile Gloves and Gown
      via the Closed Method   103
2-10 Emergency Airway Management   105
2-11 Administering Cardiopulmonary
      Resuscitation (CPR)   107
2-12 Performing the Heimlich Maneuver   113
2-13 Responding to Accidental Poisoning   119
2-14 Emergency Client Transport   121

CHAPTER 3 • CLIENT CARE AND COMFORT

3-1   The Effective Communication Process   127
3-2   Guided Imagery   131
3-3   Progressive Muscle Relaxation   133
3-4   Therapeutic Massage   135
3-5   Applying Moist Heat   139
3-6   Warm Soaks and Sitz Baths   143
3-7   Applying Dry Heat   145
3-8   Using a Thermal Blanket and an
      Infant Radiant Heat Warmer   149
3-9   Applying Cold Treatment   153
3-10 Assisting with a Transcutaneous Electrical
      Nerve Stimulation (TENS) Unit   155

CHAPTER 4 • BASIC CARE

4-1   Changing Linens in an Unoccupied Bed   159
4-2   Changing Linens in an Occupied Bed   165
4-3   Turning and Positioning a Client   167
4-4   Moving a Client in Bed   171
4-5   Assisting with a Bedpan or Urinal   175
4-6   Assisting with Feeding   179
4-7   Bathing a Client in Bed   181
4-8   Oral Care   185
4-9   Perineal and Genital Care   191
4-10   Eye Care   195
4-11   Hair and Scalp Care   201
4-12   Hand and Foot Care   205
4-13   Shaving a Client   209
4-14   Giving a Back Rub   211
4-15   Changing the IV Gown   213
4-16   Assisting from Bed to Stretcher   217
4-17   Assisting from Bed to Wheelchair, Commode, or Chair   221
4-18   Assisting from Bed to Walking   225
4-19   Using a Hydraulic Lift   227
4-20   Administering Preoperative Care   231
4-21   Preparing a Surgical Site   235
4-22   Administering Immediate Postoperative Care   239
4-23   Postoperative Exercise Instruction   243
4-24   Administering Passive Range of Motion (ROM) Exercises   247
4-25   Postmortem Care   251

CHAPTER 5 • MEDICATION ADMINISTRATION

5-1   Administering Oral, Sublingual, and Buccal Medications   255
5-2   Administering Eye and Ear Medications   259
5-3   Administering Skin/Topical Medications   265
5-4   Administering Nasal Medications   269
5-5   Administering Rectal Medications   271
5-6   Administering Vaginal Medications   275
5-7   Administering Nebulized Medications   279
5-8   Administering an Intradermal Injection   285
5-9   Administering a Subcutaneous Injection   289
5-10   Administering an Intramuscular Injection   293
5-11   Administering Medication via Z-track Injection   297
5-12   Withdrawing Medication from a Vial   301
5-13   Withdrawing Medication from an Ampule   305
5-14   Mixing Medications from Two Vials into One Syringe   309
5-15   Preparing an IV Solution   313
5-16   Adding Medications to an IV Solution   317
5-17   Administering Medications via Secondary Administration Sets (Piggyback)   321
5-18   Administering Medications via IV Bolus or IV Push   325
5-19   Administering Medications via Volume-Control Sets   329
5-20   Administering Medication via a Cartridge System   333
5-21   Administering Patient-Controlled Analgesia (PCA)   335
5-22   Administering Epidural Analgesia   337
5-23   Managing Controlled Substances   341

CHAPTER 6 • NUTRITION AND ELIMINATION

6-1   Inserting and Maintaining a Nasogastric Tube   345
6-2   Assessing Placement of a Large-Bore Feeding Tube   349
6-3   Assessing Placement of a Small-Bore Feeding Tube   351
6-4   Removing a Nasogastric Tube   353
6-5   Feeding and Medicating via a Gastrostomy Tube   357
6-6   Maintaining Gastrointestinal Suction Devices   361
6-7   Applying a Condom Catheter   363
6-8   Inserting an Indwelling Catheter: Male   367
6-9   Inserting an Indwelling Catheter: Female   371
6-10   Routine Catheter Care   375
6-11   Obtaining a Residual Urine Specimen from an Indwelling Catheter   377
6-12   Irrigating a Urinary Catheter   379
6-13   Irrigating the Bladder Using a Closed-System Catheter   383
6-14   Removing an Indwelling Catheter   387
6-15   Catheterizing a Noncontinent Urinary Diversion   391
6-16   Maintaining a Continent Urinary Diversion   395
6-17   Pouching a Noncontinent Urinary Diversion   399
6-18   Administering Peritoneal Dialysis   403
6-19   Administering an Enema   407

6-20   Digital Removal of Fecal Impaction   413
6-21   Inserting a Rectal Tube   417
6-22   Irrigating and Cleaning a Stoma   419
6-23   Changing a Bowel Diversion Ostomy
Appliance: Pouching a Stoma   423

CHAPTER 7 • OXYGENATION

7-1   Administering Oxygen Therapy   427
7-2   Assisting a Client with Controlled
Coughing and Deep Breathing   431
7-3   Assisting a Client with an Incentive
Spirometer   435
7-4   Administering Pulmonary Therapy and
Postural Drainage   437
7-5   Administering Pulse Oximetry   439
7-6   Measuring Peak Expiratory Flow Rates   441
7-7   Administering Intermittent Positive-
Pressure Breathing (IPPB)   445
7-8   Assisting with Continuous Positive
Airway Pressure (CPAP)   447
7-9   Preparing the Chest Drainage System   449
7-10   Maintaining the Chest Tube and Chest
Drainage System   453
7-11   Measuring the Output from a Chest
Drainage System   457
7-12   Obtaining a Specimen from a Chest
Drainage System   459
7-13   Removing a Chest Tube   461
7-14   Ventilating the Client with an Ambu Bag®   463
7-15   Inserting the Pharyngeal Airway   467
7-16   Maintaining Mechanical Ventilation   469
7-17   Suctioning Endotracheal and Tracheal
Tubes   471
7-18   Maintaining and Cleaning Endotracheal
Tubes   475
7-19   Maintaining and Cleaning the
Tracheostomy Tube   477
7-20   Maintaining a Double Cannula
Tracheostomy Tube   481
7-21   Plugging the Tracheostomy Tube   485

CHAPTER 8 • CIRCULATORY

8-1   Performing Venipuncture (Blood Drawing)   487
8-2   Starting an IV   491
8-3   Inserting a Butterfly Needle   495
8-4   Preparing the IV Bag and Tubing   499
8-5   Setting the IV Flow Rate   503
8-6   Assessing and Maintaining an IV
Insertion Site   505
8-7   Changing the IV Solution   509
8-8   Discontinuing the IV and Changing to a
Saline or Heparin Lock   511
8-9   Administering a Blood Transfusion   515
8-10   Assessing and Responding to Transfusion
Reactions   519
8-11   Assisting with the Insertion of a
Central Venous Catheter   523
8-12   Changing the Central Venous Dressing   525
8-13   Changing the Central Venous Tubing   529
8-14   Flushing a Central Venous Catheter   531
8-15   Measuring Central Venous
Pressure (CVP)   533
8-16   Drawing Blood from a Central
Venous Catheter   537
8-17   Infusing Total Parenteral Nutrition
(TPN) and Fat Emulsion through a
Central Venous Catheter   541
8-18   Removing the Central Venous Catheter   543
8-19   Inserting a Peripherally Inserted Central
Catheter (PICC)   545
8-20   Administering Peripheral Vein Total
Parenteral Nutrition   551
8-21   Hemodialysis Site Care   555
8-22   Using an Implantable Venous Access
Device   559
8-23   Caring for an Implanted Venous Access
Device   563
8-24   Obtaining an Arterial Blood Gas
Specimen   567
8-25   Assisting with the Insertion and
Maintenance of an Epidural Catheter   571

CHAPTER 9 • SKIN INTEGRITY AND WOUND CARE

9-1   Bandaging   573
9-2   Applying a Dry Dressing   577
9-3   Applying a Wet to Damp Dressing
(Wet to Dry to Moist Dressing)   581
9-4   Applying a Transparent Dressing   585
9-5   Applying a Pressure Bandage   587
9-6   Changing Dressings around Therapeutic
Puncture Sites   589
9-7   Irrigating a Wound   593
9-8   Packing a Wound   595

9-9   Cleaning and Dressing a Wound
with an Open Drain 599

9-10 Dressing a Wound with Retention Sutures 603

9-11 Obtaining a Wound Drainage Specimen
for Culturing 607

9-12 Maintaining a Closed Wound
Drainage System 609

9-13 Care of the Jackson-Pratt (JP) Drain Site
and Emptying the Drain Bulb 613

9-14 Removing Skin Sutures and Staples 617

9-15 Preventing and Managing the
Pressure Ulcer 621

9-16 Managing Irritated Peristomal Skin 625

9-17 Pouching a Draining Wound 629

CHAPTER 10 • IMMOBILIZATION AND SUPPORT

10-1 Applying an Elastic Bandage 633

10-2 Applying a Splint 635

10-3 Applying an Arm Sling 637

10-4 Applying Antiembolic Stockings 639

10-5 Applying a Pneumatic Compression
Device 641

10-6 Applying Abdominal, T-, or Breast Binders 643

10-7 Applying Skin Traction—Adhesive and
Nonadhesive 645

10-8 Maintaining and Monitoring
Skeletal Traction 649

10-9 External Fixation or Skeletal
Pin Care 653

10-10 Assisting with Casting—Plaster and
Fiberglass 655

10-11 Cast Care and Comfort 659

10-12 Cast Bivalving and Windowing 661

10-13 Cast Removal 663

10-14 Assisting with a Continuous Passive
Motion Device 665

10-15 Assisting with Crutches, Cane,
or Walker 669

CHAPTER 11 • SPECIAL PROCEDURE

11-1 Administering an Electrocardiogram 675

11-2 Magnetic Resonance Imaging (MRI) 677

11-3 Assisting with Computed Tomography
(CT) Scanning 679

11-4 Assisting with a Liver Biopsy 681

11-5 Assisting with a Thoracentesis 685

11-6 Assisting with an Abdominal
Paracentesis 689

11-7 Assisting with a Bone Marrow Biopsy/
Aspiration 693

11-8 Assisting with a Lumbar Puncture 695

11-9 Assisting with Amniocentesis 699

11-10 Assisting with Bronchoscopy 701

11-11 Assisting with Gastrointestinal
Endoscopy 707

11-12 Assisting with a Proctosigmoidoscopy 711

11-13 Assisting with Arteriography 715

11-14 Positron-Emission Tomography
Scanning 717

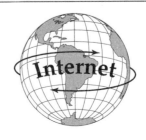

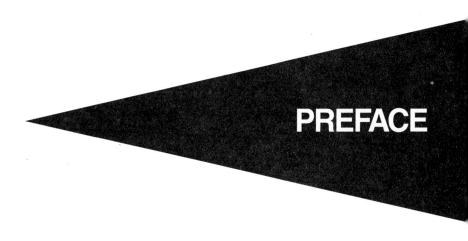

PREFACE

The skills checklists in this manual are summaries of the step-by-step procedures in *Delmar's Fundamental & Advanced Nursing Skills 2e* textbook. They are arranged according to the first three steps of the nursing process:

- Assessment
- Planning/Expected Outcomes
- Implementation

Each checklist follows the procedure as described in the textbook. To use the skills checklists more effectively, the student should refer to the procedure first, then "practice," referring to the checklist.

When students are evaluated using the checklists, there are three categories to document their performances of the skills: "Able to Perform," "Able to Perform with Assistance," or "Unable to Perform." These categories lend themselves to the college laboratory setting as well as to the clinical setting, where students may perform procedures with faculty assistance.

Checklist for Procedure 1-1   Physical Assessment

Name _____ Date _____

School _____

Instructor _____

Course _____

Procedure 1-1 Physical Assessment	Able to Perform	Able to Perform with Assistance	Unable to Perform	Initials and Date
Assessment				
1. Assess the environment, resources, and client's medical condition. *Comments:*	☐	☐	☐	
2. Assess the client's history of previous physical assessments and the availability of previous data. *Comments:*	☐	☐	☐	
3. Assess the client's receptiveness to being examined. *Comments:*	☐	☐	☐	
4. Assess the client's understanding of the procedure. *Comments:*	☐	☐	☐	
Planning/Expected Outcomes				
1. Identify health parameters. *Comments:*	☐	☐	☐	
2. Identify findings that require immediate attention. *Comments:*	☐	☐	☐	
3. Identify abnormalities that need planned intervention. *Comments:*	☐	☐	☐	
4. Monitor chronic stable problems to detect changes. *Comments:*	☐	☐	☐	
5. Identify health risks, concerns, or needs. *Comments:*	☐	☐	☐	
6. Respond to health maintenance needs. *Comments:*	☐	☐	☐	

continued on the following page

continued from the previous page

Procedure 1-1	Able to Perform	Able to Perform with Assistance	Unable to Perform	Initials and Date
Implementation				
Preparation				
1. Organize equipment. *Comments:*	☐	☐	☐	
2. Review client medical history. *Comments:*	☐	☐	☐	
3. Wash hands, preferably in front of client. *Comments:*	☐	☐	☐	
4. Explain the plan and procedure. *Comments:*	☐	☐	☐	
5. Assist client to sitting position, if possible. *Comments:*	☐	☐	☐	
6. Examine client. *Comments:*	☐	☐	☐	
7. Present findings, if appropriate. Ask for additional information. Answer client's questions. *Comments:*	☐	☐	☐	
8. Schedule follow-up assessments, tests, or other appointments as needed. *Comments:*	☐	☐	☐	
9. Clean, replace, and discard equipment appropriately. *Comments:*	☐	☐	☐	
10. Wash hands. *Comments:*	☐	☐	☐	
Measurements and Overall Observations 11. Obtain baseline measurements and compare with normal data. Check height, weight, head circumference (for infants to 24 months), and temperature. *Comments:*	☐	☐	☐	

Procedure 1-1	Able to Perform	Able to Perform with Assistance	Unable to Perform	Initials and Date
12. Measure the heart rate, rhythm, and volume, the respiratory rate and rhythm, and the blood pressure bilaterally. *Comments:*	☐	☐	☐	
13. Check anthropometric measurements prn, body mass index (BMI), etc. *Comments:*	☐	☐	☐	
14. Assess the overall appearance of the client in a "once over" evaluation. *Comments:*	☐	☐	☐	
Skin, Hair, and Nails Examination 15. • Inspect: color, vascularity, lesions, ulcers, scars, hair distribution, nail shape and configuration, and nail bed angles. Measure, describe, draw, and/or stage abnormals. • Palpate: moisture, temperature, texture, turgor, capillary refill, and edema. *Comments:*	☐	☐	☐	
Head, Face, and Lymphatic Examination 16. Inspect and palpate the head, face, and lymph nodes. Proceed front to back. *Comments:*	☐	☐	☐	
17. Head: Examine scalp, hair, and cranium. Examine fontanelles and sutures in infants to 24 months. *Comments:*	☐	☐	☐	
18. Lymph nodes: Examine lymph nodes in head and neck. *Comments:*	☐	☐	☐	
19. Temporomandibular joint: Observe the motion of opening and closing the jaw. *Comments:*	☐	☐	☐	
20. Face: Observe for shape, symmetry, and expression. Assess tactile sensation over the trigeminal nerve sites and mandible bilaterally. *Comments:*	☐	☐	☐	

continued on the following page

continued from the previous page

Procedure 1-1	Able to Perform	Able to Perform with Assistance	Unable to Perform	Initials and Date
Eye, Ear, Nose, Mouth, and Throat Examination				
21. Examine the eyes. Inspect and palpate external structures. Inspect eye position and palpebral fissures. Examine conjunctivae, sclera, cornea, and iris. Assess for a corneal touch reflex. *Comments:*	☐	☐	☐	
22. Extraocular mobility: Check for Hirschberg's corneal light reflex. Check the six cardinal fields of gaze. Examine pupils, lens, and retinal structures. *Comments:*	☐	☐	☐	
23. Have the client identify an object, such as your finger, as it enters the visual fields from each of four directions. *Comments:*	☐	☐	☐	
24. Check for visual acuity, including near and far sight, primary colors, and Ishihara plates. *Comments:*	☐	☐	☐	
25. Examine the ears. Inspect and palpate the external ear. Observe the shape, color, and size of the ear. *Comments:*	☐	☐	☐	
26. Proceed with an otoscopic assessment, starting with the ear canal. Observe tympanic membrane movement. Use tympanometry, if needed, to confirm visual findings. *Comments:*	☐	☐	☐	
27. Check the client's hearing acuity. *Comments:*	☐	☐	☐	
28. Examine the nose. Inspect and palpate for nasal patency. Observe the external surface, nasal mucosa, turbinates, and septum. *Comments:*	☐	☐	☐	
29. Have the client identify common odors. *Comments:*	☐	☐	☐	

Procedure 1-1	Able to Perform	Able to Perform with Assistance	Unable to Perform	Initials and Date
30. Examine the mouth, including the teeth, tongue, and throat. *Comments:*	☐	☐	☐	
31. Inspect and count teeth. *Comments:*	☐	☐	☐	
32. Inspect and palpate lips and frenula, gums, buccal mucosa, tongue protrusion, salivary glands, hard and soft palates, tonsils, uvula position and movement, and arches. Inspect the naso-oropharynx. *Comments:*	☐	☐	☐	
33. Conduct gag reflex response, and taste tests for sweet, sour, bitter, and salt. *Comments:*	☐	☐	☐	
34. Examine the neck. Inspect and palpate the trachea. *Comments:*	☐	☐	☐	
35. Examine the thyroid. Identify tracheal rings, isthmus, thyroid cartilage, and gland lobes as the client is swallowing. *Comments:*	☐	☐	☐	
36. Palpate the temporal and carotid pulses. Assess the quality, character, rhythm, and strength of the pulse. *Comments:*	☐	☐	☐	
Upper Neuromuscular Examination 37. Inspect and palpate muscles, bones, and joints. *Comments:*	☐	☐	☐	
38. Examine the cervical spine. Flex, extend, move lateral, and rotate the spine. Examine the spine for resistive strength. *Comments:*	☐	☐	☐	
39. Examine shoulders. Flex, hyperextend, abduct, adduct, turn in internal and external rotation, shrug, and push/pull against the shoulders. *Comments:*	☐	☐	☐	

continued on the following page

continued from the previous page

Procedure 1-1	Able to Perform	Able to Perform with Assistance	Unable to Perform	Initials and Date
40. Examine elbows. Flex, extend, rotate, push, and pull each elbow. *Comments:*	☐	☐	☐	
41. Examine wrists. Flex, extend, and rotate each wrist. *Comments:*	☐	☐	☐	
42. Examine hand strength by having the client grasp your hands with his/hers. *Comments:*	☐	☐	☐	
43. Examine fingers. Abduct, adduct the fingers. Perform finger thumb opposition with counting and position sense. *Comments:*	☐	☐	☐	
44. Examine the epitrochlear lymph nodes, brachial and radial pulses, and bicep, tricep, and brachioradialis reflexes. *Comments:*	☐	☐	☐	
Chest and Breast Examination 45. Inspect and palpate the breast, nipple, and areola. Palpate the axillary lymph nodes. *Comments:*	☐	☐	☐	
46. Calculate the Tanner stage of sexual maturity, if appropriate. *Comments:*	☐	☐	☐	
47. Repeat breast and axillae examination while the client is in the supine position. *Comments:*	☐	☐	☐	
Back and Posterior Lung Examination 48. Inspect and palpate the skin. *Comments:*	☐	☐	☐	
49. Recheck the thyroid from the posterior position. *Comments:*	☐	☐	☐	

Procedure 1-1	Able to Perform	Able to Perform with Assistance	Unable to Perform	Initials and Date
50. Examine the cervical and thoracic spine, the scapulae, and the rib cage. Observe the posterior thoracic expansion. Estimate the anteroposterior to transverse chest ratio. *Comments:*	☐	☐	☐	
51. Feel for the presence of fremitus posteriorly and laterally. Compare sides. *Comments:*	☐	☐	☐	
52. Use indirect percussion at a minimum of four sites. *Comments:*	☐	☐	☐	
53. Auscultate the lungs. Listen to inspiration and expiration at each site. Listen for vocal fremitus. *Comments:*	☐	☐	☐	
Thorax, Lungs, and Respiratory Examination 54. Stand in front of the client. *Comments:*	☐	☐	☐	
55. Inspect and palpate the anterior chest. Observe position, chest movement, size, shape, and symmetry of the clavicles and ribs. *Comments:*	☐	☐	☐	
56. Listen to the respiratory rate, including rhythm and depth of respirations. *Comments:*	☐	☐	☐	
57. Observe the diaphragmatic excursion, intercostal spaces (ICS), respiratory muscles, respiratory effort, and expansion. *Comments:*	☐	☐	☐	
58. Feel for fremitus along the lung apexes and bases. *Comments:*	☐	☐	☐	
59. Use indirect percussion at intervals over intercostal spaces. Percuss lung apexes and bases, and the cardiac border, if appropriate. *Comments:*	☐	☐	☐	

continued on the following page

continued from the previous page

Procedure 1-1	Able to Perform	Able to Perform with Assistance	Unable to Perform	Initials and Date
60. Auscultate the anterior lung fields. Observe intensity, pitch, ratio, and quality. Listen for vocal fremitus. *Comments:*	☐	☐	☐	
Heart and Cardiovascular System Examination 61. Inspect and palpate the precordium. Identify the point of maximal intensity (PMI) and confirm synchrony with the carotid pulse. *Comments:*	☐	☐	☐	
62. Auscultate with the client sitting, then leaning forward. Listen with the diaphragm and then the bell. *Comments:*	☐	☐	☐	
63. Auscultate the apical heart rate and feel the radial pulse at the same time. Identify rate, rhythm, regularity, amplitude, and difference between apical and radial pulses. Note carotid impulse with apical sound. *Comments:*	☐	☐	☐	
64. Examine all valvular landmarks at least twice. Locate and identify the heart sounds. Listen for other sounds. Auscultate in an orderly fashion. *Comments:*	☐	☐	☐	
65. In the mitral area identify that S_1 is louder than S_2 with the diaphragm of the stethoscope. Use the bell to listen for a possible S_3 sound. *Comments:*	☐	☐	☐	
66. In the tricuspid area identify that S_1 is louder than S_2 with the diaphragm, but that it is softer than at the mitral area. Listen for a possible S_1 split that disappears when the client holds his breath. Listen for the S_3 sound with the bell. *Comments:*	☐	☐	☐	
67. In the pulmonic area identify that S_2 is louder than S_1, but softer than at aortic area. In the aortic area identify that S_2 is louder than S_1 with the diaphragm. *Comments:*	☐	☐	☐	
68. Assess the epigastric, axillary, and Erb's point areas. *Comments:*	☐	☐	☐	

Procedure 1-1	Able to Perform	Able to Perform with Assistance	Unable to Perform	Initials and Date
69. Summarize the character of the heart sounds including any abnormal sounds. *Comments:*	☐	☐	☐	
70. Assist client to left lateral position to continue the cardiac examination. *Comments:*	☐	☐	☐	
71. Auscultate mitral and tricuspid sites with the bell. *Comments:*	☐	☐	☐	
72. Assist client to return to supine position and continue cardiac examination. *Comments:*	☐	☐	☐	
73. • Inspect and palpate the precordium. Identify the PMI and confirm synchrony with carotid pulse. • Assess all pulses. • Percuss the cardiac borders if needed. • Auscultate the heart in supine position with bell and diaphragm. Auscultate with bell for bruits at carotid and temporal pulse sites. *Comments:*	☐	☐	☐	
74. Raise head to 30–45° angle and inspect the jugular vein distention (JVD). *Comments:*	☐	☐	☐	
Abdominal Examination 75. Inspect the size, contour, and symmetry of the abdomen. Note the condition of the umbilicus, and any respiratory or peristaltic movement. Check the rectus abdominus muscle. *Comments:*	☐	☐	☐	
76. Auscultate with the diaphragm and then the bell. Listen for bowel sounds in each of the four quadrants. *Comments:*	☐	☐	☐	
77. Percuss all four quadrants, gastric bubble, spleen, bladder, and liver span. Percuss the kidney posteriorly while the client is sitting, if needed. *Comments:*	☐	☐	☐	

continued on the following page

continued from the previous page

Procedure 1-1	Able to Perform	Able to Perform with Assistance	Unable to Perform	Initials and Date
78. Palpate all four quadrants superficially first, then deeply, and check rebound palpations. Check superficial abdominal reflexes in all four quadrants, spleen, liver, aorta, kidney, and bladder. Evaluate for guarding on expiration. *Comments:*	☐	☐	☐	
79. Check femoral pulses and superficial and deep inguinal nodes. *Comments:*	☐	☐	☐	
External Genitalia Examination 80. Assist client to modified or full lithotomy position. *Comments:*	☐	☐	☐	
81. Inspect and palpate deep inguinal nodes. *Comments:*	☐	☐	☐	
82. Observe pubic hair distribution, color, and texture. Check the femoral and inguinal areas for hernias. *Comments:*	☐	☐	☐	
83. Calculate the Tanner stage of sexual maturity, if appropriate. *Comments:*	☐	☐	☐	
84. Check skin and look for abnormalities. In women, examine the mons pubis, labia, clitoris, urethral meatus, vaginal introitus, and perineum. *Comments:*	☐	☐	☐	
85. In men, check the cremasteric reflex (in infants), urethral meatus, penis, scrotum, scrotal rugae, testicles, epididymis, spermatic cord, and external inguinal ring. *Comments:*	☐	☐	☐	
86. Examine the anus. Inspect and palpate the sacrococcygeal area and anal mucosa. *Comments:*	☐	☐	☐	

Procedure 1-1	Able to Perform	Able to Perform with Assistance	Unable to Perform	Initials and Date
87. Assist the client down from the table to a standing position. *Comments:*	☐	☐	☐	
88. Have the client walk across the room while observing his or her gait. *Comments:*	☐	☐	☐	
Lower Extremity and Musculoskeletal Examination 89. Assist client to supine position. *Comments:*	☐	☐	☐	
90. • Inspect and palpate the skin. Look at the skin color, check capillary refill, observe hair distribution, veins, temperature, and texture of skin. • Observe the size, shape, isometric muscle contraction, tone, and strength of muscles. *Comments:*	☐	☐	☐	
91. • Inspect the joints. Observe contour, periarticular tissue, neutral anatomic position, range of motion (ROM), and strength. Evaluate the hips. • Assess the knees. Check knee flexion, extension, and strength. • For the ankles and feet, palpate the Achilles tendon, at rest, in dorsiflexion and plantar flexion, eversion and inversion. Check toe flexion, abduction, and adduction. Palpate metatarsophalangeal joints and interphalangeal joints. • Check popliteal, posterior tibial, and dorsalis pedis pulses. *Comments:*	☐	☐	☐	
Neurological Examination 92. Assist client to sitting position. *Comments:*	☐	☐	☐	
93. • Check for deep tendon reflexes. • Check infantile reflexes. • Check the Babinski's reflex. *Comments:*	☐	☐	☐	

continued on the following page

continued from the previous page

Procedure 1-1	Able to Perform	Able to Perform with Assistance	Unable to Perform	Initials and Date
94. • Examine the client's sensory abilities. Check for responses to skin sensations. • Check exteroceptive sensation, including light touch, and sharp and dull. If the sharp/dull evaluation was abnormal, check temperature sensation as well. • Check the proprioceptive sensations of vibration, motion, and position. • Check the cortical sensations of stereognosis and graphesthesia. If needed, examine two-point discrimination and extinction. *Comments:*	☐	☐	☐	
95. Review and recheck the cranial nerves. *Comments:*	☐	☐	☐	
96. Evaluate the client's mental status: • Check level of consciousness. • Check orientation to person, time, place. • Check general appearance, behavior, affect, speech, content, memory. • Check logic and abstract reasoning, judgment, and spatial perception. *Comments:*	☐	☐	☐	
97. Examine cerebellar status: • Conduct a finger-to-nose test. Repeat with the other hand. • Conduct a RAHM (rapid alternating hand movements). • Have the client touch fingers-to-thumb. • Have the client touch heel-to-shin, foot tapping (rapid alternating foot movements), and foot "figure 8" movement tests. Determine if the client can run heel down the shin of the opposite leg. *Comments:*	☐	☐	☐	
98. Assist client to standing position. *Comments:*	☐	☐	☐	
99. • Inspect and/or palpate posture, weight-bearing and standing spine alignment, spinous processes, paravertebral muscles, and ROM. Do a Romberg test. • Have the client balance on one foot for 10 seconds. • Repeat heel-to-shin test, and have client hop on each foot and do shallow knee bends. *Comments:*	☐	☐	☐	

Procedure 1-1	Able to Perform	Able to Perform with Assistance	Unable to Perform	Initials and Date
100. Assess mobility by having the client perform a casual gait, toe and heel walk, tandem walk (forward and backward), step right, step left, walk briskly, and do jumping jacks (if client's condition permits). *Comments:*	☐	☐	☐	
101. Recheck heart and respiratory sounds after exercising. *Comments:*	☐	☐	☐	
102. Compare the client's status to age-appropriate standards. *Comments:*	☐	☐	☐	
103. Evaluate for psychiatric symptoms. *Comments:*	☐	☐	☐	

Checklist for Procedure 1-2   Taking a Temperature

Name _____ Date _____

School _____

Instructor _____

Course _____

Procedure 1-2 Taking a Temperature	Able to Perform	Able to Perform with Assistance	Unable to Perform	Initials and Date
Assessment				
1. Assess body temperature for changes due to exposure to pyrogens or to extreme hot or cold external environments. *Comments:*	☐	☐	☐	
2. Assess the client for the most appropriate site to check his temperature. *Comments:*	☐	☐	☐	
3. Confirm that the client has not smoked or consumed hot or cold foods just before the measurement of an oral temperature. *Comments:*	☐	☐	☐	
4. Assess for mouth breathing and tachypnea. *Comments:*	☐	☐	☐	
5. Assess for oral lesions. *Comments:*	☐	☐	☐	
Planning/Expected Outcomes				
1. An accurate temperature reading will be obtained. *Comments:*	☐	☐	☐	
2. The client will verbalize understanding of the reason for the procedure. *Comments:*	☐	☐	☐	
Implementation				
Preparation 1. Review medical record for baseline data and factors that influence vital signs. *Comments:*	☐	☐	☐	

continued on the following page

continued from the previous page

Procedure 1-2	Able to Perform	Able to Perform with Assistance	Unable to Perform	Initials and Date
2. Explain to the client that vital signs will be assessed. *Comments:*	☐	☐	☐	
3. Assess client's toileting needs and proceed as appropriate. *Comments:*	☐	☐	☐	
4. Gather equipment. *Comments:*	☐	☐	☐	
5. Provide for privacy. *Comments:*	☐	☐	☐	
6. Wash hands and apply gloves, when appropriate. *Comments:*	☐	☐	☐	
Oral Temperature: Electronic Thermometer 7. Repeat Actions 1–6. *Comments:*	☐	☐	☐	
8. Place disposable protective sheath over probe. *Comments:*	☐	☐	☐	
9. Grasp top of the probe's stem. *Comments:*	☐	☐	☐	
10. Place tip of thermometer under the client's tongue and along the gumline. *Comments:*	☐	☐	☐	
11. Instruct client to keep mouth closed around thermometer. *Comments:*	☐	☐	☐	
12. Thermometer will signal (beep) when a constant temperature registers. *Comments:*	☐	☐	☐	
13. Read measurement on digital display. Push ejection button to discard disposable sheath and return probe to storage well. *Comments:*	☐	☐	☐	

Procedure 1-2	Able to Perform	Able to Perform with Assistance	Unable to Perform	Initials and Date
14. Inform client of temperature reading. *Comments:*	☐	☐	☐	
15. Remove gloves and wash hands. *Comments:*	☐	☐	☐	
16. Record reading. *Comments:*	☐	☐	☐	
17. Return electronic thermometer unit to charging base. *Comments:*	☐	☐	☐	
18. Wash hands. *Comments:*	☐	☐	☐	
Tympanic Temperature: Infrared Thermometer 19. Repeat Actions 1–6. *Comments:*	☐	☐	☐	
20. Position client in Sims' position or sitting position. *Comments:*	☐	☐	☐	
21. Remove probe from container and attach probe cover to tympanic thermometer unit. *Comments:*	☐	☐	☐	
22. Turn client's head to one side. For an adult, pull pinna upward and back; for a child, pull down and back. Gently insert probe with firm pressure into ear canal. *Comments:*	☐	☐	☐	
23. Remove probe after the reading is displayed on digital unit. *Comments:*	☐	☐	☐	
24. Remove probe cover and replace in storage container. *Comments:*	☐	☐	☐	
25. Return tympanic thermometer to storage unit. *Comments:*	☐	☐	☐	

continued on the following page

continued from the previous page

Procedure 1-2	Able to Perform	Able to Perform with Assistance	Unable to Perform	Initials and Date
26. Record reading. *Comments:*	☐	☐	☐	
27. Wash hands. *Comments:*	☐	☐	☐	
Using a Tempa-Dot 28. Repeat Actions 1–6. *Comments:*	☐	☐	☐	
29. Position the client in a sitting or lying position. *Comments:*	☐	☐	☐	
30. Prepare Tempa-Dot according to directions. *Comments:*	☐	☐	☐	
31. Record temperature, indicate the method, and discard the thermometer. *Comments:*	☐	☐	☐	
32. Wash hands. *Comments:*	☐	☐	☐	
33. Repeat Actions 1–6. *Comments:*	☐	☐	☐	
34. Position the client in a sitting or lying position with the head of the bed elevated from 45–60° for measurement of all vital signs except those designated otherwise. *Comments:*	☐	☐	☐	
Oral Temperature: Glass Thermometer 35. Repeat Steps 1–6 then select correct color tip of thermometer from client's bedside container. *Comments:*	☐	☐	☐	
36. Remove the thermometer from storage container, hold at end away from bulb and cleanse under cool water. *Comments:*	☐	☐	☐	

Procedure 1-2	Able to Perform	Able to Perform with Assistance	Unable to Perform	Initials and Date
37. Use a tissue to dry thermometer from the bulb toward fingertips. *Comments:*	☐	☐	☐	
38. Read thermometer by locating colored solution or mercury level. It should read 35.5°C (96°F). *Comments:*	☐	☐	☐	
39. If thermometer is not below a normal body temperature, grasp at end away from bulb with thumb and forefinger and shake vigorously. *Comments:*	☐	☐	☐	
40. Place thermometer in client's mouth under the tongue and along the gumline. Instruct client to hold lips closed. *Comments:*	☐	☐	☐	
41. Leave in place 3–5 minutes. *Comments:*	☐	☐	☐	
42. Remove thermometer and wipe with a tissue away from fingers toward the bulb. *Comments:*	☐	☐	☐	
43. Read at eye level, rotating slowly until mercury level is visualized. *Comments:*	☐	☐	☐	
44. Shake thermometer down, cleanse, rinse, and return to storage. *Comments:*	☐	☐	☐	
45. Remove and dispose of gloves in appropriate receptacle. *Comments:*	☐	☐	☐	
46. Record reading. *Comments:*	☐	☐	☐	
47. Wash hands. *Comments:*	☐	☐	☐	

continued on the following page

continued from the previous page

Procedure 1-2	Able to Perform	Able to Perform with Assistance	Unable to Perform	Initials and Date
Rectal Temperature				
48. Repeat Actions 1–6. *Comments:*	☐	☐	☐	
49. Place client in the Sims' position with upper knee flexed. Expose only anal area. *Comments:*	☐	☐	☐	
50. Place tissues within easy reach. Apply gloves. *Comments:*	☐	☐	☐	
51 Prepare the thermometer. *Comments:*	☐	☐	☐	
52. Lubricate tip of rectal thermometer or probe. *Comments:*	☐	☐	☐	
53. With dominant hand, grasp thermometer. With other hand, separate buttocks to expose anus. *Comments:*	☐	☐	☐	
54. Instruct client to take a deep breath. Insert thermometer or probe gently into anus. *Comments:*	☐	☐	☐	
55. Hold in place for 2 minutes. *Comments:*	☐	☐	☐	
56. Wipe secretions off glass thermometer with a tissue. Dispose of electronic thermometer cover in waste receptacle. *Comments:*	☐	☐	☐	
57. Read measurement and inform client of temperature reading. *Comments:*	☐	☐	☐	
58. While holding glass thermometer in one hand, use other hand to wipe anal area with tissue to remove lubricant or feces. Dispose of soiled tissue. Cover client. *Comments:*	☐	☐	☐	

Procedure 1-2	Able to Perform	Able to Perform with Assistance	Unable to Perform	Initials and Date
59. Cleanse thermometer. *Comments:*	☐	☐	☐	
60. Remove and dispose of gloves in appropriate receptacle. Wash hands. *Comments:*	☐	☐	☐	
61. Record reading. *Comments:*	☐	☐	☐	
Axillary Temperature 62. Repeat Actions 1–6. *Comments:*	☐	☐	☐	
63. Remove client's arm and shoulder from sleeve of gown. Avoid exposing chest. *Comments:*	☐	☐	☐	
64. Make sure axillary skin is dry; if necessary, pat dry. *Comments:*	☐	☐	☐	
65. Prepare thermometer. *Comments:*	☐	☐	☐	
66. Place thermometer or probe into center of axilla. Fold client's arm across chest. *Comments:*	☐	☐	☐	
67. Leave glass thermometer in place 6–8 minutes. Leave an electronic thermometer in place until signal is heard. *Comments:*	☐	☐	☐	
68. Remove and read thermometer. *Comments:*	☐	☐	☐	
69. Inform client of temperature reading. *Comments:*	☐	☐	☐	

continued on the following page

continued from the previous page

Procedure 1-2	Able to Perform	Able to Perform with Assistance	Unable to Perform	Initials and Date
70. Cleanse glass thermometer. Shake down thermometer, cleanse thermometer with soapy water, rinse under cold water, and return to storage container. *Comments:*	☐	☐	☐	
71. Assist client with replacing gown. *Comments:*	☐	☐	☐	
72. Record reading. *Comments:*	☐	☐	☐	
73. Wash hands. *Comments:*	☐	☐	☐	
Disposable (Chemical Strip) Thermometer 74 Repeat Actions 1–6. *Comments:*	☐	☐	☐	
75. Apply tape to appropriate skin area, usually forehead. *Comments:*	☐	☐	☐	
76. Observe tape for color changes. *Comments:*	☐	☐	☐	
77. Record reading and indicate method. *Comments:*	☐	☐	☐	
78. Wash hands. *Comments:*	☐	☐	☐	

Checklist for Procedure 1-3 Taking a Pulse

Name _____ Date _____

School _____

Instructor _____

Course _____

Procedure 1-3 Taking a Pulse	Able to Perform	Able to Perform with Assistance	Unable to Perform	Initials and Date
Assessment				
1. Assess client for need to monitor pulse. *Comments:*	☐	☐	☐	
2. Assess the pulse for rate, amplitude, contour, and regularity. *Comments:*	☐	☐	☐	
3. Assess for signs of cardiovascular alterations. *Comments:*	☐	☐	☐	
4. Assess for factors that may affect the character of the pulse. *Comments:*	☐	☐	☐	
5. Assess for the appropriate site for measuring pulse. *Comments:*	☐	☐	☐	
6. Assess baseline heart rate and rhythm in the client's chart. *Comments:*	☐	☐	☐	
7. Assess circulatory status by using appropriate site. *Comments:*	☐	☐	☐	
Planning/Expected Outcomes				
1. Pulse rate, quality, rhythm, and volume will be within normal range. *Comments:*	☐	☐	☐	
2. The client will be comfortable with the procedure. *Comments:*	☐	☐	☐	

continued on the following page

continued from the previous page

Procedure 1-3	Able to Perform	Able to Perform with Assistance	Unable to Perform	Initials and Date
Implementation				
Taking a Radial (Wrist) Pulse				
1. Wash hands. *Comments:*	☐	☐	☐	
2. Inform client of the site(s) at which you will measure pulse. *Comments:*	☐	☐	☐	
3. Flex client's elbow and place lower part of arm across chest. *Comments:*	☐	☐	☐	
4. Support client's wrist by grasping outer aspect with thumb. *Comments:*	☐	☐	☐	
5. Place your index and middle finger over the radial artery and palpate pulse. *Comments:*	☐	☐	☐	
6. Identify pulse rhythm. *Comments:*	☐	☐	☐	
7. Determine pulse volume. *Comments:*	☐	☐	☐	
8. Count pulse rate by using second hand on a watch. *Comments:*	☐	☐	☐	
Taking an Apical Pulse				
9. Wash hands. *Comments:*	☐	☐	☐	
10. Raise client's gown to expose sternum and left side of chest. *Comments:*	☐	☐	☐	
11. Cleanse earpiece and diaphragm of stethoscope with an alcohol swab. *Comments:*	☐	☐	☐	

Procedure 1-3	Able to Perform	Able to Perform with Assistance	Unable to Perform	Initials and Date
12. Put stethoscope around your neck. *Comments:*	☐	☐	☐	
13. Locate apex of heart. *Comments:*	☐	☐	☐	
14. Inform client that you are going to listen to his or her heart. Instruct client to remain silent. *Comments:*	☐	☐	☐	
15. Put earpieces in your ears and warm stethoscope diaphragm in your hand. *Comments:*	☐	☐	☐	
16. Place diaphragm of stethoscope over the PMI and auscultate for sounds S_1 and S_2 to hear lub-dub sound. *Comments:*	☐	☐	☐	
17. Note regularity of rhythm. *Comments:*	☐	☐	☐	
18. Start to count while looking at second hand of watch. Count lub-dub sound as one beat: • For a regular rhythm, count rate for 30 seconds and multiply by 2. • For an irregular rhythm, count rate for a full minute, noting number of irregular beats. *Comments:*	☐	☐	☐	
19. Share your findings with client. *Comments:*	☐	☐	☐	
20. Record site, rate, rhythm, and number of irregular beats. *Comments:*	☐	☐	☐	
21. Wash hands. *Comments:*	☐	☐	☐	

Checklist for Procedure 1-4   Counting Respirations

Name _____ Date _____

School _____

Instructor _____

Course _____

Procedure 1-4 Counting Respirations	Able to Perform	Able to Perform with Assistance	Unable to Perform	Initials and Date
Assessment				
1. Assess the client's chest wall movement. *Comments:*	☐	☐	☐	
2. Assess the rate of respirations. *Comments:*	☐	☐	☐	
3. Assess the depth of the client's breaths. *Comments:*	☐	☐	☐	
4. Assess for risk factors that may alter the respirations. *Comments:*	☐	☐	☐	
5. Assess for factors that normally influence respirations. *Comments:*	☐	☐	☐	
Planning/Expected Outcomes				
1. An accurate evaluation of the respiratory rate and character will be obtained. *Comments:*	☐	☐	☐	
2. The respiratory rate and character will be normal. *Comments:*	☐	☐	☐	
Implementation				
1. Wash hands. *Comments:*	☐	☐	☐	
2. Be sure chest movement is visible. *Comments:*	☐	☐	☐	

continued on the following page

continued from the previous page

Procedure 1-4	Able to Perform	Able to Perform with Assistance	Unable to Perform	Initials and Date
3. Observe one complete respiratory cycle. *Comments:*	☐	☐	☐	
4. Start counting with first inspiration while looking at the second hand of watch. *Comments:*	☐	☐	☐	
5. Observe character of respirations. *Comments:*	☐	☐	☐	
6. Replace client's gown if needed. *Comments:*	☐	☐	☐	
7. Record rate and character of respirations. *Comments:*	☐	☐	☐	
8. Wash hands. *Comments:*	☐	☐	☐	

Checklist for Procedure 1-5   Taking Blood Pressure

Name _____ Date _____

School _____

Instructor _____

Course _____

Procedure 1-5 Taking Blood Pressure	Able to Perform	Able to Perform with Assistance	Unable to Perform	Initials and Date
Assessment				
1. Assess the condition of the potential blood pressure (BP) site. *Comments:*	☐	☐	☐	
2. Assess the artery for any compromise. *Comments:*	☐	☐	☐	
3. Assess the distal pulse to check if it is intact and palpable. *Comments:*	☐	☐	☐	
4. Assess the circumference of the extremity for the right size cuff. *Comments:*	☐	☐	☐	
5. Assess for factors that affect blood pressure. *Comments:*	☐	☐	☐	
6. Determine client's baseline blood pressure. *Comments:*	☐	☐	☐	
Planning/Expected Outcomes				
1. An accurate estimate of the arterial pressure at diastole and systole will be obtained. *Comments:*	☐	☐	☐	
2. BP is within normal range for the client. *Comments:*	☐	☐	☐	
3. Client will be able to explain why the BP is taken and what it means. *Comments:*	☐	☐	☐	

continued on the following page

continued from the previous page

Procedure 1-5	Able to Perform	Able to Perform with Assistance	Unable to Perform	Initials and Date
Implementation				
Auscultation Method Using Brachial Artery				
1. Wash hands. *Comments:*	☐	☐	☐	
2. Determine which extremity is most appropriate for reading. *Comments:*	☐	☐	☐	
3. Select a cuff size appropriate for the client. *Comments:*	☐	☐	☐	
4. Move clothing away from upper aspect of arm. Have the client's bared arm resting on a support so the midpoint of the upper arm is at the level of the heart. Extend the elbow with palm turned upward. *Comments:*	☐	☐	☐	
5. Make sure bladder cuff is fully deflated and pump valve moves freely. *Comments:*	☐	☐	☐	
6. Palpate the brachial artery in the antecubital space, and place the cuff so that the midline of the bladder is over the arterial position. *Comments:*	☐	☐	☐	
7. Inflate the cuff rapidly to 70 mm Hg and increase by 10-mm increments while palpating the radial pulse. *Comments:*	☐	☐	☐	
8. Insert earpieces of stethoscope into ears with a forward tilt. *Comments:*	☐	☐	☐	
9. Relocate brachial pulse and place bell or diaphragm directly over pulse. *Comments:*	☐	☐	☐	
10. Turn valve to close. Inflate cuff to 30 mm Hg above previously noted diminished pulse point. *Comments:*	☐	☐	☐	

Procedure 1-5	Able to Perform	Able to Perform with Assistance	Unable to Perform	Initials and Date
11. Partially unscrew (open) the valve counter-clockwise to deflate the bladder at 2 mm/sec while listening for the appearance of the five phases of the Korotkoff sounds. *Comments:*	☐	☐	☐	
12. After the last Korotkoff sound is heard, deflate the cuff slowly for at least another 10 mm Hg to ensure that no other sounds are audible; then, deflate rapidly and completely. *Comments:*	☐	☐	☐	
13. Allow the client to rest for at least 30 seconds and remove cuff. *Comments:*	☐	☐	☐	
14. Inform client of reading. *Comments:*	☐	☐	☐	
15. Record reading. *Comments:*	☐	☐	☐	
16. If appropriate, lower bed, raise side rails, place call light in easy reach. *Comments:*	☐	☐	☐	
17. Put all equipment in proper place. *Comments:*	☐	☐	☐	
18. Wash hands. *Comments:*	☐	☐	☐	

Checklist for Procedure 1-6   Weighing a Client, Mobile and Immobile

Name _____ Date _____

School _____

Instructor _____

Course _____

Procedure 1-6 Weighing a Client, Mobile and Immobile	Able to Perform	Able to Perform with Assistance	Unable to Perform	Initials and Date
Assessment				
1. Assess the client's ability to stand on a scale. *Comments:*	☐	☐	☐	
2. Determine if current clothing is similar to that worn at previous weight. *Comments:*	☐	☐	☐	
Planning/Expected Outcomes				
1. Health care provider obtains accurate weight. *Comments:*	☐	☐	☐	
2. Client incurs no injuries. *Comments:*	☐	☐	☐	
3. Client maintains privacy. *Comments:*	☐	☐	☐	
Implementation				
Standing Scale 1. Wash hands. *Comments:*	☐	☐	☐	
2. Introduce yourself to client and explain what you would like him or her to do. *Comments:*	☐	☐	☐	
3. Place scale near client. *Comments:*	☐	☐	☐	
4. Turn on scale and calibrate scale to zero. *Comments:*	☐	☐	☐	

continued on the following page

continued from the previous page

Procedure 1-6	Able to Perform	Able to Perform with Assistance	Unable to Perform	Initials and Date
5. Ask client to remove shoes (if necessary) step up on the scale, and stand still. Electronic scale: Read weight after digital numbers have stopped fluctuating. Balance scale: Slide the larger weight into the notch most closely approximating the client's weight. Slide the smaller weight to the notch such that the balance rests in the middle. Add the two numbers to read the client's weight. *Comments:*	☐	☐	☐	
6. Ask client to step down. Assist client if necessary. *Comments:*	☐	☐	☐	
7. Wipe scale with appropriate disinfectant. *Comments:*	☐	☐	☐	
8. Wash hands. *Comments:*	☐	☐	☐	
Sling Scale 9. Wash hands and put on gloves if appropriate. *Comments:*	☐	☐	☐	
10. Introduce yourself to client and explain what you would like him or her to do. *Comments:*	☐	☐	☐	
11. Place plastic covering on sling, if available. *Comments:*	☐	☐	☐	
12. Remove pillow. Turn client to one side and place sling on bed next to client with one-half rolled up against client's back. *Comments:*	☐	☐	☐	
13. Turn client to other side, and unroll rest of sling so it lays flat beneath client. *Comments:*	☐	☐	☐	

Procedure 1-6	Able to Perform	Able to Perform with Assistance	Unable to Perform	Initials and Date
14. Roll the scale over the bed. Open and lock the legs of the scale. *Comments:*	☐	☐	☐	
15. Turn on scale and calibrate to zero. *Comments:*	☐	☐	☐	
16. Lower arms of the scale and slip hooks through holes in sling. *Comments:*	☐	☐	☐	
17. Pump scale until sling rests completely off the bed. *Comments:*	☐	☐	☐	
18. Read weight after digital numbers have stopped fluctuating. *Comments:*	☐	☐	☐	
19. Lower client back onto bed and remove arms of scale from sling. *Comments:*	☐	☐	☐	
20. Unlock legs, return to their original position, and remove scale from bed. *Comments:*	☐	☐	☐	
21. Turn client from side to side to remove sling. *Comments:*	☐	☐	☐	
22. Realign client with pillows and covers. *Comments:*	☐	☐	☐	
23. Remove plastic covering from sling and discard. *Comments:*	☐	☐	☐	
24. Remove gloves. *Comments:*	☐	☐	☐	
25. Wash hands. *Comments:*	☐	☐	☐	

Checklist for Procedure 1-7   Measuring Intake and Output

Name _____ Date _____

School _____

Instructor _____

Course _____

Procedure 1-7 **Measuring Intake and Output**	Able to Perform	Able to Perform with Assistance	Unable to Perform	Initials and Date
Assessment				
1. Assess the client's risk factors for fluid overload. *Comments:*	☐	☐	☐	
2. Determine if the client is receiving fluids or medications that would predispose him or her to fluid overload. *Comments:*	☐	☐	☐	
3. Assess the client's risk factors for fluid loss. *Comments:*	☐	☐	☐	
4. Determine if the client's urine output is in excess of fluid intake. *Comments:*	☐	☐	☐	
5. Assess the client's ability to understand and cooperate with intake and output measurement. *Comments:*	☐	☐	☐	
Planning/Expected Outcomes				
1. The client's fluid intake and output will be accurately measured and recorded. *Comments:*	☐	☐	☐	
2. The client will participate in the recording of fluid intake and output to the best of his or her ability. *Comments:*	☐	☐	☐	
Implementation				
Intake 1. Wash hands. *Comments:*	☐	☐	☐	

continued on the following page

continued from the previous page

Procedure 1-7	Able to Perform	Able to Perform with Assistance	Unable to Perform	Initials and Date
2. Explain rules of intake and output (I&O) record. *Comments:*	☐	☐	☐	
3. Measure all oral fluids in accord with agency policy. Record all IV fluids as they are infused. *Comments:*	☐	☐	☐	
4. Record time and amount of all fluid intake in the designated space on bedside form. *Comments:*	☐	☐	☐	
5. Transfer 8-hour total fluid intake from bedside I&O record to graphic sheet or 24-hour I&O record on client's chart. *Comments:*	☐	☐	☐	
6. Record all forms of intake, except blood and blood products, in the appropriate column. *Comments:*	☐	☐	☐	
7. Complete 24-hour intake record by adding all 8-hour totals. *Comments:*	☐	☐	☐	
Output 8. Apply nonsterile gloves. *Comments:*	☐	☐	☐	
9. Empty urinal, bedpan, or Foley drainage bag into graduated container or commode "hat." *Comments:*	☐	☐	☐	
10. Remove gloves and wash hands. *Comments:*	☐	☐	☐	
11. Record time and amount of output on bedside I&O record. *Comments:*	☐	☐	☐	
12. Transfer 8-hour output totals to graphic sheet or 24-hour I&O record on the client's chart. *Comments:*	☐	☐	☐	

continued from the previous page

Procedure 1-7	Able to Perform	Able to Perform with Assistance	Unable to Perform	Initials and Date
13. Complete 24-hour output record by totaling all 8-hour totals. *Comments:*	☐	☐	☐	
14. Wash hands. *Comments:*	☐	☐	☐	

Checklist for Procedure 1-8 Breast Self-Examination

Name _____ Date _____

School _____

Instructor _____

Course _____

Procedure 1-8 Breast Self-Examination	Able to Perform	Able to Perform with Assistance	Unable to Perform	Initials and Date
Assessment				
1. Assess client's musculoskeletal and range of motion ability. *Comments:*	☐	☐	☐	
2. Assess demonstrated health-seeking behaviors. *Comments:*	☐	☐	☐	
3. Assess client's knowledge of breast self-examination. *Comments:*	☐	☐	☐	
4. Assess client's personal and family history. *Comments:*	☐	☐	☐	
5. Assess if the client's health history reveals past or present use of hormonal medications. A thorough follow-up may be necessary if any abnormalities are found because hormone use may increase the risk for breast cancer. *Comments:*	☐	☐	☐	
6. Assess if the client's family history includes breast cancer in first-degree (mother or sister) or second-degree (aunt or grandmother) relatives. A thorough follow-up may be necessary as this is a known risk factor. *Comments:*	☐	☐	☐	
7. Assess if the woman is postmenopausal because breasts in postmenopausal women may show normal atrophy of glandular tissue and increased striations. *Comments:*	☐	☐	☐	
8. Assess age for a male with enlarged breasts because breast enlargement in adolescent males is usually normal during puberty and is common when a boy is overweight. *Comments:*	☐	☐	☐	

continued on the following page

continued from the previous page

Procedure 1-8	Able to Perform	Able to Perform with Assistance	Unable to Perform	Initials and Date
Planning/Expected Outcomes				
1. Normal breast examination. *Comments:*	☐	☐	☐	
2. Client is able to demonstrate proper procedure for breast self-examination and offer a plan of when it will be performed monthly. *Comments:*	☐	☐	☐	
3. Client will identify when next screening should be performed. *Comments:*	☐	☐	☐	
Implementation				
1. Review personal history, medications, allergies, and family health history. *Comments:*	☐	☐	☐	
2. Ask client to disrobe to the waist and to put on a gown with the opening in the front. *Comments:*	☐	☐	☐	
3. Wash hands. Apply gloves if required by institutional policy. *Comments:*	☐	☐	☐	
4. Assist client to sitting position and expose chest and breasts. *Comments:*	☐	☐	☐	
5. Inspect breasts, areola, and nipples with client's arms at her sides, arms overhead, hands pressed on hips, and with arms extended. *Comments:*	☐	☐	☐	
6. Palpate adjacent lymph nodes. *Comments:*	☐	☐	☐	
7. Palpate breast using the palmar surfaces of the fingers. *Comments:*	☐	☐	☐	

Procedure 1-8	Able to Perform	Able to Perform with Assistance	Unable to Perform	Initials and Date
8. Explain and teach breast self-examination as you proceed. *Comments:*	☐	☐	☐	
9. Palpate areola and nipple. *Comments:*	☐	☐	☐	
10. Palpate into axilla. *Comments:*	☐	☐	☐	
11. Repeat Actions 7–9 on the left breast, areola, nipple, and axilla. *Comments:*	☐	☐	☐	
12. Assist client to supine position. Place arm on examination side under head and place a small pillow under the same side scapula. *Comments:*	☐	☐	☐	
13. Palpate breast, areola, and nipple as in Actions 7–9. *Comments:*	☐	☐	☐	
14. Assist client to sitting position. Review steps and ask client to demonstrate the breast self-examination. *Comments:*	☐	☐	☐	
15. Allow client to dress. *Comments:*	☐	☐	☐	
16. Remove gloves and wash hands. *Comments:*	☐	☐	☐	
17. Give client written materials to reinforce teaching. *Comments:*	☐	☐	☐	

Checklist for Procedure 1-9   Male Genitalia, Hernia, and Rectal Examination

Name _____ Date _____

School _____

Instructor _____

Course _____

Procedure 1-9 Male Genitalia, Hernia, and Rectal Examination	Able to Perform	Able to Perform with Assistance	Unable to Perform	Initials and Date
Assessment				
1. Assess the sexual maturation of the client, the size and shape of the penis, and skin integrity. *Comments:*	☐	☐	☐	
2. Note the color and texture of scrotal skin. *Comments:*	☐	☐	☐	
3. Note Tanner stage for children and adolescents. *Comments:*	☐	☐	☐	
4. Assess testicular size and adnexal structures. *Comments:*	☐	☐	☐	
5. Inspect the inguinal areas and groin for nodules, swelling, or bulges. *Comments:*	☐	☐	☐	
6. Assess the cremaster reflex. *Comments:*	☐	☐	☐	
7. Assess the prostate gland for size, shape, consistency, sensitivity, and mobility of the prostate. *Comments:*	☐	☐	☐	
8. Assess the seminal vesicles for tenderness and masses. *Comments:*	☐	☐	☐	
Planning/Expected Outcomes				
1. Normal penile exam. *Comments:*	☐	☐	☐	

continued on the following page

continued from the previous page

Procedure 1-9	Able to Perform	Able to Perform with Assistance	Unable to Perform	Initials and Date
2. Normal exam of the scrotum, with normal size, contour, and symmetry. *Comments:*	☐	☐	☐	
3. Tanner stage is appropriate for age. *Comments:*	☐	☐	☐	
4. Testicular size and adnexal structures are within normal limits. *Comments:*	☐	☐	☐	
5. Inguinal areas and groin are free of nodules, swelling, and bulges. *Comments:*	☐	☐	☐	
6. The prostate gland is within normal limits for size, shape, consistency, sensitivity, and mobility. *Comments:*	☐	☐	☐	

Implementation

Penile Examination

	Able to Perform	Able to Perform with Assistance	Unable to Perform	Initials and Date
1. Ask the client to disrobe completely and put on a gown. *Comments:*	☐	☐	☐	
2. Explain the procedure to the client. *Comments:*	☐	☐	☐	
3. Wash hands and apply clean gloves. *Comments:*	☐	☐	☐	
4. Have the client stand and hold up gown to expose his genitalia. *Comments:*	☐	☐	☐	
5. Inspect the penis and pubic hair distribution. *Comments:*	☐	☐	☐	
6. Retract or have client retract the prepuce (foreskin), if present. *Comments:*	☐	☐	☐	

Procedure 1-9	Able to Perform	Able to Perform with Assistance	Unable to Perform	Initials and Date
7. Observe the glans penis and the urethral meatus. *Comments:*	☐	☐	☐	
8. Palpate the entire length of the penis between your thumb and first two fingers. *Comments:*	☐	☐	☐	
9. Inspect the scrotum for erythema, discoloration, swelling, and skin integrity. *Comments:*	☐	☐	☐	
10. Elicit the cremaster reflex on both sides. *Comments:*	☐	☐	☐	
11. Palpate each testis and epididymis between the thumb and first two fingers. *Comments:*	☐	☐	☐	
12. Palpate each spermatic cord, including the vas deferens within the cord, between your thumb and fingers. *Comments:*	☐	☐	☐	
Hernia Examination 13. Inspect the inguinal and femoral areas. Ask client to strain down or cough. *Comments:*	☐	☐	☐	
14. Palpate for a femoral hernia by placing your fingers on the anterior thigh in the region of the femoral canal. Ask the client to bear down and cough. *Comments:*	☐	☐	☐	
15. Palpate for an inguinal hernia. *Comments:*	☐	☐	☐	
Rectal Examination 16. Use standing or left lateral decubitis position. If the client is on their left side flex their hips and knees to stabilize the client and improve visibility. *Comments:*	☐	☐	☐	

continued from the previous page

Procedure 1-9	Able to Perform	Able to Perform with Assistance	Unable to Perform	Initials and Date
17. Provide a warm quiet environment. *Comments:*	☐	☐	☐	
18. Wash hands and apply clean gloves. *Comments:*	☐	☐	☐	
19. Spread apart buttocks and examine anus, perianal area, and sacral region. *Comments:*	☐	☐	☐	
20. Lubricate the gloved index finger and slowly insert finger into anal canal. *Comments:*	☐	☐	☐	
21. Insert finger as far as possible into the rectum. *Comments:*	☐	☐	☐	
22. Anterioraly palpate the two lobes of the prostate gland and its sulcus. *Comments:*	☐	☐	☐	
23. If possible, extend fingers above the prostate region and palpate the superior portion of the lateral lobe to the region of the seminal vesicles and the peritoneal cavity. *Comments:*	☐	☐	☐	
24. Gently withdraw your finger. *Comments:*	☐	☐	☐	
25. Offer client tissue or wipe excess lubricant /stool from anus. *Comments:*	☐	☐	☐	

Checklist for Procedure 1-10 Collecting a Clean-Catch, Midstream Urine Specimen

Name _____ Date _____

School _____

Instructor _____

Course _____

Procedure 1-10 Collecting a Clean-Catch, Midstream Urine Specimen	Able to Perform	Able to Perform with Assistance	Unable to Perform	Initials and Date
Assessment				
1. Evaluate the client's ability to obtain a clean-catch specimen. *Comments:*	☐	☐	☐	
2. Assess for signs and symptoms of urinary tract infections or other abnormalities. *Comments:*	☐	☐	☐	
Planning/Expected Outcomes				
1. Client will be able to obtain a clean, midstream specimen. *Comments:*	☐	☐	☐	
2. Client will have absence of urinary abnormalities. *Comments:*	☐	☐	☐	
3. Client will understand procedure. *Comments:*	☐	☐	☐	
Implementation				
1. Check orders and assess need for procedure. *Comments:*	☐	☐	☐	
2. Gather equipment. *Comments:*	☐	☐	☐	
3. Assess the client's ability to complete the procedure. *Comments:*	☐	☐	☐	
4. Assess the client for signs and symptoms of urinary abnormalities. *Comments:*	☐	☐	☐	

continued on the following page

continued from the previous page

Procedure 1-10	Able to Perform	Able to Perform with Assistance	Unable to Perform	Initials and Date
5. Check the client's identification. *Comments:*	☐	☐	☐	
6. If client is to complete procedure in privacy, explain procedure, give equipment to client, and wait for specimen. *Comments:*	☐	☐	☐	
7. If nurse is to perform procedure, wash hands and apply gloves. If the client is to perform procedure, instruct client to wash hands before and after the procedure, or allow client to wear gloves. *Comments:*	☐	☐	☐	
8. Provide privacy. *Comments:*	☐	☐	☐	
9. Instruct the client. Female client: Sit with legs separated on the toilet. Male client: Sit down on toilet. *Comments:*	☐	☐	☐	
10. Using sterile procedure, open kit or towelettes. Open sterile container, placing the lid with sterile side up. *Comments:*	☐	☐	☐	
11. Female client: Use thumb and forefinger to separate labia, or have client separate labia with fingers. With the labia separated, use a downward stroke to cleanse each side of the labia and the urethral opening. Use a new towelette each time. *Comments:*	☐	☐	☐	
12. Male client: Pull back the foreskin (if present in uncircumcised male) and clean with a single stroke around meatus and glans. Use a circular motion starting at the urethral opening, moving down the glans shaft. Discard the towelette. Cleanse the head of the penis three times in a circular motion using a new towelette each time. *Comments:*	☐	☐	☐	

Procedure 1-10	Able to Perform	Able to Perform with Assistance	Unable to Perform	Initials and Date
13. Ask the client to begin to urinate into the toilet. After the stream starts with good flow, place the collection cup under the stream of urine. Fill the container with 30–60 cc of urine and remove the container before urination ceases. *Comments:*	☐	☐	☐	
14. Place the sterile lid back onto the container and close tightly. Clean and dry the outside of the container. Label and enclose in a biohazard bag and transport specimen to the laboratory. *Comments:*	☐	☐	☐	
15. Remove and dispose of gloves and wash hands. *Comments:*	☐	☐	☐	

Checklist for Procedure 1-11 Testing Urine for Specific Gravity, Ketones, Glucose, and Occult Blood

Name _____ Date _____

School _____

Instructor _____

Course _____

Procedure 1-11 Testing Urine for Specific Gravity, Ketones, Glucose, and Occult Blood	Able to Perform	Able to Perform with Assistance	Unable to Perform	Initials and Date
Assessment				
1. Assess the client's understanding of the urine test to be performed. *Comments:*	☐	☐	☐	
2. Assess the client's hydration. *Comments:*	☐	☐	☐	
3. Assess the client's history for renal function. *Comments:*	☐	☐	☐	
4. If measuring glucose, assess the client for symptoms of increased glucose. *Comments:*	☐	☐	☐	
5. If the client is to perform long-term tests, assess the client's ability to perform the tests. *Comments:*	☐	☐	☐	
Planning/Expected Outcomes				
1. Normal specific gravity. *Comments:*	☐	☐	☐	
2. Absence of glucose and ketones in the urine. *Comments:*	☐	☐	☐	
3. The client understands the purpose of the test. *Comments:*	☐	☐	☐	
4. The client understands how to perform the test (if needed). *Comments:*	☐	☐	☐	

continued on the following page

continued from the previous page

Procedure 1-11	Able to Perform	Able to Perform with Assistance	Unable to Perform	Initials and Date
Implementation				
Overview—Measuring Specific Gravity				
1. Wash hands. Apply nonsterile gloves. *Comments:*	☐	☐	☐	
2. Obtain urine from client either via clean catch or from catheter. *Comments:*	☐	☐	☐	
3. Measure specific gravity using equipment available in your facility. *Comments:*	☐	☐	☐	
4. Discard urine according to standard precautions. *Comments:*	☐	☐	☐	
5. Remove gloves and wash hands. *Comments:*	☐	☐	☐	
6. Clean equipment. *Comments:*	☐	☐	☐	
7. Record results and compare with previous recording. *Comments:*	☐	☐	☐	
Using a Digital Clinical Refractometer to Measure Specific Gravity				
8. Become familiar with the manufacturer's instructions. *Comments:*	☐	☐	☐	
9. Use an eye dropper to drip urine onto the prism at the center of the stainless steel stage until the prism is covered. *Comments:*	☐	☐	☐	
10. Press the button designated by the manufacturer to activate the meter. The specific gravity reading is displayed. *Comments:*	☐	☐	☐	

Procedure 1-11	Able to Perform	Able to Perform with Assistance	Unable to Perform	Initials and Date
Using a Nondigital Refractometer to Measure Specific Gravity				
11. Collect a few drops of urine. *Comments:*	☐	☐	☐	
12. Place a drop of urine on the horizontal glass slide at the top of the scope. *Comments:*	☐	☐	☐	
13. Close the cover over the slide and turn on the light. *Comments:*	☐	☐	☐	
14. Look through the scope. *Comments:*	☐	☐	☐	
15. Read the number at the line where the top black and lower white circle meet. Write down the number. *Comments:*	☐	☐	☐	
16. Clean the slide. *Comments:*	☐	☐	☐	
Using a Urinometer to Measure Specific Gravity				
17. Pour fresh urine into glass cylinder to indicated line on urinometer. *Comments:*	☐	☐	☐	
18. Place urinometer on flat surface and insert weighted glass stem. Gently spin the top of the glass stem. *Comments:*	☐	☐	☐	
19. When the stem stops moving, read at lowest point of meniscus at eye level. *Comments:*	☐	☐	☐	
Using a Dipstick to Test Urine for Glucose, Ketones, Occult Blood, or Specific Gravity				
20. Collect a clean voided specimen. *Comments:*	☐	☐	☐	

continued on the following page

continued from the previous page

Procedure 1-11	Able to Perform	Able to Perform with Assistance	Unable to Perform	Initials and Date
21. Obtain the correct product for testing. Check expiration date. *Comments:*	☐	☐	☐	
22. Review the instructions on the label. *Comments:*	☐	☐	☐	
23. The dipstick is dipped into the container of urine and read at a specified time interval. *Comments:*	☐	☐	☐	
24. Record the results. *Comments:*	☐	☐	☐	
25. Discard the urine and strip according to standard precautions. *Comments:*	☐	☐	☐	
26. Remove gloves and wash hands. *Comments:*	☐	☐	☐	

Checklist for Procedure 1-12   Performing a Skin Puncture

Name _____ Date _____

School _____

Instructor _____

Course _____

Procedure 1-12 Performing a Skin Puncture	Able to Perform	Able to Perform with Assistance	Unable to Perform	Initials and Date
Assessment				
1. Assess the condition of the client's skin at the potential puncture site. *Comments:*	☐	☐	☐	
2. Assess the circulation at the potential puncture site. *Comments:*	☐	☐	☐	
3. Assess the client's comfort level regarding the procedure. *Comments:*	☐	☐	☐	
4. Assess the cleanliness of the client's skin. *Comments:*	☐	☐	☐	
Planning/Expected Outcomes				
1. An adequate blood specimen will be obtained. *Comments:*	☐	☐	☐	
2. The client will suffer minimal trauma during specimen collection. *Comments:*	☐	☐	☐	
3. The specimen will be collected and stored in a manner compatible with the ordered tests. *Comments:*	☐	☐	☐	
Implementation				
1. Wash hands. *Comments:*	☐	☐	☐	
2. Check client's identification band, if appropriate. *Comments:*	☐	☐	☐	

continued on the following page

continued from the previous page

Procedure 1-12	Able to Perform	Able to Perform with Assistance	Unable to Perform	Initials and Date
3. Explain procedure to client. *Comments:*	☐	☐	☐	
4. Prepare supplies, open packages, and label specimen tubes. *Comments:*	☐	☐	☐	
5. Apply gloves. *Comments:*	☐	☐	☐	
6. Select site. *Comments:*	☐	☐	☐	
7. Place the hand or heel in a dependent position. *Comments:*	☐	☐	☐	
8. Place hand towel or absorbent pad under the extremity. *Comments:*	☐	☐	☐	
9. Cleanse puncture site with an antiseptic and allow to dry. *Comments:*	☐	☐	☐	
10. Apply gentle milking pressure above or around the puncture site. Identify whether the client has received recent antimicrobials and obtain a specimen prior to treatment, if possible. *Comments:*	☐	☐	☐	
11. • With the sterile lancet at a 90° angle to the skin, use a quick stab to puncture the skin (about 2 mm deep). • With the automatic unistik, push the lancet into the body of unistik until it clicks. Hold the body of the unistik and twist off the lancet cap. Place the end of the unistik tightly against the client's finger and press the lever. The needle automatically retracts after use. *Comments:*	☐	☐	☐	
12. Wipe off the first drop of blood with sterile gauze; allow the blood to flow freely. *Comments:*	☐	☐	☐	

Procedure 1-12	Able to Perform	Able to Perform with Assistance	Unable to Perform	Initials and Date
13. Collect the blood into the appropriate tube(s). *Comments:*	☐	☐	☐	
14. Apply pressure to the puncture site with sterile gauze. *Comments:*	☐	☐	☐	
15. Place contaminated articles into a sharps container. *Comments:*	☐	☐	☐	
16. Remove and dispose of gloves. Wash hands. *Comments:*	☐	☐	☐	
17. Position client for comfort with call light in reach. *Comments:*	☐	☐	☐	
18. Wash hands. *Comments:*	☐	☐	☐	

Checklist for Procedure 1-13   Measuring Blood Glucose Levels

Name _____ Date _____

School _____

Instructor _____

Course _____

Procedure 1-13 Measuring Blood Glucose Levels	Able to Perform	Able to Perform with Assistance	Unable to Perform	Initials and Date
Assessment				
1. Review the health care provider's order for glucose monitoring. *Comments:*	☐	☐	☐	
2. Identify which type of equipment is available. *Comments:*	☐	☐	☐	
3. Review the client's medical history for diabetes. *Comments:*	☐	☐	☐	
4. Determine if the test requires special timing. *Comments:*	☐	☐	☐	
5. Assess the client's or caregiver's ability to manage the equipment and perform the test accurately if the care will be provided at home. *Comments:*	☐	☐	☐	
6. Assess the client's understanding of and willingness to perform the test independently. *Comments:*	☐	☐	☐	
7. Assess the client's sites for skin puncture. *Comments:*	☐	☐	☐	
Planning/Expected Outcomes				
1. Blood glucose level is maintained within a normal range. *Comments:*	☐	☐	☐	
2. Client or caregiver demonstrates accurate performance of the procedure. *Comments:*	☐	☐	☐	

continued on the following page

continued from the previous page

Procedure 1-13	Able to Perform	Able to Perform with Assistance	Unable to Perform	Initials and Date
3. Client verbalizes an understanding of the importance of the test and the need for accurate results. *Comments:*	☐	☐	☐	
4. Client verbalizes minimal anxiety associated with the procedure. *Comments:*	☐	☐	☐	
5. Skin puncture sites remain free of signs and symptoms of infection. *Comments:*	☐	☐	☐	
Implementation				
1. Review orders, identify client, and review instructions for meter usage. *Comments:*	☐	☐	☐	
2. Wash hands. *Comments:*	☐	☐	☐	
3. Assemble the equipment at the bedside. *Comments:*	☐	☐	☐	
4. Have client wash hands with soap and water and position client in a semi-Fowler's position. *Comments:*	☐	☐	☐	
5. Remove a reagent strip from the container and reseal the container cap. Turn on meter. *Comments:*	☐	☐	☐	
6. Calibrate meter following manufacturer's instructions. *Comments:*	☐	☐	☐	
7. Place unused reagent strip on a clean, dry surface with the test pad facing up. *Comments:*	☐	☐	☐	
8. Apply disposable gloves. *Comments:*	☐	☐	☐	

Procedure 1-13	Able to Perform	Able to Perform with Assistance	Unable to Perform	Initials and Date
9. Select appropriate puncture site, and perform skin puncture. *Comments:*	☐	☐	☐	
10. Wipe away the first drop of blood from the site. *Comments:*	☐	☐	☐	
11. Gently squeeze the site to produce a large droplet of blood. *Comments:*	☐	☐	☐	
12. Transfer the drop of blood to the reagent strip. *Comments:*	☐	☐	☐	
13. Press the timer on the meter. *Comments:*	☐	☐	☐	
14. Apply pressure to the puncture site. *Comments:*	☐	☐	☐	
15. After 60 seconds, wipe the blood from the test pad; place the strip into the meter. (Note: This step may vary with meter.) *Comments:*	☐	☐	☐	
16. Read the meter for results found on the unit display when the time is up. *Comments:*	☐	☐	☐	
17. Turn meter off and dispose of test strip, cotton ball, and lancet properly. *Comments:*	☐	☐	☐	
18. Remove disposable gloves and place them in appropriate receptacle. *Comments:*	☐	☐	☐	
19. Wash hands. *Comments:*	☐	☐	☐	

continued on the following page

continued from the previous page

Procedure 1-13	Able to Perform	Able to Perform with Assistance	Unable to Perform	Initials and Date
20. Review test results with client. *Comments:*	☐	☐	☐	
21. Notify physician or qualified practitioner of results. *Comments:*	☐	☐	☐	
22. Wash hands. *Comments:*	☐	☐	☐	

Checklist for Procedure 1-14   Collecting Nose, Throat, and Sputum Specimens

Name _____ Date _____

School _____

Instructor _____

Course _____

Procedure 1-14 Collecting Nose, Throat, and Sputum Specimens	Able to Perform	Able to Perform with Assistance	Unable to Perform	Initials and Date
Assessment				
1. Assess the client's understanding of the purpose of the procedure. *Comments:*	☐	☐	☐	
2. Assess the type of nasal or sinus drainage. *Comments:*	☐	☐	☐	
3. Review the health care provider's orders for the cultures requested. *Comments:*	☐	☐	☐	
4. Assess the client for postnasal drip, sinus headache, tenderness, nasal congestion, or sore throat. *Comments:*	☐	☐	☐	
5. Identify whether the client has received recent antimicrobials and obtain a specimen prior to treatment, if possible. *Comments:*	☐	☐	☐	
Planning/Expected Outcomes				
1. An adequate specimen will be obtained. *Comments:*	☐	☐	☐	
2. The procedure will be performed with a minimum of trauma to the client. *Comments:*	☐	☐	☐	
Implementation				
1. Wash hands and put on clean gloves. *Comments:*	☐	☐	☐	
2. Ask client to sit erect in bed or on chair facing nurse. *Comments:*	☐	☐	☐	

continued on the following page

continued from the previous page

Procedure 1-14	Able to Perform	Able to Perform with Assistance	Unable to Perform	Initials and Date
3. Prepare sterile swab for use by loosening top from container. *Comments:*	☐	☐	☐	
Collect Throat Culture 4. Ask client to tilt head backward, open mouth, and say "ah." *Comments:*	☐	☐	☐	
5. Depress anterior one-third of tongue with tongue blade. *Comments:*	☐	☐	☐	
6. Insert the swab without touching the cheek, lips, teeth, or tongue. *Comments:*	☐	☐	☐	
7. Swab tonsillar area from side to side in a quick, gentle motion. *Comments:*	☐	☐	☐	
8. Withdraw swab and place in culture tube. Crush ampule at bottom of tube and push swab into liquid medium. *Comments:*	☐	☐	☐	
9. Secure top to culture tube and label with client's name. *Comments:*	☐	☐	☐	
10. Discard tongue depressor. Remove and discard gloves. Wash hands. *Comments:*	☐	☐	☐	
Collect Nose Culture 11. Instruct client to blow nose and check nostrils for patency with penlight. *Comments:*	☐	☐	☐	
12. Ask client to occlude one nostril, then the other, and exhale. *Comments:*	☐	☐	☐	

Procedure 1-14	Able to Perform	Able to Perform with Assistance	Unable to Perform	Initials and Date
13. Ask client to tilt head back. *Comments:*	☐	☐	☐	
14. Insert swab into nostril until it reaches the inflamed mucosa and rotate the swab. *Comments:*	☐	☐	☐	
15. Withdraw the swab and place in culture tube. Crush ampule at bottom of tube and push swab into liquid medium. *Comments:*	☐	☐	☐	
16. Secure top to culture tube and label with client's name. *Comments:*	☐	☐	☐	
17. Remove gloves and discard. Wash hands. *Comments:*	☐	☐	☐	
Collection of Nasopharyngeal Culture 18. Follow Actions 11–17 above except use a swab on a flexible wire that can reach the nasopharynx via the nose. *Comments:*	☐	☐	☐	
Collecting a Sputum Culture 19. Explain to the client that the specimen must be sputum coughed up from the back of the throat or lungs. *Comments:*	☐	☐	☐	
20. Have a sterile specimen cup ready for the sample and some tissue at hand. *Comments:*	☐	☐	☐	
21. Have the client take several deep breaths and then cough deeply. *Comments:*	☐	☐	☐	
22. Have the client expectorate the sputum into the sterile cup without touching the inside of the cup. *Comments:*	☐	☐	☐	

continued on the following page

continued from the previous page

Procedure 1-14	Able to Perform	Able to Perform with Assistance	Unable to Perform	Initials and Date
23. Place the lid on the specimen container without touching the inside of the lid or the container. *Comments:*	☐	☐	☐	
24. Provide the client with a tissue and make him or her comfortable. *Comments:*	☐	☐	☐	
Alternative Sputum Collection Method 25. Obtain a sterile suction catheter and an inline sputum collection container. *Comments:*	☐	☐	☐	
26. Provide the client with warm humidified air for about 20 minutes if it is not contraindicated by his condition. *Comments:*	☐	☐	☐	
27. Hook the sputum collector up to suction tubing and a suction device. Hook the suction catheter to the sputum collector. *Comments:*	☐	☐	☐	
28. If the client is able to cooperate, have him or her take several deep breaths and cough. *Comments:*	☐	☐	☐	
29. As the client is coughing up sputum, carefully insert the catheter either orally or nasopharyngeally into the back of the client's throat and suction the sputum into the specimen container. *Comments:*	☐	☐	☐	
30. Safely dispose of the suction catheter. *Comments:*	☐	☐	☐	
31. Close the specimen container. *Comments:*	☐	☐	☐	
32. Provide tissue or other measures for client comfort. *Comments:*	☐	☐	☐	

Procedure 1-14	Able to Perform	Able to Perform with Assistance	Unable to Perform	Initials and Date
33. Wash hands. *Comments:*	☐	☐	☐	
34. Label each specimen with client's name. *Comments:*	☐	☐	☐	
35. Send specimen to laboratory. *Comments:*	☐	☐	☐	

Checklist for Procedure 1-15   Testing for Occult Blood with a Hemoccult Slide

Name _____ Date _____

School _____

Instructor _____

Course _____

Procedure 1-15 Testing for Occult Blood with a Hemoccult Slide	Able to Perform	Able to Perform with Assistance	Unable to Perform	Initials and Date
Assessment				
1. Assess the client's or family member's understanding of the need for this test. *Comments:*	☐	☐	☐	
2. Assess the client's ability to cooperate with the procedure. *Comments:*	☐	☐	☐	
3. Assess the client's medical history for bleeding disorders. *Comments:*	☐	☐	☐	
4. Assess any medications the client receives that can cause gastrointestinal bleeding. *Comments:*	☐	☐	☐	
Planning/Expected Outcomes				
1. The client will understand the purpose of the test. *Comments:*	☐	☐	☐	
2. The client will be able to collect the specimen, or allow the specimen to be collected. *Comments:*	☐	☐	☐	
3. The test for occult blood will be conducted properly and results will be recorded. *Comments:*	☐	☐	☐	
Implementation				
1. Wash hands and apply clean gloves. *Comments:*	☐	☐	☐	

continued on the following page

continued from the previous page

Procedure 1-15	Able to Perform	Able to Perform with Assistance	Unable to Perform	Initials and Date
2. Obtain stool specimen from client, commode, specimen cup, or bedpan. *Comments:*	☐	☐	☐	
3. Obtain small portion of feces with wooden applicator. *Comments:*	☐	☐	☐	
4. Read and follow the manufacturer's instructions. *Comments:*	☐	☐	☐	
Perform Hemoccult Slide Test 5. Open flap of slide and smear thin sample of feces on paper in first box. *Comments:*	☐	☐	☐	
6. Apply feces from a different area of the specimen to the second box. *Comments:*	☐	☐	☐	
7. Close slide cover and turn to reverse side. Open flap and apply two drops of developing solution on each sample box and on each control box. *Comments:*	☐	☐	☐	
8. Note color change after 60 seconds. *Comments:*	☐	☐	☐	
9. Dispose of slide and applicator in proper receptacle. Remove gloves and wash hands. *Comments:*	☐	☐	☐	
Perform Hematest 10. Apply small amount of feces on guaiac-impregnated paper. *Comments:*	☐	☐	☐	
11. Place Hematest tablet on top of stool specimen. *Comments:*	☐	☐	☐	

Procedure 1-15	Able to Perform	Able to Perform with Assistance	Unable to Perform	Initials and Date
12. Apply 2–3 drops of tap water on tablet. *Comments:*	☐	☐	☐	
13. Note color change after 2 minutes. *Comments:*	☐	☐	☐	
14. Dispose of tablet, paper, and applicator in proper receptacle. *Comments:*	☐	☐	☐	
15. Remove gloves and wash hands. *Comments:*	☐	☐	☐	

Checklist for Procedure 2-1 Proper Body Mechanics, Safe Lifting, and Transferring

Name _____ Date _____

School _____

Instructor _____

Course _____

Procedure 2-1 **Proper Body Mechanics, Safe Lifting,** **and Transferring** Assessment	Able to Perform	Able to Perform with Assistance	Unable to Perform	Initials and Date
1. Assess the need and degree to which the client requires assistance. *Comments:*	☐	☐	☐	
2. Identify the type of physical movement required. *Comments:*	☐	☐	☐	
3. Identify the potential need for assistive equipment. *Comments:*	☐	☐	☐	
4. Identify any unusual risks to safe lifting. *Comments:*	☐	☐	☐	
5. Assess the client's vital signs, pain status, and need for pain medications prior to ambulating. Assess incisional areas and/or areas of injury. *Comments:*	☐	☐	☐	
6. Check equipment to ensure that it is in working order to facilitate a safe and uninterrupted transfer. Especially check locks on wheelchair. *Comments:*	☐	☐	☐	
7. Identify all equipment and tubes connected to the client and take appropriate preventive measures. Frequently, clients that require lifting or transfer have intravenous tubing, other tubing, and/or orthopedic equipment. *Comments:*	☐	☐	☐	
8. Assess the client's understanding of the steps required to achieve the goal of a safe transfer and the ability to assist. Explanation of the steps in a clear, concise fashion will decrease anxiety, secure cooperation, and ease physical requirements for both the client and the nurse/caregiver. *Comments:*	☐	☐	☐	

continued on the following page

continued from the previous page

Procedure 2-1	Able to Perform	Able to Perform with Assistance	Unable to Perform	Initials and Date
Planning/Expected Outcomes				
1. Clients will be safely lifted by staff. *Comments:*	☐	☐	☐	
2. Accidents during lifting of clients will be avoided. *Comments:*	☐	☐	☐	
3. Heavy lifting will be facilitated by mechanical devices and a team effort. *Comments:*	☐	☐	☐	
4. Clients and families will be taught safe lifting techniques. *Comments:*	☐	☐	☐	
5. The nurse will practice safe lifting and proper body mechanics. *Comments:*	☐	☐	☐	
Implementation				
1. Wash hands. *Comments:*	☐	☐	☐	
2. Assess the situation for obstacles. Reduce or remove safety hazards prior to lifting the client or object. *Comments:*	☐	☐	☐	
3. Assess the situation for slippery surfaces. Resolve the slippery surface prior to lifting the client or object. *Comments:*	☐	☐	☐	
4. Assess the situation for hidden risks. *Comments:*	☐	☐	☐	
5. Maintain low center of gravity by bending at the hips and knees, not at the waist. Squat down rather than bend over to lift and lower. *Comments:*	☐	☐	☐	
6. Establish a wide support base with feet spread apart. *Comments:*	☐	☐	☐	

Procedure 2-1	Able to Perform	Able to Perform with Assistance	Unable to Perform	Initials and Date
7. Use feet to move, not a twisting or bending motion from the waist. *Comments:*	☐	☐	☐	
8. When pushing or pulling, stand near the object and stagger one foot partially ahead of the other. *Comments:*	☐	☐	☐	
9. When pushing a client or an object, lean into the client or object and apply continuous light pressure. When pulling an object, lean away and grasp with light pressure. Never jerk or twist your body to force a weight to move. *Comments:*	☐	☐	☐	
10. When stooping to move an object, maintain a wide base of support with feet, flex knees to lower, and maintain straight upper body. *Comments:*	☐	☐	☐	
11. When lifting an object, squat down in front of the object, take a firm hold, and assume a standing position by using the leg muscles, keeping the back straight. *Comments:*	☐	☐	☐	
12. When raising up from a squatting position, arch your back slightly. Keep the buttocks and abdomen tucked in and raise up with your head first. *Comments:*	☐	☐	☐	
13. When lifting or carrying heavy objects, keep the weight as close to your center of gravity as possible. *Comments:*	☐	☐	☐	
14. When reaching for an object, keep the back straight. *Comments:*	☐	☐	☐	
15. Use safety aids and equipment. *Comments:*	☐	☐	☐	

Checklist for Procedure 2-2   Assisting with Ambulation and Safe Falling

Name _____ Date _____

School _____

Instructor _____

Course _____

Procedure 2-2 Assisting with Ambulation and Safe Falling	Able to Perform	Able to Perform with Assistance	Unable to Perform	Initials and Date
Assessment				
1. Determine the client's most recent activity level and tolerance. *Comments:*	☐	☐	☐	
2. Assess the client's current status, including vital signs, fatigue, pain, and medications to identify conditions that might adversely affect ambulation. *Comments:*	☐	☐	☐	
3. Check for handrails, a clean and level floor, and adequate lighting. *Comments:*	☐	☐	☐	
4. Assess the client's ambulation equipment. *Comments:*	☐	☐	☐	
5. Check the client's clothing to determine that the client's shoes or slippers are safe to walk in and that he or she has adequate covering for warmth and privacy. *Comments:*	☐	☐	☐	
6. While the client is ambulating, assess gait and bearing. *Comments:*	☐	☐	☐	
7. After ambulation, assess the client's ability to recover from the activity. *Comments:*	☐	☐	☐	
Planning/Expected Outcomes				
1. The client will be able to walk a predetermined distance, with assistance as needed, and return to the starting point. *Comments:*	☐	☐	☐	

continued on the following page

continued from the previous page

Procedure 2-2	Able to Perform	Able to Perform with Assistance	Unable to Perform	Initials and Date
2. While walking, the client will not suffer any injury. *Comments:*	☐	☐	☐	
3. The client will be able to increase the distance he or she can walk and/or will require less assistance to accomplish the distance. *Comments:*	☐	☐	☐	
Implementation				
1. Place the IV pole with wheels, if present, at the head of the bed before having the client dangle the legs. *Comments:*	☐	☐	☐	
2. Transfer the IV infusion from the bed IV pole to the portable IV pole. *Comments:*	☐	☐	☐	
3. When assisting the client with a urinary drainage bag, empty the drainage bag prior to ambulation. Remove the urinary drainage bag from the bed. *Comments:*	☐	☐	☐	
4. When the client has a drainage tube, be sure to secure the drainage tube and bag prior to ambulation. *Comments:*	☐	☐	☐	
5. Ambulating the client with a closed chest tube drainage system often requires two nurses. Remove the drainage system from the bed. Hold the closed chest tube drainage system upright at all times to maintain the water seal. *Comments:*	☐	☐	☐	
6. Use a transfer belt or gait belt when ambulating a client who is weak. *Comments:*	☐	☐	☐	
7. If a client feels faint or dizzy during dangling, return the client to a supine position in bed and lower the head of the bed. Monitor the client's blood pressure and pulse. *Comments:*	☐	☐	☐	

continued from the previous page

Procedure 2-2	Able to Perform	Able to Perform with Assistance	Unable to Perform	Initials and Date
8. If the client feels faint or dizzy during ambulation, allow the client to sit in a chair. Stay with the client for safety. Request another nurse to secure a wheelchair to return the client to bed. *Comments:*	☐	☐	☐	
9. If the client feels faint or dizzy during the ambulation and starts to fall, ease the client to the floor while supporting and protecting the client's head. Ask other personnel to assist you in returning the client to bed. Assess orthostatic blood pressures. *Comments:*	☐	☐	☐	
10. Encourage the client to void before ambulating, especially with elderly clients. *Comments:*	☐	☐	☐	
Safe Walking 11. Inform client of the purposes and distance of the walking exercise. *Comments:*	☐	☐	☐	
12. Elevate the head of the bed and wait several minutes. *Comments:*	☐	☐	☐	
13. Lower the bed height. *Comments:*	☐	☐	☐	
14. With one arm on the client's back and one arm under the client's upper legs, move the client into the dangling position. *Comments:*	☐	☐	☐	
15. Encourage the client dangle for several minutes. *Comments:*	☐	☐	☐	
16. Place gait belt around client's waist; secure the buckle in front. *Comments:*	☐	☐	☐	

continued on the following page

continued from the previous page

Procedure 2-2	Able to Perform	Able to Perform with Assistance	Unable to Perform	Initials and Date
17. Stand in front of client with your knees touching client's knees. *Comments:*	☐	☐	☐	
18. Place arms under client's axilla. *Comments:*	☐	☐	☐	
19. Assist client to a standing position, allowing client time to balance. *Comments:*	☐	☐	☐	
20. Help the client ambulate. *Comments:*	☐	☐	☐	
21. Help the client back to the bed or chair. Make the client comfortable, and make sure all lines and tubes are secure. *Comments:*	☐	☐	☐	
22. Wash hands. *Comments:*	☐	☐	☐	

Checklist for Procedure 2-3   Applying Restraints

Name _____ Date _____

School _____

Instructor _____

Course _____

Procedure 2-3 Applying Restraints	Able to Perform	Able to Perform with Assistance	Unable to Perform	Initials and Date
Assessment				
1. Assess the client's level of consciousness. *Comments:*	☐	☐	☐	
2. Assess the client's degree of orientation. *Comments:*	☐	☐	☐	
3. Assess the client's physical condition. *Comments:*	☐	☐	☐	
4. Assess the client's history. *Comments:*	☐	☐	☐	
5. Assess the client's intent. *Comments:*	☐	☐	☐	
6. Assess the need for restraints. *Comments:*	☐	☐	☐	
7. Assess client and family knowledge regarding the use of and rationale for restraints or protective devices. *Comments:*	☐	☐	☐	
Planning/Expected Outcomes				
1. The client will remain uninjured. *Comments:*	☐	☐	☐	
2. The client will not suffer injury or impairment from the restraints. *Comments:*	☐	☐	☐	
3. The client's therapeutic equipment will remain intact and functional. *Comments:*	☐	☐	☐	

continued on the following page

continued from the previous page

Procedure 2-3	Able to Perform	Able to Perform with Assistance	Unable to Perform	Initials and Date
4. Others will not be harmed by the client. *Comments:*	☐	☐	☐	
5. The client will be restrained just enough to prevent injury. *Comments:*	☐	☐	☐	

Implementation

Chest Restraint

1. Explain that the client will be wearing a jacket attached to the bed for his or her safety. *Comments:*	☐	☐	☐	
2. Place the restraint over the client's hospital gown or clothing. *Comments:*	☐	☐	☐	
3. Place the restraint with the opening in the front. *Comments:*	☐	☐	☐	
4. Overlap the front pieces, threading the ties through the appropriate slots. *Comments:*	☐	☐	☐	
5. If the client is in bed, secure the ties to the movable part of the mattress frame with a half-knot. *Comments:*	☐	☐	☐	
6. If the client is in a chair, cross the straps behind the seat and secure to the chair's lower legs. *Comments:*	☐	☐	☐	
7. Step back and assess the client's overall safety. *Comments:*	☐	☐	☐	
8. Wash your hands. *Comments:*	☐	☐	☐	

Procedure 2-3	Able to Perform	Able to Perform with Assistance	Unable to Perform	Initials and Date
Applying Wrist or Ankle Restraints 9. Explain that you will be placing a wrist or ankle band that will restrict movement. *Comments:*	☐	☐	☐	
10. Place padding around the client's wrist/ankle. *Comments:*	☐	☐	☐	
11. Wrap the restraint around the wrist/ankle pulling the tie through the appropriate loops. *Comments:*	☐	☐	☐	
12. Fasten the restraint ties to the movable portion of the mattress frame with a secure knot. *Comments:*	☐	☐	☐	
13. Slip two fingers under the restraint to check for tightness. *Comments:*	☐	☐	☐	
14. Step back and assess the client's overall safety. *Comments:*	☐	☐	☐	
15. Place the call light within the client's reach. *Comments:*	☐	☐	☐	
16. Check on the client every half-hour while restrained. *Comments:*	☐	☐	☐	
17. Wash your hands. *Comments:*	☐	☐	☐	

Checklist for Procedure 2-4   Handwashing

Name _____ Date _____

School _____

Instructor _____

Course _____

Procedure 2-4 Handwashing	Able to Perform	Able to Perform with Assistance	Unable to Perform	Initials and Date
Assessment				
1. Assess the environment to establish if facilities are adequate for cleansing the hands. *Comments:*	☐	☐	☐	
2. Assess your hands. *Comments:*	☐	☐	☐	
Planning/Expected Outcomes				
1. The caregiver's hands will be cleansed adequately to remove microorganisms, transient flora, and soil from the skin. *Comments:*	☐	☐	☐	
Implementation				
1. Remove jewelry. Wristwatch may be pushed up above the wrist (midforearm). Push sleeves of uniform or shirt up above the wrist at midforearm level. *Comments:*	☐	☐	☐	
2. Assess hands for hangnails, cuts or breaks in the skin, and areas that are heavily soiled. *Comments:*	☐	☐	☐	
3. Turn on the water. Adjust the flow and temperature. *Comments:*	☐	☐	☐	
4. Wet hands and lower forearms thoroughly by holding under running water. Keep hands and forearms in the down position with elbows straight. *Comments:*	☐	☐	☐	
5. Apply about 5 ml (1 teaspoon) of liquid soap. Lather thoroughly. *Comments:*	☐	☐	☐	

continued on the following page

continued from the previous page

Procedure 2-4	Able to Perform	Able to Perform with Assistance	Unable to Perform	Initials and Date
6. Thoroughly rub hands together for about 10–15 seconds. *Comments:*	☐	☐	☐	
7. Rinse with hands in the down position, elbows straight. Rinse in the direction of forearm to wrist to fingers. *Comments:*	☐	☐	☐	
8. Blot hands and forearms to dry thoroughly. Dry in the direction of fingers to wrist and forearms. Discard the paper towels in the proper receptacle. *Comments:*	☐	☐	☐	
9. Turn off the water faucet with a clean, dry paper towel. *Comments:*	☐	☐	☐	

Checklist for Procedure 2-5 Donning and Removing Clean and Contaminated Gloves, Cap, and Mask

Name _____ Date _____

School _____

Instructor _____

Course _____

Procedure 2-5 **Donning and Removing Clean** **and Contaminated Gloves, Cap, and Mask**	Able to Perform	Able to Perform with Assistance	Unable to Perform	Initials and Date
Assessment				
1. Assess the specific isolation precautions needed for the client's condition. *Comments:*	☐	☐	☐	
2. Assess the client's laboratory results. *Comments:*	☐	☐	☐	
3. Assess what nursing measures are required. *Comments:*	☐	☐	☐	
4. Assess the client's knowledge for the need to wear a cap, mask, and gloves during care. *Comments:*	☐	☐	☐	
5. Assess whether the isolation is airborne, droplet, or contact, and which isolation attire is necessary. *Comments:*	☐	☐	☐	
Planning/Expected Outcomes				
1. The client will remain free of nosocomial infections. *Comments:*	☐	☐	☐	
2. The health care provider will be protected from infection when caring for the client. *Comments:*	☐	☐	☐	
3. The staff will avoid transmitting microorganisms to others. *Comments:*	☐	☐	☐	
4. The client will interact on a social level with the nurse, family members, and other visitors. *Comments:*	☐	☐	☐	

continued on the following page

continued from the previous page

Procedure 2-5	Able to Perform	Able to Perform with Assistance	Unable to Perform	Initials and Date
Implementation				
1. Wash hands. *Comments:*	☐	☐	☐	
2. The first item of apparel donned should be the cap or surgical hat/hood. *Comments:*	☐	☐	☐	
3. Apply a mask around the mouth and nose. Secure the mask in a manner that prevents venting. *Comments:*	☐	☐	☐	
4. Open gown, slip arms into sleeves, and secure at neck and side. *Comments:*	☐	☐	☐	
5. Protective eyewear should be worn whenever the health care provider or client are at risk for splash and contamination. *Comments:*	☐	☐	☐	
6. Don clean gloves. If sterile gloves are required for a procedure use open or closed method. *Comments:*	☐	☐	☐	
7. The open glove technique: • Slide the hands into the gown all the way through the cuffs on the gown. • Pick up the cuff of the left glove using the thumb and index finger of the right hand. • Pull the glove onto the left hand, leaving the cuff of the glove turned down. • Take the gloved left hand and slide the fingers inside the cuff of the right glove keeping the gloved fingers under the folded cuff. • Pull the glove onto the right hand. • Rotate the arm as the cuff of the glove is pulled over the gown. *Comments:*	☐	☐	☐	

Procedure 2-5	Able to Perform	Able to Perform with Assistance	Unable to Perform	Initials and Date
8. The closed glove technique: • Slide the hands into the gown all the way through the cuffs on the gown. • Use right hand to pick up left glove. • Place the glove on the upward-turned left hand—palm side down thumb to thumb with the fingers extending along the forearm pointing toward the elbow. • Hold the glove cuff and sleeve cuff together with the thumb of the left hand. • The right hand stretches the cuff of the left glove over the opened end of the sleeve. • Work the fingers into the glove as the cuff is pulled onto the wrist. • The left glove is done in the same manner. *Comments:*	☐	☐	☐	
9. Enter the client's room and explain the rationale for wearing isolation attire. *Comments:*	☐	☐	☐	
10. After performing necessary tasks, remove gown, gloves, mask, and cap before leaving the room. *Comments:*	☐	☐	☐	
11. Removal of gown: untie gown and remove from shoulders. Fold and roll gown down in front into a ball, so contaminated area is rolled into center of gown. *Comments:*	☐	☐	☐	
12. • Grasp outside cuff of one glove and pull off, turning inside out. • Pull the second glove off without touching the outside of the second glove. *Comments:*	☐	☐	☐	

Checklist for Procedure 2-6   Removing Contaminated Items

Name _____ Date _____

School _____

Instructor _____

Course _____

Procedure 2-6 Removing Contaminated Items	Able to Perform	Able to Perform with Assistance	Unable to Perform	Initials and Date
Assessment				
1. Assess the client's disease process and medical condition. *Comments:*	☐	☐	☐	
2. Assess the client's level of understanding regarding infection precautions. *Comments:*	☐	☐	☐	
Planning/Expected Outcomes				
1. Client will demonstrate an understanding regarding infection control procedures. *Comments:*	☐	☐	☐	
2. Client will demonstrate self-care measures related to infection prevention. *Comments:*	☐	☐	☐	
3. All contaminated items within the client's environment will be disposed of in an appropriate manner. *Comments:*	☐	☐	☐	
4. Personnel caring for the client will use appropriate infection prevention measures. *Comments:*	☐	☐	☐	
Implementation				
Removal of Soiled Linen 1. Wash hands when entering the client's room. *Comments:*	☐	☐	☐	
2. Wear disposable gloves and other protective items as needed. *Comments:*	☐	☐	☐	

continued on the following page

continued from the previous page

Procedure 2-6	Able to Perform	Able to Perform with Assistance	Unable to Perform	Initials and Date
3. Place labeled linen bag in stand. *Comments:*	☐	☐	☐	
4. Gather linen and separate from disposable items. *Comments:*	☐	☐	☐	
5. Do not allow any linen to touch the floor. *Comments:*	☐	☐	☐	
6. Place soiled linen in the linen bag; keep clean linen in a different area. *Comments:*	☐	☐	☐	
7. Take care not to shake the linen when removing items. *Comments:*	☐	☐	☐	
8. Do not allow the soiled linen to come in contact with your clothing. Carry linens with arms extended in front of you. *Comments:*	☐	☐	☐	
9. Do not overfill the bag. *Comments:*	☐	☐	☐	
10. Tie ends of the bag securely. *Comments:*	☐	☐	☐	
11. Check for any punctures or tears in the bag. *Comments:*	☐	☐	☐	
12. Double bag items if there is concern that the outside of the bag is contaminated or torn. *Comments:*	☐	☐	☐	
13. Wash hands. *Comments:*	☐	☐	☐	

Procedure 2-6	Able to Perform	Able to Perform with Assistance	Unable to Perform	Initials and Date
Double-Bagging Technique 14. When double bagging linens, follow Actions 1–11. Then place the first bag into a second bag. *Comments:*	☐	☐	☐	
15. The second bag is properly labeled and secured. *Comments:*	☐	☐	☐	
16. The linens are then ready for the laundry. *Comments:*	☐	☐	☐	
17. Wash hands thoroughly upon leaving the room. *Comments:*	☐	☐	☐	
Removal of Other Contaminated Items 18. Removal and bagging of trash bags follows the same procedure as for linens. *Comments:*	☐	☐	☐	
19. Sharps containers need to be removed when three-fourths full or if the outside of the container becomes contaminated. *Comments:*	☐	☐	☐	
20. Always wash hands when entering or leaving the client's room. *Comments:*	☐	☐	☐	
21. Use disposable equipment when possible. *Comments:*	☐	☐	☐	
22. Properly bag, label, and remove any nondisposable equipment that will require special cleaning. *Comments:*	☐	☐	☐	
23. Disassemble special procedure trays into disposable and nondisposable parts. Send both to the proper area. *Comments:*	☐	☐	☐	

continued on the following page

continued from the previous page

Procedure 2-6	Able to Perform	Able to Perform with Assistance	Unable to Perform	Initials and Date
24. Laboratory specimens should be placed in a leakproof container and require no other precautions. *Comments:*	☐	☐	☐	
25. Wash hands. *Comments:*	☐	☐	☐	

Checklist for Procedure 2-7   Applying Sterile Gloves via the Open Method

Name _____ Date _____

School _____

Instructor _____

Course _____

Procedure 2-7 Applying Sterile Gloves via the Open Method	Able to Perform	Able to Perform with Assistance	Unable to Perform	Initials and Date
Assessment				
1. Assess the glove package. *Comments:*	☐	☐	☐	
2. Assess the local environment. *Comments:*	☐	☐	☐	
3. Assess the correct glove size for proper fit. *Comments:*	☐	☐	☐	
Planning/Expected Outcomes				
1. Sterility of the gloves will be maintained while they are being applied. *Comments:*	☐	☐	☐	
2. Sterility of the procedure will be maintained. *Comments:*	☐	☐	☐	
Implementation				
1. Wash hands. *Comments:*	☐	☐	☐	
2. Remove the outer wrapper from the package, place the inner wrapper onto a clean, dry surface. Open inner wrapper to expose gloves. *Comments:*	☐	☐	☐	
3. Identify right and left hand; glove dominant hand first. *Comments:*	☐	☐	☐	
4. Grasp the 2-inch (5-cm)-wide cuff with the thumb and first two fingers of the nondominant hand, touching only the inside of the cuff. *Comments:*	☐	☐	☐	

continued on the following page

continued from the previous page

Procedure 2-7	Able to Perform	Able to Perform with Assistance	Unable to Perform	Initials and Date
5. Gently pull the glove over the dominant hand. *Comments:*	☐	☐	☐	
6. With the gloved dominant hand, slip your fingers under the cuff of the other glove. *Comments:*	☐	☐	☐	
7. Gently slip the glove onto your nondominant hand. *Comments:*	☐	☐	☐	
8. With gloved hands, interlock fingers to fit the gloves onto each finger. *Comments:*	☐	☐	☐	
9. If the gloves are soiled, remove as follows: Slip gloved fingers of the dominant hand under the cuff of the opposite hand, or grasp the outer part of the glove at the wrist if there is no cuff. *Comments:*	☐	☐	☐	
10. Pull the glove down to the fingers, exposing the thumb. *Comments:*	☐	☐	☐	
11. Slip the uncovered thumb into the opposite glove at the wrist. *Comments:*	☐	☐	☐	
12. Pull the glove down over the dominant hand almost to the fingertips and slip the glove onto the other hand. *Comments:*	☐	☐	☐	
13. Pull the glove over the dominant hand so that only the inside is exposed. *Comments:*	☐	☐	☐	
14. Dispose of soiled gloves and wash hands. *Comments:*	☐	☐	☐	

Checklist for Procedure 2-8   Surgical Scrub

Name _____ Date _____

School _____

Instructor _____

Course _____

Procedure 2-8 Surgical Scrub	Able to Perform	Able to Perform with Assistance	Unable to Perform	Initials and Date
Assessment				
1. Assess the scrub environment for equipment and cleanliness. *Comments:*	☐	☐	☐	
2. Assess your preparedness. *Comments:*	☐	☐	☐	
Planning/Expected Outcomes				
1. Hands and forearms will be adequately cleansed for applying sterile gloves and gown. *Comments:*	☐	☐	☐	
Implementation				
Preparation 1. Rings, watches, and bracelets should be removed prior to beginning the surgical scrub. *Comments:*	☐	☐	☐	
2. Use a deep sink with side or foot pedal to dispense soap and control water flow. *Comments:*	☐	☐	☐	
3. Have two surgical scrub brushes and nail file available. *Comments:*	☐	☐	☐	
4. Apply surgical shoe covers and cap. *Comments:*	☐	☐	☐	
5. Apply mask. *Comments:*	☐	☐	☐	

continued on the following page

continued from the previous page

Procedure 2-8	Able to Perform	Able to Perform with Assistance	Unable to Perform	Initials and Date
6. • Open the sterile package containing the gown and form a sterile field. • Open the sterile towel and drop it onto the center of field. • Open the sterile gloves and drop the inner package of gloves onto the sterile field. *Comments:*	☐	☐	☐	
Surgical Handwashing 7. At a deep sink, under flowing water, wet forearms and hands. *Comments:*	☐	☐	☐	
8. Apply soap and rub hands and arms to 2 inches above elbows. *Comments:*	☐	☐	☐	
9. Clean under each nail of both hands and drop file into sink. *Comments:*	☐	☐	☐	
10. Wet and apply soap to scrub brush, if needed. Open prepackaged scrub brush if available. With brush in your dominant hand using a circular motion, scrub nails and all skin areas of nondominant hand and arm (10 strokes in each of the following areas): • Nails • Palm of hand and anterior side of fingers. *Comments:*	☐	☐	☐	
11. Rinse brush thoroughly; reapply soap. *Comments:*	☐	☐	☐	
12. Continue with scrub of nondominant arm. Drop brush into the sink. *Comments:*	☐	☐	☐	
13. Maintaining the hands and arms above elbow level, place the fingertips under running water and thoroughly rinse the fingers, hands, and arms (allow the water to run off your elbow into the sink); take care not to get your uniform wet. *Comments:*	☐	☐	☐	

Procedure 2-8	Able to Perform	Able to Perform with Assistance	Unable to Perform	Initials and Date
14. With the second scrub brush, repeat Actions 10–13 on your dominant hand and arm. *Comments:*	☐	☐	☐	
15. Keep arms flexed and proceed to area with sterile field. *Comments:*	☐	☐	☐	
16. Secure sterile towel by grasping it on one edge and opening the towel full length, making sure it does not touch your uniform. *Comments:*	☐	☐	☐	
17. Dry each hand and arm separately with a rotating motion up to the elbow. *Comments:*	☐	☐	☐	
18. Reverse the towel and repeat the same action on the other hand and arm, thoroughly drying the skin. *Comments:*	☐	☐	☐	
19. Discard the towel into a linen hamper. *Comments:*	☐	☐	☐	

Checklist for Procedure 2-9   Applying Sterile Gloves and Gown via the Closed Method

Name _____ Date _____

School _____

Instructor _____

Course _____

Procedure 2-9 **Applying Sterile Gloves and Gown via the Closed Method**	Able to Perform	Able to Perform with Assistance	Unable to Perform	Initials and Date
Assessment				
1. Assess the surrounding environment. *Comments:*	☐	☐	☐	
2. Assess the condition of your hands. *Comments:*	☐	☐	☐	
Planning/Expected Outcomes				
1. The caregiver will don a sterile gown and gloves without compromising their sterility. *Comments:*	☐	☐	☐	
Implementation				
Gowning 1. The sterile gown comes folded inside out. *Comments:*	☐	☐	☐	
2. Grasp the gown inside the neckline, step back, and allow it to fall open. *Comments:*	☐	☐	☐	
3. Slip both arms into the gown; keep your hands inside the sleeves of the gown. *Comments:*	☐	☐	☐	
4. The circulating nurse will secure the ties at the neck and waist. *Comments:*	☐	☐	☐	
Closed Gloving 5. With hands still inside the gown sleeves, open the inner wrapper of the sterile gloves. *Comments:*	☐	☐	☐	

continued on the following page

continued from the previous page

Procedure 2-9	**Able to Perform**	**Able to Perform with Assistance**	**Unable to Perform**	**Initials and Date**
6. With your nondominant sleeved hand, place the palm of the dominant hand glove against the sleeved palm of the dominant hand. *Comments:*	☐	☐	☐	
7. Manipulate the glove cuff with your dominant, sleeved thumb. With your nondominant hand, turn the cuff over the end of dominant hand and gown's cuff. *Comments:*	☐	☐	☐	
8. With sleeved nondominant hand, grasp the cuff of the glove and the gown's sleeve of the dominant hand; slowly extend the fingers into the glove, making sure the cuff of the glove remains above the cuff of the gown's sleeve. *Comments:*	☐	☐	☐	
9. With the gloved dominant hand, repeat Actions 7 and 8. *Comments:*	☐	☐	☐	
10. Interlock gloved fingers and secure fit. *Comments:*	☐	☐	☐	

Checklist for Procedure 2-10 Emergency Airway Management

Name _____ Date _____

School _____

Instructor _____

Course _____

Procedure 2-10 Emergency Airway Management	Able to Perform	Able to Perform with Assistance	Unable to Perform	Initials and Date
Assessment				
1. Assess for visible respirations. *Comments:*	☐	☐	☐	.
2. Assess the client's mental status. *Comments:*	☐	☐	☐	
3. Assess for stridor, ability to speak or cough effectively, or clutching of the throat. *Comments:*	☐	☐	☐	
4. Assess for the presence of obstruction, such as thick secretions, food, or other foreign bodies to avoid advancing the obstruction deeper into the respiratory system. If appropriate, consult with staff, client, or family to determine knowledge of foreign object aspirated. *Comments:*	☐	☐	☐	
Planning/Expected Outcomes				
1. The client will breathe effectively through an open airway. *Comments:*	☐	☐	☐	
Implementation				
1. Wash hands and apply gloves if available. *Comments:*	☐	☐	☐	
2. Assess airway. Call for assistance. *Comments:*	☐	☐	☐	
3. If the mouth is unopened, gently tilt the head backward. *Comments:*	☐	☐	☐	
4. Assess for spontaneous respirations. *Comments:*	☐	☐	☐	

continued on the following page

continued from the previous page

Procedure 2-10	Able to Perform	Able to Perform with Assistance	Unable to Perform	Initials and Date
5. Turn the client on the side and clear the mouth of secretions or obstructions. *Comments:*	☐	☐	☐	
6. Insert oropharyngeal airway if available. *Comments:*	☐	☐	☐	
7. If spontaneous respirations occur, maintain head in proper position. *Comments:*	☐	☐	☐	
8. If respirations do not resume, initiate artificial respiration. *Comments:*	☐	☐	☐	
9. Assess client for presence of cardiac arrest. If present follow steps for Skill 2-11. *Comments:*	☐	☐	☐	
10. Continue efforts until assistance arrives. *Comments:*	☐	☐	☐	
11. When client is stable, remove gloves and wash hands. *Comments:*	☐	☐	☐	
12. Document interventions in the appropriate manner. *Comments:*	☐	☐	☐	

Checklist for Procedure 2-11   Administering Cardiopulmonary Resuscitation (CPR)

Name _____ Date _____

School _____

Instructor _____

Course _____

Procedure 2-11 Administering Cardiopulmonary Resuscitation (CPR)	Able to Perform	Able to Perform with Assistance	Unable to Perform	Initials and Date
Assessment				
1. Assess responsiveness and level of consciousness. *Comments:*	☐	☐	☐	
2. Assess the amount and abilities of any available assistance. *Comments:*	☐	☐	☐	
3. Assess the client's position. *Comments:*	☐	☐	☐	
4. Assess respiratory status. *Comments:*	☐	☐	☐	
5. Assess circulatory status. *Comments:*	☐	☐	☐	
Planning/Expected Outcomes				
1. Client will experience improved clinical status. *Comments:*	☐	☐	☐	
2. Client does not experience negative sequela related to hypoxic event. *Comments:*	☐	☐	☐	
3. Client does not have damage inflicted secondary to CPR. *Comments:*	☐	☐	☐	
4. Cardiopulmonary resuscitation was terminated appropriately. *Comments:*	☐	☐	☐	

continued on the following page

continued from the previous page

Procedure 2-11	Able to Perform	Able to Perform with Assistance	Unable to Perform	Initials and Date
Implementation				
CPR: One Rescuer—Adult, Adolescent				
1. Assess responsiveness. *Comments:*	☐	☐	☐	
2. Activate emergency medical system. *Comments:*	☐	☐	☐	
3. Position client in a supine position on a hard, flat surface. *Comments:*	☐	☐	☐	
4. Apply appropriate body substance isolation items, if available. *Comments:*	☐	☐	☐	
5. Position self. *Comments:*	☐	☐	☐	
6. Open airway. *Comments:*	☐	☐	☐	
7. Assess for respirations. *Comments:*	☐	☐	☐	
8. If respirations are absent: • Occlude nostrils with the thumb and index finger. • Form a seal over the client's mouth with your mouth or the appropriate device. Give two full breaths. • Mouth-to-nose ventilation may be used. *Comments:*	☐	☐	☐	
9. Assess for the rise and fall of the chest: • If present, continue to Action 10. • If absent, assess for airway obstruction. *Comments:*	☐	☐	☐	
10. Palpate the carotid pulse: • If present, continue rescue breathing. • If absent, begin cardiac compressions. *Comments:*	☐	☐	☐	

Procedure 2-11	Able to Perform	Able to Perform with Assistance	Unable to Perform	Initials and Date
11. Cardiac compressions are performed as follows: • Maintain a position on knees parallel to sternum. • Position hands for compressions. • Extend or interlace fingers. • Keep arms straight and lock elbows. • Compress at the age-appropriate rate. • Ventilate client as described in Action 8. *Comments:*	☐	☐	☐	
12. Maintain the compression rate for approximately 100 times/min, interjecting 2 ventilations after every 15 compressions. (compression:ventilation rate at 15:2) *Comments:*	☐	☐	☐	
13. Reassess the client after four cycles. *Comments:*	☐	☐	☐	

CPR: Two Rescuers—Adult, Adolescent

14. Follow the steps above with the following changes:
   - One rescuer is positioned facing the client parallel to the head while the other rescuer is positioned on the opposite side facing the client parallel to the sternum next to the trunk.
   - The rescuer positioned at the client's trunk is responsible for performing cardiac compressions and maintaining the verbal mnemonic count. This is rescuer 1.
   - The rescuer positioned at the client's head is responsible for monitoring respirations, assessing the carotid pulse, establishing an open airway, and performing rescue breathing. This is rescuer two.
   - Maintain the compression rate for approximately 100 times/min, interjecting two ventilations after every 15 compressions. (compression:ventilation rate at 15:2)
   - Rescuer 2 palpates the carotid pulse with each chest compression during the first full minute.
   - Rescuer 2 is responsible for calling for a change when fatigued, following this protocol.
   - Rescuer 1 calls for a change and completes the 15 chest compressions.
   - Rescuer 2 administers two breaths and then moves to a position parallel to the client's sternum and assumes the proper hand position.
   - Rescuer 1 moves to the rescue breathing position and checks the carotid pulse for 5 seconds. If cardiac arrest persists, rescuer 1 says, "continue CPR" and delivers one breath. Rescuer 2 resumes cardiac compressions immediately after the breath.

   Comments: ☐   ☐   ☐

continued on the following page

continued from the previous page

Procedure 2-11	Able to Perform	Able to Perform with Assistance	Unable to Perform	Initials and Date
CPR: One Rescuer—Child (1–7 years)				
15. Follow Actions 1–7. *Comments:*	☐	☐	☐	
16. If respirations are absent, begin rescue breathing. *Comments:*	☐	☐	☐	
17. Palpate the carotid pulse (5–10 seconds): • If present, continue ventilation. • If absent, begin cardiac compressions. *Comments:*	☐	☐	☐	
18. Cardiac compressions (child 1–7 years): • Maintain a position on knees parallel to child's sternum. • Place a small towel under the child's shoulders. • Position the hands for compressions. • At the end of every fifth compression, administer a ventilation. • Reevaluate child after ten cycles. *Comments:*	☐	☐	☐	
CPR: One Rescuer—Infant (1–12 months)				
19. Follow Actions 1–7. *Comments:*	☐	☐	☐	
20. If respirations are absent, begin rescue breathing. *Comments:*	☐	☐	☐	
21. Assess circulatory status using the brachial pulse: • If a pulse is palpated, continue rescue breathing. • If a pulse is absent, begin cardiac compressions. *Comments:*	☐	☐	☐	
22. Cardiac compressions (infant 1–12 months): • Maintain a position parallel to the infant. • Place a small towel under the infant's shoulders/neck. • Position the hands for compressions. • Reevaluate infant after ten cycles. *Comments:*	☐	☐	☐	

Procedure 2-11	Able to Perform	Able to Perform with Assistance	Unable to Perform	Initials and Date

CPR: Two Rescuers—Child (1–7 years) and Infant (1–12 months)
23. Follow Action 14 except:
  • Utilize the child or infant procedure for chest compressions.
  • Change the ratio of compressions to ventilation to 3:1.
  • Deliver the ventilation on the upstroke of the third compression.
  Comments:
	☐	☐	☐	

CPR: Neonate or Premature Infant
24. Follow the infant guidelines except:
  • Encircle the chest with both hands.
  • Position thumbs over the midsternum.
  • Compress the midsternum with both thumbs.
  Comments:
	☐	☐	☐	

25. If properly trained use an automated external defibrillator (AED). *Comments:*	☐	☐	☐	

Checklist for Procedure 2-12   Performing the Heimlich Maneuver

Name _____ Date _____

School _____

Instructor _____

Course _____

Procedure 2-12 Performing the Heimlich Maneuver	Able to Perform	Able to Perform with Assistance	Unable to Perform	Initials and Date
Assessment				
1. Assess air exchange. *Comments:*	☐	☐	☐	
2. Establish airway obstruction. *Comments:*	☐	☐	☐	
3. In the pediatric client, differentiate between infection and airway obstruction. *Comments:*	☐	☐	☐	
Planning/Expected Outcomes				
1. The client's clinical status will improve. *Comments:*	☐	☐	☐	
2. The client's gas exchange will improve. *Comments:*	☐	☐	☐	
3. The client will experience minimal discomfort during airway clearance. *Comments:*	☐	☐	☐	
4. The client will not experience complications. *Comments:*	☐	☐	☐	
Implementation				
Foreign Body Obstruction—All Clients 1. Assess airway for complete or partial blockage. *Comments:*	☐	☐	☐	
2. Activate emergency response assistance. *Comments:*	☐	☐	☐	

continued on the following page

continued from the previous page

Procedure 2-12	Able to Perform	Able to Perform with Assistance	Unable to Perform	Initials and Date
Conscious Adult Client—Sitting or Standing (Heimlich Maneuver)				
3. Stand behind the client. *Comments:*	☐	☐	☐	
4. Wrap your arms around the client's waist. *Comments:*	☐	☐	☐	
5. Make a fist with one hand and grasp it with your other hand, placing the thumb side of the fist against the client's abdomen. *Comments:*	☐	☐	☐	
6. Perform a quick upward thrust into the client's abdomen. *Comments:*	☐	☐	☐	
7. Repeat this process six to ten times until the client either expels the foreign body or loses consciousness. *Comments:*	☐	☐	☐	
Adult Client Who Is or Becomes Unconscious				
8. Repeat Actions 1 and 2. *Comments:*	☐	☐	☐	
9. Position the client supine, kneel astride the client's abdomen. *Comments:*	☐	☐	☐	
10. Place the heel of one hand below the xiphoid process and above the navel. Place the second hand on top of the first hand. *Comments:*	☐	☐	☐	
11. Perform a quick upward thrust into the diaphragm, repeating six to ten times. *Comments:*	☐	☐	☐	
12. Perform a finger sweep. *Comments:*	☐	☐	☐	
13. Open the client's airway and attempt ventilation. *Comments:*	☐	☐	☐	

Procedure 2-12	Able to Perform	Able to Perform with Assistance	Unable to Perform	Initials and Date
14. Continue sequence of Heimlich maneuver, finger sweep, and rescue breathing as long as necessary. *Comments:*	☐	☐	☐	
Conscious Adult Sitting or Standing—Chest Thrusts 15. Repeat Actions 1 and 2. *Comments:*	☐	☐	☐	
16. Stand behind the client and encircle the chest with arms under the axilla. *Comments:*	☐	☐	☐	
17. Make a fist and place the thumb side of the fist on the middle of the client's sternum and grasp the fist with the second hand. *Comments:*	☐	☐	☐	
18. Perform backward thrusts until the client either becomes unconscious or the foreign body is expelled. *Comments:*	☐	☐	☐	
Unconscious Adult—Chest Thrusts 19. Repeat Actions 1 and 2. *Comments:*	☐	☐	☐	
20. Place client supine and kneel at the client's side. *Comments:*	☐	☐	☐	
21. Place the heel of one hand on the lower half of the sternum. *Comments:*	☐	☐	☐	
22. Perform each thrust in a slow, separate, and distinct manner. *Comments:*	☐	☐	☐	
23. Follow Actions 9–12 for the adult Heimlich maneuver, unconscious client. *Comments:*	☐	☐	☐	

continued on the following page

continued from the previous page

Procedure 2-12	Able to Perform	Able to Perform with Assistance	Unable to Perform	Initials and Date
Airway Obstruction—Infants and Small Children				
24. Differentiate between infection and airway obstruction. *Comments:*	☐	☐	☐	
Infant Airway Obstruction				
25. Straddle infant over forearm in the prone position with the head lower than the trunk. Support the infant's head. *Comments:*	☐	☐	☐	
26. Deliver four back blows between the infant's shoulder blades. *Comments:*	☐	☐	☐	
27. Keeping the infant's head down, turn the infant over. *Comments:*	☐	☐	☐	
28. Deliver four thrusts as in infant external cardiac compressions. *Comments:*	☐	☐	☐	
29. Assess for a foreign body in an unconscious infant. Utilize the finger sweep only if a foreign body is visualized. *Comments:*	☐	☐	☐	
30. Open airway and assess for respiration. If respirations are absent, attempt rescue breathing. *Comments:*	☐	☐	☐	
31. Repeat the entire sequence as long as necessary. *Comments:*	☐	☐	☐	
Small Child—Airway Obstruction (Conscious, Standing or Sitting)				
32. Assess air exchange and encourage coughing and breathing. *Comments:*	☐	☐	☐	

Procedure 2-12	Able to Perform	Able to Perform with Assistance	Unable to Perform	Initials and Date
33. Ask the child if he or she is choking. If the response is affirmative, follow the steps outlined below. In addition, if the child has poor air exchange (and infection has been ruled out), initiate the following steps: • Stand behind the child with your arms wrapped around the waist and administer six to ten subdiaphragmatic abdominal thrusts. • Continue until foreign object is expelled or the child becomes unconscious. *Comments:*	☐	☐	☐	
Small Child—Airway Obstruction (Conscious or Unconscious, Lying) 34. Position the child supine and kneel at the child's feet. Gently deliver six to ten subdiaphragmatic abdominal thrusts. *Comments:*	☐	☐	☐	
35. Open airway. Perform a finger sweep only if a foreign body is visualized. *Comments:*	☐	☐	☐	
36. If breathing is absent, begin rescue breathing. *Comments:*	☐	☐	☐	
37. Repeat this sequence as long as necessary. *Comments:*	☐	☐	☐	
38. Wash hands. *Comments:*	☐	☐	☐	

Checklist for Procedure 2-13   Responding to Accidental Poisoning

Name _____ Date _____

School _____

Instructor _____

Course _____

Procedure 2-13 Responding to Accidental Poisoning	Able to Perform	Able to Perform with Assistance	Unable to Perform	Initials and Date
Assessment				
Prevention 1. Assess the environment. *Comments:*	☐	☐	☐	
2. Assess if client is able to read medicine labels accurately. *Comments:*	☐	☐	☐	
Response 1. Assess for signs of poisoning. *Comments:*	☐	☐	☐	
2. Assess what, when, and how much of the harmful substance was taken. *Comments:*	☐	☐	☐	
Planning/Expected Outcomes				
1. Accidental poisoning will be prevented. *Comments:*	☐	☐	☐	
2. If accidental poisoning occurs, the client will experience a minimum of trauma. *Comments:*	☐	☐	☐	
Implementation				
When a Potential Poisoning Victim Is Discovered 1. Be familiar with the emergency procedures needed. *Comments:*	☐	☐	☐	
2. Call for help. Assess the client. If the client does not have a pulse and/or is not breathing, intervene with appropriate lifesaving measures. *Comments:*	☐	☐	☐	

continued on the following page

continued from the previous page

Procedure 2-13	Able to Perform	Able to Perform with Assistance	Unable to Perform	Initials and Date
3. If the client is conscious and breathing, call 911 or poison control for assistance. *Comments:*	☐	☐	☐	
4. Determine what substance and how much was ingested. Keep the container if available. *Comments:*	☐	☐	☐	
5. If you are talking to poison control, have them determine what treatment is appropriate. *Comments:*	☐	☐	☐	
6. If appropriate, give syrup of ipecac or activated charcoal. *Comments:*	☐	☐	☐	
7. Follow the instructions of the emergency providers. *Comments:*	☐	☐	☐	
8. Wash hands. *Comments:*	☐	☐	☐	

Checklist for Procedure 2-14   Emergency Client Transport

Name _____ Date _____

School _____

Instructor _____

Course _____

Procedure 2-14 Emergency Client Transport	Able to Perform	Able to Perform with Assistance	Unable to Perform	Initials and Date
Assessment				
1. Determine the nature of the disaster and where the danger is located. *Comments:*	☐	☐	☐	
2. Determine who is in charge of the evacuation. *Comments:*	☐	☐	☐	
3. Determine obstacles to the evacuation. *Comments:*	☐	☐	☐	
4. Determine your current client's medical needs, activity level, and tolerance. *Comments:*	☐	☐	☐	
5. Review what equipment will be needed to ensure client safety. *Comments:*	☐	☐	☐	
Planning/Expected Outcomes				
1. Client will be evacuated to a safe environment without injury. *Comments:*	☐	☐	☐	
2. Client will have essential medical support restored after the evacuation. *Comments:*	☐	☐	☐	
Implementation				
1. Remain calm; do not panic. *Comments:*	☐	☐	☐	

continued on the following page

continued from the previous page

Procedure 2-14	Able to Perform	Able to Perform with Assistance	Unable to Perform	Initials and Date
2. Assess the source of the danger. *Comments:*	☐	☐	☐	
3. Assess for the increasing risk of danger from secondary source. *Comments:*	☐	☐	☐	
4. Determine the immediate risk to yourself and your ability to handle the situation. *Comments:*	☐	☐	☐	
5. Check the condition of the clients and staff. *Comments:*	☐	☐	☐	
6. Determine who is in charge of the evacuation. *Comments:*	☐	☐	☐	
7. Determine the safe location where clients will be transported. *Comments:*	☐	☐	☐	
8. Determine who needs to be transported. *Comments:*	☐	☐	☐	
9. Determine what mode of transport will be used. *Comments:*	☐	☐	☐	
10. Inform the client about what is happening and how he or she will be transported. *Comments:*	☐	☐	☐	
11. Gather equipment and personnel. *Comments:*	☐	☐	☐	
12. Make sure the escape route is clear and you know where to go. *Comments:*	☐	☐	☐	

Procedure 2-14	Able to Perform	Able to Perform with Assistance	Unable to Perform	Initials and Date
13. Make sure you have a light source. *Comments:*	☐	☐	☐	
14. Transport the client as predetermined. *Comments:*	☐	☐	☐	
15. Recheck the client after evacuation and provide intervention as needed. *Comments:*	☐	☐	☐	
16. If the evacuation location is outdoors, protect the client from the elements. *Comments:*	☐	☐	☐	
17. Continue to monitor the situation. *Comments:*	☐	☐	☐	
18. Continue with the disaster protocol. *Comments:*	☐	☐	☐	
Emergency Transfer for Evacuation 19. Put the head of the bed up. *Comments:*	☐	☐	☐	
20. Pull covers down past the feet. *Comments:*	☐	☐	☐	
21. Put slippers or shoes on feet if time permits. *Comments:*	☐	☐	☐	
22. Put on robe, coat, or blanket if needed. *Comments:*	☐	☐	☐	
23. Disconnect medical equipment. Reconnect to portable device if time permits. *Comments:*	☐	☐	☐	
24. Assist the client to stand and help with wheelchair or walker if needed. *Comments:*	☐	☐	☐	

continued on the following page

continued from the previous page

Procedure 2-14	Able to Perform	Able to Perform with Assistance	Unable to Perform	Initials and Date
25. Walk with the client to the safe location. *Comments:*	☐	☐	☐	
Emergency One-Person and Two-Person Evacuations 26. Support-walk with the client. *Comments:*	☐	☐	☐	
27. *One person.* Assist the client to a standing position. Grasp the client's wrist and wrap the client's arm around the back of your neck. Place your arm around the client's waist and walk with the client. *Comments:*	☐	☐	☐	
28. *Two people.* Each person grasps one of the client's wrists and wraps the client's arm around the back of the rescuer's neck. Each person places an arm around the client's waist; the rescuers walk the client. *Comments:*	☐	☐	☐	
29. *Piggyback carry (one person).* Have the client stand or sit. Turn your back to him or her. Bend your knees and have the client place hands on your shoulders. Lift the client and grab the legs behind the knees. *Comments:*	☐	☐	☐	
30. *Cradle arms carry (one person).* Have the client stand. Place one arm under the client's knees and the other arm around the client's back and lift. *Comments:*	☐	☐	☐	
31. *Drag (one or two people).* Place the client on his or her back and kneel at the head. Slide your hands under the client's shoulders and grasp the rib cage under the armpits. Rise and drag the client backward. • Use clothing as a handhold. • Use a blanket or mattress to support the client as you drag him or her. • *On stairs.* Back down or climb up the steps. Let the hips and legs slide and drop from step to step. *Comments:*	☐	☐	☐	

Procedure 2-14	Able to Perform	Able to Perform with Assistance	Unable to Perform	Initials and Date
32. *Chair drag (one or two people).* Place the client securely in a chair. Drag the chair and the client to safety. *Comments:*	☐	☐	☐	
33. *Fireman's carry (one person).* Have the client stand facing you. Grab the client's wrist furthest from your body. Squat/lean and grab the client's thigh closest to your body. Hoist the weight of the client over your shoulder and lift. *Comments:*	☐	☐	☐	
34. *Two-person packsaddle carry (two people).* Each rescuer grasps their own wrist and the other bearer's wrist, forming a seat. Lower the seat. Have the client sit and wrap each of his or her arms around a rescuer. *Comments:*	☐	☐	☐	
35. *Cradle carry (two people).* Lay client on his or her back; kneel on each side. Each rescuer slides one arm under the client's thighs and the other under the client's back. Each rescuer grasps the other's wrists. On a signal, they rise together. *Comments:*	☐	☐	☐	

Checklist for Procedure 3-1   The Effective Communication Process

Name _____ Date _____

School _____

Instructor _____

Course _____

Procedure 3-1 The Effective Communication Process	Able to Perform	Able to Perform with Assistance	Unable to Perform	Initials and Date
Assessment				
1. Assess the client's ability to send clear messages. *Comments:*	☐	☐	☐	
2. Check the ability to receive messages. Check for physical, emotional, or mental barriers. *Comments:*	☐	☐	☐	
3. Assess for the amount of information that may effectively be delivered or received and processed in a time block. *Comments:*	☐	☐	☐	
4. Check for impediments to communication in the surrounding environment. *Comments:*	☐	☐	☐	
5. Assess your own ability to receive and send messages. *Comments:*	☐	☐	☐	
Planning/Expected Outcomes				
1. The client's environment will be as free from barriers to communication as is possible. *Comments:*	☐	☐	☐	
2. The nurse will communicate successfully. *Comments:*	☐	☐	☐	
3. The client or health care team member will communicate successfully. *Comments:*	☐	☐	☐	
Implementation				
1. Wash hands. *Comments:*	☐	☐	☐	

continued on the following page

continued from the previous page

Procedure 3-1	Able to Perform	Able to Perform with Assistance	Unable to Perform	Initials and Date
2. Arrange for an uninterrupted time block. *Comments:*	☐	☐	☐	
3. Prepare to be an effective communicator: • Decide what information you wish to communicate or solicit. • Determine the appropriate difficulty level for your language and how much information you should attempt to communicate at any one time. • Decide how long the session will be and at what pace to provide messages. • Review the tenets of active listening. • Do a quick internal check for beliefs or prejudices that might affect your ability to communicate. *Comments:*	☐	☐	☐	
4. Assess the environment for barriers to communication. *Comments:*	☐	☐	☐	
5. Assess the client for barriers to communication, and intervene where possible. *Comments:*	☐	☐	☐	
6. Sit in a comfortable chair, or squat close to the client. You should be at eye level to allow you to make eye contact, to hear and be heard, and to use touch if appropriate. *Comments:*	☐	☐	☐	
7. Provide similar seating to an interpreter or other person participating in the communication. *Comments:*	☐	☐	☐	
8. Introduce yourself and state the purpose of your communication. *Comments:*	☐	☐	☐	
9. Using the purpose of the communication as a guide, draw the client into the communication session with you. *Comments:*	☐	☐	☐	
10. Regularly request feedback from the client to assess if your communication is being received as you intended it. *Comments:*	☐	☐	☐	

Procedure 3-1	Able to Perform	Able to Perform with Assistance	Unable to Perform	Initials and Date
11. Regularly provide feedback to the client that states what you are hearing the client communicate. *Comments:*	☐	☐	☐	
12. Monitor yourself and your client for nonverbal messages. *Comments:*	☐	☐	☐	
13. Assess for signs of boredom, distraction, confusion, or emotional responses. Adjust your communication or terminate the session, if needed. *Comments:*	☐	☐	☐	
14. Terminate the session if interrupted by a higher priority, or at the client's request. Identify a time and place to resume. *Comments:*	☐	☐	☐	
15. When the information has been communicated by the client, nurse, or family and adequate feedback has been obtained on both sides, terminate the communication session. Confirm follow-up actions or third-party communications as planned. If information to be passed along is confidential, verify the client's consent. *Comments:*	☐	☐	☐	

Checklist for Procedure 3-2   Guided Imagery

Name _____ Date _____

School _____

Instructor _____

Course _____

Procedure 3-2 Guided Imagery	Able to Perform	Able to Perform with Assistance	Unable to Perform	Initials and Date
Assessment				
1. Assess the client's mental status. *Comments:*	☐	☐	☐	
2. Assess the client's sensory or cognitive deficits. *Comments:*	☐	☐	☐	
3. Discuss the procedure with the client. *Comments:*	☐	☐	☐	
4. Have clients describe their current problem. *Comments:*	☐	☐	☐	
5. Identify your own feelings regarding imagery's effectiveness. *Comments:*	☐	☐	☐	
Planning/Expected Outcomes				
1. Reduced pain. *Comments:*	☐	☐	☐	
2. Reduced anxiety. *Comments:*	☐	☐	☐	
3. Increased coping methods. *Comments:*	☐	☐	☐	
4. Increased sense of self-control. *Comments:*	☐	☐	☐	
Implementation				
1. Wash hands. *Comments:*	☐	☐	☐	

continued on the following page

continued from the previous page

Procedure 3-2	Able to Perform	Able to Perform with Assistance	Unable to Perform	Initials and Date
2. Explain the procedure to the client. *Comments:*	☐	☐	☐	
3. Select a comfortable environment that will be free of distraction for approximately 20 minutes. *Comments:*	☐	☐	☐	
4. With the client in a comfortable position, turn on either background music or prerecorded audiotape. *Comments:*	☐	☐	☐	
5. Begin the session with a few relaxing breaths, then proceed to guide the client to a pleasing, restful place. *Comments:*	☐	☐	☐	
6. Slowly bring the client back to the present. *Comments:*	☐	☐	☐	

Checklist for Procedure 3-3   Progressive Muscle Relaxation

Name _____ Date _____

School _____

Instructor _____

Course _____

Procedure 3-3 **Progressive Muscle Relaxation**	Able to Perform	Able to Perform with Assistance	Unable to Perform	Initials and Date
Assessment				
1. Check the client's mental status. *Comments:*	☐	☐	☐	
2. Check for any sensory deficits. *Comments:*	☐	☐	☐	
3. Determine the client's willingness to participate. *Comments:*	☐	☐	☐	
4. Check the nature of the medical or emotional problem. *Comments:*	☐	☐	☐	
5. Have the client quantify the problem. *Comments:*	☐	☐	☐	
Planning/Expected Outcomes				
1. Reduced client anxiety. *Comments:*	☐	☐	☐	
2. Reduced pain. *Comments:*	☐	☐	☐	
3. Reduced nausea. *Comments:*	☐	☐	☐	
4. Reduced insomnia. *Comments:*	☐	☐	☐	
5. Increased sense of self-control. *Comments:*	☐	☐	☐	

continued on the following page

continued from the previous page

Procedure 3-3	Able to Perform	Able to Perform with Assistance	Unable to Perform	Initials and Date
Implementation				
1. Wash hands. *Comments:*	☐	☐	☐	
2. Arrange for an uninterrupted 15–30 minute time block. *Comments:*	☐	☐	☐	
3. Lower lighting level and turn on music to desirable level. *Comments:*	☐	☐	☐	
4. Make client warm and comfortable. *Comments:*	☐	☐	☐	
5. Have client take 3–6 breaths, relaxing with each breath. *Comments:*	☐	☐	☐	
6. Keep your voice calm and smooth. Provide gentle correction if needed. *Comments:*	☐	☐	☐	
7. Begin the tensing-relaxation process, coordinating inhalation, and slow exhalation with relaxation. *Comments:*	☐	☐	☐	
8. Have client finish with 3–6 additional relaxation breaths. *Comments:*	☐	☐	☐	
9. Have client slowly move feet, hands, arms, legs, reopen eyes, and reorient him- or herself. *Comments:*	☐	☐	☐	

Checklist for Procedure 3-4   Therapeutic Massage

Name _____ Date _____

School _____

Instructor _____

Course _____

Procedure 3-4 **Therapeutic Massage**	Able to Perform	Able to Perform with Assistance	Unable to Perform	Initials and Date
Assessment				
1. Assess the client's current emotional and physical condition. *Comments:*	☐	☐	☐	
2. Review the client's current diagnosis. *Comments:*	☐	☐	☐	
3. Assess the client's current physical surroundings. *Comments:*	☐	☐	☐	
4. Assess the client's acceptance of touch and past experience with touch. *Comments:*	☐	☐	☐	
5. Assess for allergies to lotion. *Comments:*	☐	☐	☐	
Planning/Expected Outcomes				
1. Client's relaxation will be increased. *Comments:*	☐	☐	☐	
2. Circulation to the massaged area will be increased. *Comments:*	☐	☐	☐	
Implementation				
1. Provide low or indirect lighting, privacy, background music, and a warm room. *Comments:*	☐	☐	☐	
2. Place a clean sheet on the table or bed. Adjust the surface height. *Comments:*	☐	☐	☐	
3. Remove your rings and watches. Wash hands. *Comments:*	☐	☐	☐	

continued on the following page

continued from the previous page

Procedure 3-4	Able to Perform	Able to Perform with Assistance	Unable to Perform	Initials and Date
4. Explain the procedure to the client. *Comments:*	☐	☐	☐	
5. Help the client assume either a prone, supine, or sitting position. *Comments:*	☐	☐	☐	
6. Loosen or remove client's clothing. Drape the areas not being treated directly with a sheet. *Comments:*	☐	☐	☐	
7. Warm a small amount of lotion or oil between your palms. *Comments:*	☐	☐	☐	
8. Begin with light to medium effleurage at lower back and continue upward following muscle groups. Continue the effleurage for approximately 3 minutes. *Comments:*	☐	☐	☐	
9. Continue treatment, if appropriate, with gentle petrissage. *Comments:*	☐	☐	☐	
10. Use friction on particular muscle groups where tension is being held. *Comments:*	☐	☐	☐	
11. Use tapotement to stimulate any muscle groups that may be fatigued. *Comments:*	☐	☐	☐	
12. Finish treatment with effleurage. *Comments:*	☐	☐	☐	
13. Wipe any excess lotion or oil from skin with a towel or soap and water. *Comments:*	☐	☐	☐	
14. Assist client into a comfortable position for a period of rest or sleep. *Comments:*	☐	☐	☐	

Procedure 3-4	Able to Perform	Able to Perform with Assistance	Unable to Perform	Initials and Date
15. Document treatment. *Comments:*	☐	☐	☐	
16. Wash hands. *Comments:*	☐	☐	☐	

Checklist for Procedure 3-5   Applying Moist Heat

Name _____ Date _____

School _____

Instructor _____

Course _____

Procedure 3-5 Applying Moist Heat	Able to Perform	Able to Perform with Assistance	Unable to Perform	Initials and Date
Assessment				
1. Assess the area to receive heat treatment for circulation. *Comments:*	☐	☐	☐	
2. Assess the skin sensation and integrity around the area to be treated. *Comments:*	☐	☐	☐	
3. Assess for open wounds in the area to be treated. *Comments:*	☐	☐	☐	
Planning/Expected Outcomes				
1. The client will experience a decrease in pain and tension. *Comments:*	☐	☐	☐	
2. Circulation will improve. *Comments:*	☐	☐	☐	
3. The client will experience a decrease in swelling in the area being treated. *Comments:*	☐	☐	☐	
Implementation				
1. Check the physician's order and the reason for the warm compress. Explain to the client. *Comments:*	☐	☐	☐	
2. Wash hands. *Comments:*	☐	☐	☐	
3. Assess the client's skin. *Comments:*	☐	☐	☐	

continued on the following page

continued from the previous page

Procedure 3-5	Able to Perform	Able to Perform with Assistance	Unable to Perform	Initials and Date
4. Determine the client's medical condition. *Comments:*	☐	☐	☐	
5. Warm the container of sterile saline or tap water. Follow the manufacturer's directions for heating a commercial compress. *Comments:*	☐	☐	☐	
6. Place a waterproof pad under the body area that needs the warm compress. *Comments:*	☐	☐	☐	
7. A thin layer of petroleum jelly may be placed on the area to be treated. *Comments:*	☐	☐	☐	
8. Pour the sterile saline into the sterile basin. Soak an appropriate-size piece of gauze or a towel, wring out the excess saline, and place it on the affected area. *Comments:*	☐	☐	☐	
9. Wrap the area with a waterproof pad or apply heat pad. *Comments:*	☐	☐	☐	
10. Check the client's skin periodically for signs of heat intolerance. Tell the client to report any discomfort immediately. *Comments:*	☐	☐	☐	
11. Leave the compress in place for approximately 30 minutes and then remove it. *Comments:*	☐	☐	☐	
12. Dry the affected area with sterile or clean towels, as appropriate. *Comments:*	☐	☐	☐	
13. Properly dispose of all single-use equipment. *Comments:*	☐	☐	☐	
14. Clean bath basin and thermometer. *Comments:*	☐	☐	☐	

Procedure 3-5	Able to Perform	Able to Perform with Assistance	Unable to Perform	Initials and Date
15. Remove gloves and wash your hands. *Comments:*	☐	☐	☐	
16. Reassess the condition of the client's skin. *Comments:*	☐	☐	☐	
17. Record the procedure. *Comments:*	☐	☐	☐	

Checklist for Procedure 3-6   Warm Soaks and Sitz Baths

Name _____   Date _____

School _____

Instructor _____

Course _____

Procedure 3-6 Warm Soaks and Sitz Baths	Able to Perform	Able to Perform with Assistance	Unable to Perform	Initials and Date
Assessment				
1. Assess the client for conditions that may require alteration to the treatment plan. *Comments:*	☐	☐	☐	
2. Assess ability of the client to participate in treatment. *Comments:*	☐	☐	☐	
3. Assess the area of injury for drainage, edema, or redness. *Comments:*	☐	☐	☐	
4. Assess the availability of appropriate equipment and clean hot water. *Comments:*	☐	☐	☐	
5. Assess each client's experience of using warm soaks before teaching. *Comments:*	☐	☐	☐	
Planning/Expected Outcomes				
1. Client will experience decrease in pain. *Comments:*	☐	☐	☐	
2. Affected area will heal. *Comments:*	☐	☐	☐	
Implementation				
1. Wash hands and assemble equipment. *Comments:*	☐	☐	☐	
2. Run tap water to preferred temperature. *Comments:*	☐	☐	☐	

continued on the following page

continued from the previous page

Procedure 3-6	Able to Perform	Able to Perform with Assistance	Unable to Perform	Initials and Date
3. For toilet insert model, raise the seat of the toilet. Set the basin on the rim of the toilet bowl. • Fill water bag and prime tubing. Close the clamp. • Hang the water bag above the toilet. Thread the tubing through the front of the basin. Secure the tubing in the notch in the bottom of the basin. *Comments:*	☐	☐	☐	
4. For stand-alone model, fill basin with water. *Comments:*	☐	☐	☐	
5. Pad the seat with a towel. *Comments:*	☐	☐	☐	
6. Have client remove peri-pad and dispose of properly. *Comments:*	☐	☐	☐	
7. Ensure that the floor is dry. Assist client if necessary. *Comments:*	☐	☐	☐	
8. Have client sit in the basin. For toilet insert model, demonstrate unclamping the tubing to start the water flow. *Comments:*	☐	☐	☐	
9. Cover the client's lap for warmth and modesty. *Comments:*	☐	☐	☐	
10. Place call button within reach. Instruct the client to call before standing up. *Comments:*	☐	☐	☐	
11. After 20 minutes, assist client to dry the area. *Comments:*	☐	☐	☐	
12. Assist client to bed. *Comments:*	☐	☐	☐	
13. For toilet insert model, empty remaining water into toilet. Rinse basin and bag and allow to air dry. For stand-alone model, empty water from drain tap into basin. Clean and dry equipment. *Comments:*	☐	☐	☐	

Checklist for Procedure 3-7 Applying Dry Heat

Name _____ Date _____

School _____

Instructor _____

Course _____

Procedure 3-7 Applying Dry Heat	Able to Perform	Able to Perform with Assistance	Unable to Perform	Initials and Date
Assessment				
1. Assess the skin integrity in the area where heat is to be applied. *Comments:*	☐	☐	☐	
2. Assess the client's tolerance of heat. *Comments:*	☐	☐	☐	
3. Assess the client's vascular status. *Comments:*	☐	☐	☐	
4. Assess the client's preexisting illness. *Comments:*	☐	☐	☐	
5. Assess the skin for the presence of any lotion or ointments. *Comments:*	☐	☐	☐	
Planning/Expected Outcomes				
1. The client will derive the planned benefits of the heat treatment. *Comments:*	☐	☐	☐	
2. The client will not experience any injury to skin integrity. *Comments:*	☐	☐	☐	
Implementation				
1. Check the order and the purpose of the heat treatment. *Comments:*	☐	☐	☐	
2. Determine if there are any underlying problems that may affect the use of heat treatment. *Comments:*	☐	☐	☐	

continued on the following page

continued from the previous page

Procedure 3-7	Able to Perform	Able to Perform with Assistance	Unable to Perform	Initials and Date
3. Wash hands. *Comments:*	☐	☐	☐	
4. Check the skin for lotions or ointments and remove if present. *Comments:*	☐	☐	☐	
5. Teach the client about the heat treatment. *Comments:*	☐	☐	☐	
6. Gather equipment and complete as follows: For a disposable heat pack: • Activate the pack according to the manufacturer's directions. • Wrap the pack in a towel or protective covering. • Discard after use. For a heating pad: • Note: Heating pads are generally not used in hospital facilities. • Place a formed cover over the pad. • Instruct the client not to lie on the heating pad. • Turn the switch to low and place the heating pad on the affected area. • Generally, the highest setting is not used. • Set a timer and remove the pad after 20 minutes. • Clean appropriately after use. For an aquathermia pad: • Follow manufacturer's directions. • Fill the control unit with distilled water. • Check the control unit and tubing for leaks. Turn on the unit and check the temperature of the water with a thermometer. For a heat lamp with a 60-watt or infrared bulb: • Expose the area to be treated and drape the client to protect privacy. • Place the lamp 18–24 inches from the client. • Check the area after 5 minutes of heat. Remove the lamp after 20 minutes and check for any adverse reaction. • Reposition the client in a comfortable position. • Clean equipment. For a heat cradle: • Use a 25-watt bulb. Place the cradle over the client, but not touching the client. Cover both with a bath blanket. • Check the client in 5 minutes and remove the cradle after 10–15 minutes. • Assess the skin for any adverse reaction. • Reposition the client. • Clean the equipment.				

Procedure 3-7	Able to Perform	Able to Perform with Assistance	Unable to Perform	Initials and Date
For a hot water bottle: • Note: Hot water bottles are usually used only in home care settings. • Fill the bottle with tap water, tighten the cap, turn the bottle upside down, then open the cap and empty. • Fill the bottle or bag two-thirds full with hot water. Expel air, and secure cap. Wipe off excess moisture. • Cover with protective cover or towel. • Have the client keep the bottle in place for 20–30 minutes. For diathermy: • Diathermy is usually used in physical therapy. • Have client remove metal objects such as pins, rings, or watches. • Transport client to physical therapy. *Comments:*	☐	☐	☐	
7. Wash hands. *Comments:*	☐	☐	☐	

Checklist for Procedure 3-8   Using a Thermal Blanket and an Infant Radiant Heat Warmer

Name _____ Date _____

School _____

Instructor _____

Course _____

Procedure 3-8 Using a Thermal Blanket and an Infant Radiant Heat Warmer	Able to Perform	Able to Perform with Assistance	Unable to Perform	Initials and Date
Assessment				
1. Assess the client's temperature. *Comments:*	☐	☐	☐	
2. Assess the client's skin condition and integrity. *Comments:*	☐	☐	☐	
3. Assess client's knowledge regarding treatment. *Comments:*	☐	☐	☐	
4. Assess the client's mental status. *Comments:*	☐	☐	☐	
Planning/Expected Outcomes				
1. Core temperature will be maintained within the desired range. *Comments:*	☐	☐	☐	
2. The client will not incur any skin or tissue damage. *Comments:*	☐	☐	☐	
3. The client will be as comfortable as possible during the treatment. *Comments:*	☐	☐	☐	
4. The client's core temperature will not change rapidly enough to cause chilling or diaphoresis. *Comments:*	☐	☐	☐	
Implementation				
1. Wash hands. *Comments:*	☐	☐	☐	

continued on the following page

continued from the previous page

Procedure 3-8	Able to Perform	Able to Perform with Assistance	Unable to Perform	Initials and Date
2. Assemble equipment. Check that equipment is functioning properly. *Comments:*	☐	☐	☐	
3. Check orders for desired systemic temperature. *Comments:*	☐	☐	☐	
4. Check the client's vital signs, especially temperature. *Comments:*	☐	☐	☐	
5. Explain the procedure to the client. *Comments:*	☐	☐	☐	
6. If necessary, add solution to the machine. *Comments:*	☐	☐	☐	
Hypothermia Blanket 7. Place the blanket according to the manufacturer's instructions. Place a sheet between the blanket and the client and connect the machine. *Comments:*	☐	☐	☐	
8. Insert the rectal probe and tape it in place. *Comments:*	☐	☐	☐	
9. Set the machine on the desired temperature and turn on. *Comments:*	☐	☐	☐	
10. Check the client's temperature every 15 minutes and vital signs every 30 minutes. *Comments:*	☐	☐	☐	
11. Perform comparison check with another thermometer periodically. *Comments:*	☐	☐	☐	
12. When the client's temperature is close to the desired temperature, turn off the machine and assess the client. *Comments:*	☐	☐	☐	

Procedure 3-8	Able to Perform	Able to Perform with Assistance	Unable to Perform	Initials and Date
13. While the blanket is on, turn the client every hour and assess the skin condition. *Comments:*	☐	☐	☐	
An Infant Radiant Warmer 14. Check the operating instructions and equipment. *Comments:*	☐	☐	☐	
15. Prepare the parents and inform them of the purpose of the warmer. *Comments:*	☐	☐	☐	
16. Plug electrical cord in a three-wire grounded receptacle. Turn on the equipment. *Comments:*	☐	☐	☐	
17. Turn on the alarm switch and test alarm system. Turn on temperature settings. *Comments:*	☐	☐	☐	
18. Prewarm the isolette to the prescribed temperature. *Comments:*	☐	☐	☐	
19. Put on nonsterile gloves. *Comments:*	☐	☐	☐	
20. Place infant in warmer. Insert a rectal or skin temperature probe and activate an audible alarm. *Comments:*	☐	☐	☐	
21. For skin probe: Place probe with surface next to skin. *Comments:*	☐	☐	☐	
22. For rectal probe: Use lubricant and insert. *Comments:*	☐	☐	☐	
23. Check the infant's temperature with another thermometer. Inspect probe at regular intervals. *Comments:*	☐	☐	☐	

continued on the following page

continued from the previous page

Procedure 3-8	Able to Perform	Able to Perform with Assistance	Unable to Perform	Initials and Date
24. If skin irritation appears, reposition the probe. *Comments:*	☐	☐	☐	
25. The infant may be kept in the warmer until the core temperature is stabilized. *Comments:*	☐	☐	☐	
26. After the infant is removed, clean the equipment. *Comments:*	☐	☐	☐	
27. Wash hands. *Comments:*	☐	☐	☐	

Checklist for Procedure 3-9 Applying Cold Treatment

Name _____ Date _____

School _____

Instructor _____

Course _____

Procedure 3-9 Applying Cold Treatment	Able to Perform	Able to Perform with Assistance	Unable to Perform	Initials and Date
Assessment				
1. Ascertain the client's sensation of hot and cold changes. Comments:	☐	☐	☐	
2. Assess if decreased circulation is present at the site. Comments:	☐	☐	☐	
3. Check the client's systemic temperature. Comments:	☐	☐	☐	
4. Assess age. Comments:	☐	☐	☐	
Planning/Expected Outcomes				
1. The client will experience decreased bleeding. Comments:	☐	☐	☐	
2. The client will have decreased inflammation and/or edema. Comments:	☐	☐	☐	
3. The client will experience decreased pain or discomfort. Comments:	☐	☐	☐	
Implementation				
1. Wash hands. Comments:	☐	☐	☐	
2. Assess the site for sensation, skin color, and integrity. Comments:	☐	☐	☐	
3. Determine the diagnosis. Comments:	☐	☐	☐	

continued on the following page

continued from the previous page

Procedure 3-9	Able to Perform	Able to Perform with Assistance	Unable to Perform	Initials and Date
4. Check the order and the reason for the application of cold. *Comments:*	☐	☐	☐	
5. If using ice bag with moist gauze or towels: Fill the bag three-fourths full with ice and remove the air from the bag. Check for leaks. Wrap the bag in a protective cover and place on the affected area. *Comments:*	☐	☐	☐	
6. If using an ice collar: Fill the collar three-fourths full with ice and remove the air from the collar. Check for leaks. Place the collar in a protective cover and place on affected area. *Comments:*	☐	☐	☐	
7. If using a disposable cold pack: Activate the pack according to the manufacturer's directions, wrap the pack in a towel, and place it on the affected area. Secure in place. Dispose of the pack after the treatment. *Comments:*	☐	☐	☐	
8. Assess the client's skin periodically. *Comments:*	☐	☐	☐	
9. If tolerated, leave in place for approximately 20–30 minutes. *Comments:*	☐	☐	☐	
10. Reassess the condition of the site. *Comments:*	☐	☐	☐	
11. Wash hands. *Comments:*	☐	☐	☐	

Checklist for Procedure 3-10   Assisting with a Transcutaneous Electrical Nerve Stimulation (TENS) Unit

Name _____ Date _____

School _____

Instructor _____

Course _____

Procedure 3-10 Assisting with a Transcutaneous Electrical Nerve Stimulation (TENS) Unit	Able to Perform	Able to Perform with Assistance	Unable to Perform	Initials and Date
Assessment				
1. Consider the appropriateness of the treatment. Comments:	☐	☐	☐	
2. Assess the client's knowledge regarding the TENS device. Comments:	☐	☐	☐	
3. Assess client's skin condition. Comments:	☐	☐	☐	
Planning/Expected Outcomes				
1. Decreased pain sensation. Comments:	☐	☐	☐	
2. Increased comfort level. Comments:	☐	☐	☐	
3. Increased client mobility. Comments:	☐	☐	☐	
4. Increased client coping skills to pain. Comments:	☐	☐	☐	
5. Increased activities of daily living. Comments:	☐	☐	☐	
Implementation				
1. Obtain order from a physician or qualified practitioner. Comments:	☐	☐	☐	
2. Identify client. Comments:	☐	☐	☐	

continued on the following page

continued from the previous page

Procedure 3-10	Able to Perform	Able to Perform with Assistance	Unable to Perform	Initials and Date
3. Verify that the unit's internal controls are set correctly. *Comments:*	☐	☐	☐	
4. Introduce yourself and the procedure you will be doing. *Comments:*	☐	☐	☐	
5. Wash your hands. *Comments:*	☐	☐	☐	
6. Explain actions of application throughout the procedure. *Comments:*	☐	☐	☐	
7. Cleanse the area of electrode application with soap and water. *Comments:*	☐	☐	☐	
8. Rinse and dry skin in the area thoroughly. *Comments:*	☐	☐	☐	
9. Apply electrode gel between the skin and electrodes. *Comments:*	☐	☐	☐	
10. Connect the cordset to the electrodes before applying the electrodes to the skin. *Comments:*	☐	☐	☐	
11. Follow manufacturer's directions for electrode placement. *Comments:*	☐	☐	☐	
12. Place electrode on skin over or near the area of pain. *Comments:*	☐	☐	☐	
13. Hold the connector portion of the cordset, and insert into the corresponding jack. *Comments:*	☐	☐	☐	
14. Set the stimulator controls to the appropriate configurations. *Comments:*	☐	☐	☐	

Procedure 3-10	Able to Perform	Able to Perform with Assistance	Unable to Perform	Initials and Date
15. Place the protective cap over the intensity controls. *Comments:*	☐	☐	☐	
16. Turn the machine on and instruct the client to adjust the level of intensity. *Comments:*	☐	☐	☐	
17. Wash hands. *Comments:*	☐	☐	☐	
18. Record the application of TENS. *Comments:*	☐	☐	☐	

Checklist for Procedure 4-1   Changing Linens in an Unoccupied Bed

Name _____ Date _____

School _____

Instructor _____

Course _____

Procedure 4-1 Changing Linens in an Unoccupied Bed	Able to Perform	Able to Perform with Assistance	Unable to Perform	Initials and Date
Assessment				
1. Assess your equipment. *Comments:*	☐	☐	☐	
2. Assess whether the bed itself needs cleaning. *Comments:*	☐	☐	☐	
3. Assess the needs of the client in the bed. *Comments:*	☐	☐	☐	
4. Assess the client's ability to be out of bed in a safe place while changing linens. *Comments:*	☐	☐	☐	
Planning/Expected Outcomes				
1. The client will have clean linens on the bed. *Comments:*	☐	☐	☐	
2. The clean linens will be appropriate to the client's needs and condition. *Comments:*	☐	☐	☐	
Implementation				
Preparation 1. Place hamper close by. Explain procedure to client. Assess condition of blankets. *Comments:*	☐	☐	☐	
2. Gather linens and gloves. *Comments:*	☐	☐	☐	
3. Apply gloves. *Comments:*	☐	☐	☐	

continued on the following page

continued from the previous page

Procedure 4-1	Able to Perform	Able to Perform with Assistance	Unable to Perform	Initials and Date
4. Attend to the client's toileting needs as necessary. *Comments:*	☐	☐	☐	
5. Assist client to a safe, comfortable chair. *Comments:*	☐	☐	☐	
6. Position bed. *Comments:*	☐	☐	☐	
7. Remove and fold blanket and/or bedspread. *Comments:*	☐	☐	☐	
8. Remove soiled pillowcases. *Comments:*	☐	☐	☐	
9. Remove soiled linens. *Comments:*	☐	☐	☐	
10. Fold soiled linens. *Comments:*	☐	☐	☐	
11. Check the mattress. If soiled, clean appropriately. *Comments:*	☐	☐	☐	
12. Remove gloves, wash hands, and apply a second pair of clean gloves. *Comments:*	☐	☐	☐	
13. Place clean mattress pad onto the bed. Unfold half of the pad's width to the center crease. *Comments:*	☐	☐	☐	
14. Proceed with placing bottom sheet onto the mattress. *Comments:*	☐	☐	☐	
Fitted Bottom Sheet 15. Position yourself diagonally toward the head of the bed. *Comments:*	☐	☐	☐	

Procedure 4-1	Able to Perform	Able to Perform with Assistance	Unable to Perform	Initials and Date
16. Start at the head with seamed side of the fitted sheet toward the mattress. *Comments:*	☐	☐	☐	
17. Lift the mattress corner and tuck the fitted sheet over the mattress corner. Repeat for other corner. *Comments:*	☐	☐	☐	
18. Tuck the fitted sheet over the mattress corners at foot of the bed. *Comments:*	☐	☐	☐	
Flat Regular Sheet 19. Align the bottom edge of the sheet with the edge of the mattress at the foot of the bed. *Comments:*	☐	☐	☐	
20. Allow the sheet to hang over the mattress on the side and at the top of the bed. *Comments:*	☐	☐	☐	
21. Position yourself diagonally toward the head of the bed. Lift the mattress corner and smoothly tuck the sheet under the mattress. *Comments:*	☐	☐	☐	
22. Miter the corner at the head of the bed. *Comments:*	☐	☐	☐	
23. Lift and lay the top edge of the sheet onto the bed to form a triangular fold. *Comments:*	☐	☐	☐	
24. Tuck the lower edge of the sheet under the mattress. *Comments:*	☐	☐	☐	
25. Bring the triangular fold down over the side of the mattress. *Comments:*	☐	☐	☐	
26. Place the draw sheet on the bottom sheet and unfold it to the middle crease. *Comments:*	☐	☐	☐	

continued on the following page

continued from the previous page

Procedure 4-1	Able to Perform	Able to Perform with Assistance	Unable to Perform	Initials and Date
27. Tuck both the bottom and draw sheets smoothly under the mattress. *Comments:*	☐	☐	☐	
28. On the other side of the bed, repeat Actions 13–18, as used to apply the mattress pad and bottom sheet. *Comments:*	☐	☐	☐	
29. Unfold the draw sheet, and grasp both sheets. Pull toward you and tuck both sheets under the mattress. *Comments:*	☐	☐	☐	
30. Place the top sheet on the bed. Place the top edge of the sheet even with the top of the mattress. Pull the remaining length toward the bottom of the bed. *Comments:*	☐	☐	☐	
31. Unfold and apply the blanket/spread as with the top sheet. *Comments:*	☐	☐	☐	
32. Miter the bottom corners. *Comments:*	☐	☐	☐	
33. Fold the top sheet and blanket over. Fan-fold the sheet and blanket. *Comments:*	☐	☐	☐	
34. Apply clean pillowcase on each pillow. *Comments:*	☐	☐	☐	
35. Return the bed to the lowest position and elevate the head of the bed 30–45°. *Comments:*	☐	☐	☐	
36. Inquire about toileting needs of the client; assist as necessary. *Comments:*	☐	☐	☐	
37. Assist the client back into the bed and pull up the side rails; place call light within reach; take vital signs. *Comments:*	☐	☐	☐	

Procedure 4-1	Able to Perform	Able to Perform with Assistance	Unable to Perform	Initials and Date
38. Remove gloves and wash hands. *Comments:*	☐	☐	☐	
39. Document your actions and the client's response to the activity. *Comments:*	☐	☐	☐	

Checklist for Procedure 4-2   Changing Linens in an Occupied Bed

Name _____ Date _____

School _____

Instructor _____

Course _____

Procedure 4-2 Changing Linens in an Occupied Bed	Able to Perform	Able to Perform with Assistance	Unable to Perform	Initials and Date
Assessment				
1. Assess your equipment. Comments:	☐	☐	☐	
2. Assess whether the bed itself needs cleaning. Comments:	☐	☐	☐	
3. Assess the needs of the client in the bed. Comments:	☐	☐	☐	
4. Assess the client's ability to assist with the procedure. Comments:	☐	☐	☐	
Planning/Expected Outcomes				
1. The client will have clean linens on the bed. Comments:	☐	☐	☐	
2. The linens will be appropriate to the client's needs. Comments:	☐	☐	☐	
3. The linens will be changed with a minimum of trauma to the client. Comments:	☐	☐	☐	
Implementation				
1. Explain procedure to client. Comments:	☐	☐	☐	
2. Bring equipment to the bedside. Comments:	☐	☐	☐	
3. Remove top sheet and blanket. Loosen bottom sheet. Comments:	☐	☐	☐	

continued on the following page

continued from the previous page

Procedure 4-2	Able to Perform	Able to Perform with Assistance	Unable to Perform	Initials and Date
4. Position client on side, facing away from you. *Comments:*	☐	☐	☐	
5. Fan-fold or roll bottom linens toward the center of the bed. *Comments:*	☐	☐	☐	
6. Place clean bottom linens. Fan-fold or roll clean bottom linens and tuck under soiled linen. *Comments:*	☐	☐	☐	
7. Miter bottom sheet at head and foot of bed. Tuck the sides of the sheet under the mattress. *Comments:*	☐	☐	☐	
8. Fan-fold or roll draw sheet and tuck under soiled linen. Tuck draw sheet under mattress. *Comments:*	☐	☐	☐	
9. Log roll client over onto side facing you. Raise side rail. *Comments:*	☐	☐	☐	
10. At the other side of bed, remove soiled linens. *Comments:*	☐	☐	☐	
11. Unfold/unroll bottom sheet; then draw sheet. Tuck in. *Comments:*	☐	☐	☐	
12. Place top sheet and blanket over client. *Comments:*	☐	☐	☐	
13. Raise foot of mattress and miter the corner. Repeat on other side. *Comments:*	☐	☐	☐	
14. Tent top sheet and blanket over client's toes. *Comments:*	☐	☐	☐	
15. Remove and replace pillowcase. *Comments:*	☐	☐	☐	
16. Document procedure and client's condition. *Comments:*	☐	☐	☐	
17. Wash hands. *Comments:*	☐	☐	☐	

Checklist for Procedure 4-3 Turning and Positioning a Client

Name _____ Date _____

School _____

Instructor _____

Course _____

Procedure 4-3 Turning and Positioning a Client	Able to Perform	Able to Perform with Assistance	Unable to Perform	Initials and Date
Assessment				
1. Assess the client's ability to move independently. *Comments:*	☐	☐	☐	
2. Assess the client's flexibility. *Comments:*	☐	☐	☐	
3. Assess the client's overall condition. *Comments:*	☐	☐	☐	
4. Assess the orders for restrictions regarding client positioning. *Comments:*	☐	☐	☐	
Planning/Expected Outcomes				
1. The client will maintain skin integrity. *Comments:*	☐	☐	☐	
2. The client will be comfortable. *Comments:*	☐	☐	☐	
Implementation				
1. Wash hands. *Comments:*	☐	☐	☐	
2. Explain procedure to client. *Comments:*	☐	☐	☐	
3. Gather all necessary equipment. *Comments:*	☐	☐	☐	

continued on the following page

continued from the previous page

Procedure 4-3	Able to Perform	Able to Perform with Assistance	Unable to Perform	Initials and Date
4. Secure adequate assistance to safely complete task. *Comments:*	☐	☐	☐	
5. Adjust bed to comfortable working height. Lower side rail. *Comments:*	☐	☐	☐	
6. Follow proper body mechanics guidelines. *Comments:*	☐	☐	☐	
7. Position drains, tubes, and IVs to accommodate new client position. *Comments:*	☐	☐	☐	
8. Place or assist client into appropriate starting position. *Comments:*	☐	☐	☐	
Moving from Supine to Side-Lying Position 9. Move the client to one side of the bed by lifting the client's body toward you. Roll the client to side-lying position. *Comments:*	☐	☐	☐	
Maintaining Side-Lying Position 10. Follow Actions 1–8. *Comments:*	☐	☐	☐	
11. Pillows may be placed to support the client. *Comments:*	☐	☐	☐	
Moving from Side-Lying to Prone Position 12. Repeat Actions 1–8. *Comments:*	☐	☐	☐	
13. Remove positioning support devices. Move the client's inside arm next to the body. Roll the client onto the stomach. Place pillows as needed. *Comments:*	☐	☐	☐	
Maintaining Prone Position 14. Pillows or a folded towel may be used to support the client. *Comments:*	☐	☐	☐	

continued from the previous page

Procedure 4-3	Able to Perform	Able to Perform with Assistance	Unable to Perform	Initials and Date
Moving from Prone to Supine Position 15. Repeat Actions 1–8. *Comments:*	☐	☐	☐	
16. Remove supporting devices. Move the client to one side of the bed. Log roll the client toward you. *Comments:*	☐	☐	☐	
Maintaining the Supine Position 17. Pillows, a footboard, heel protectors, or a trochanter roll may be used to support the client. *Comments:*	☐	☐	☐	
18. Replace side rails to upright position and lower the bed. *Comments:*	☐	☐	☐	
19. Place call light within reach of the client. *Comments:*	☐	☐	☐	
20. Place items of frequent use within reach of the client. *Comments:*	☐	☐	☐	
21. Wash hands. *Comments:*	☐	☐	☐	

Checklist for Procedure 4-4   Moving a Client in Bed

Name _____ Date _____

School _____

Instructor _____

Course _____

Procedure 4-4 Moving a Client in Bed	Able to Perform	Able to Perform with Assistance	Unable to Perform	Initials and Date
Assessment				
1. Assess the client's ability to assist with repositioning. *Comments:*	☐	☐	☐	
2. Assess the client's ability to understand and follow directions. *Comments:*	☐	☐	☐	
3. Assess the client's environment. *Comments:*	☐	☐	☐	
Planning/Expected Outcomes				
1. The client will be moved in bed without injury. *Comments:*	☐	☐	☐	
2. The client will be moved in bed without injury to the staff. *Comments:*	☐	☐	☐	
3. The client will report an increase in comfort. *Comments:*	☐	☐	☐	
4. All tubes, lines, and drains will remain patent and intact. *Comments:*	☐	☐	☐	
Implementation				
Moving a Client Up in Bed with One Nurse 1. Wash hands. *Comments:*	☐	☐	☐	
2. Inform client of reason for the move. *Comments:*	☐	☐	☐	

continued on the following page

continued from the previous page

Procedure 4-4	Able to Perform	Able to Perform with Assistance	Unable to Perform	Initials and Date
3. Elevate bed. Lower head of bed. *Comments:*	☐	☐	☐	
4. Place pillow against the headboard. *Comments:*	☐	☐	☐	
5. Have the client fold arms across the chest, if no overhead trapeze is present. *Comments:*	☐	☐	☐	
6. Have client hold on to the overhead trapeze. *Comments:*	☐	☐	☐	
7. Have the client bend knees and place feet flat on the bed. *Comments:*	☐	☐	☐	
8. Stand at head of the bed, feet apart, knees bent. *Comments:*	☐	☐	☐	
9. Slide one hand and arm under the client's shoulder, the other under the client's thigh. *Comments:*	☐	☐	☐	
10. Lift the client while client pushes with the legs. *Comments:*	☐	☐	☐	
11. If available, have the client pull up using the trapeze as you move the client. *Comments:*	☐	☐	☐	
12. Repeat these steps until the client is high enough in bed. *Comments:*	☐	☐	☐	
13. Return the client's pillow under the head. *Comments:*	☐	☐	☐	
14. Elevate head of bed, if tolerated by client. *Comments:*	☐	☐	☐	

Procedure 4-4	Able to Perform	Able to Perform with Assistance	Unable to Perform	Initials and Date
15. Assess client for comfort. *Comments:*	☐	☐	☐	
16. Adjust the client's bedclothes as needed for comfort. *Comments:*	☐	☐	☐	
17. Lower bed and elevate side rails. *Comments:*	☐	☐	☐	
18. Wash hands. *Comments:*	☐	☐	☐	
Moving a Client Up in Bed with Two or More Nurses 19. Wash hands and apply gloves if needed. *Comments:*	☐	☐	☐	
20. Inform client of reason for the move. *Comments:*	☐	☐	☐	
21. Elevate bed. Lower head of bed. *Comments:*	☐	☐	☐	
22. Place turn/draw sheet under client's back and head. *Comments:*	☐	☐	☐	
23. Roll up the draw sheet on each side until it is next to the client. *Comments:*	☐	☐	☐	
24. Follow Actions 4–7. *Comments:*	☐	☐	☐	
25. The nurses stand on either side of the bed, with knees flexed, feet apart in a wide stance. *Comments:*	☐	☐	☐	
26. The nurses hold their elbows close to their bodies. *Comments:*	☐	☐	☐	

continued on the following page

continued from the previous page

Procedure 4-4	Able to Perform	Able to Perform with Assistance	Unable to Perform	Initials and Date
27. At the signal to move, lift up and forward in one smooth motion. *Comments:*	☐	☐	☐	
28. Repeat until the client is high enough in bed. *Comments:*	☐	☐	☐	
29. Return the client's pillow under his or her head. *Comments:*	☐	☐	☐	
30. Elevate head of bed, if tolerated by client. *Comments:*	☐	☐	☐	
31. Assess client for comfort. *Comments:*	☐	☐	☐	
32. Adjust the client's bedclothes for comfort. *Comments:*	☐	☐	☐	
33. Lower bed and elevate side rails. *Comments:*	☐	☐	☐	
34. Wash hands. *Comments:*	☐	☐	☐	

Checklist for Procedure 4-5 Assisting with a Bedpan or Urinal

Name _____ Date _____

School _____

Instructor _____

Course _____

Procedure 4-5 Assisting with a Bedpan or Urinal	Able to Perform	Able to Perform with Assistance	Unable to Perform	Initials and Date
Assessment				
1. Assess your equipment. *Comments:*	☐	☐	☐	
2. Assess how much the client can assist with the procedure. *Comments:*	☐	☐	☐	
3. Check whether the client is confused, combative, or immobile. *Comments:*	☐	☐	☐	
4. Check for casts, braces, or dressings. *Comments:*	☐	☐	☐	
5. Check for privacy and unexpected interruptions. *Comments:*	☐	☐	☐	
6. Assess if client has orders to record intake and output. If there is a need for measurement this will require a container with measurement markings. *Comments:*	☐	☐	☐	
Planning/Expected Outcomes				
1. Clients will be able to void and defecate when necessary. *Comments:*	☐	☐	☐	
2. Clients will have as much privacy and comfort as allowable. *Comments:*	☐	☐	☐	
3. Intake and output will be accurately measured as needed. *Comments:*	☐	☐	☐	
4. The urinal or bedpan will be placed without skin damage. *Comments:*	☐	☐	☐	

continued on the following page

continued from the previous page

Procedure 4-5	Able to Perform	Able to Perform with Assistance	Unable to Perform	Initials and Date
5. The bedpan will be removed and emptied without spillage. *Comments:*	☐	☐	☐	
Implementation				
Positioning a Bedpan 1. Close curtain or door. *Comments:*	☐	☐	☐	
2. Wash hands; apply gloves. *Comments:*	☐	☐	☐	
3. Lower head of bed so client is in supine position. *Comments:*	☐	☐	☐	
4. Elevate bed. *Comments:*	☐	☐	☐	
5. Assist client to side-lying position. *Comments:*	☐	☐	☐	
6. Warm and powder bedpan, if necessary. *Comments:*	☐	☐	☐	
7. Place bedpan under buttocks. *Comments:*	☐	☐	☐	
8. Help the client roll onto the back with the bedpan in place. *Comments:*	☐	☐	☐	
9. Alternate: Help the client raise the hips and slide the pan in place. Alternate: Use a fracture pan instead of a bedpan. *Comments:*	☐	☐	☐	
10. Check placement of bedpan. *Comments:*	☐	☐	☐	
11. If indicated, elevate head of bed to 45° angle. *Comments:*	☐	☐	☐	

Procedure 4-5	Able to Perform	Able to Perform with Assistance	Unable to Perform	Initials and Date
12. Place call light within reach; provide for client safety, and privacy. *Comments:*	☐	☐	☐	
13. Remove gloves; wash hands. *Comments:*	☐	☐	☐	
Positioning a Urinal 14. Close curtain or door. Wash hands; apply gloves. *Comments:*	☐	☐	☐	
15. Lift the covers. Allow client to place urinal or place it yourself. *Comments:*	☐	☐	☐	
16. Remove gloves; wash hands. *Comments:*	☐	☐	☐	
Removing a Bedpan 17. Wash hands; apply gloves. *Comments:*	☐	☐	☐	
18. Gather toilet paper and washing supplies. *Comments:*	☐	☐	☐	
19. Lower head of bed to supine position. *Comments:*	☐	☐	☐	
20. Roll client to side and remove the pan. *Comments:*	☐	☐	☐	
21. Assist with cleaning or wiping. *Comments:*	☐	☐	☐	
22. Measure output. Empty, clean, and store bedpan in proper place. *Comments:*	☐	☐	☐	
23. Remove soiled gloves. Wash hands. *Comments:*	☐	☐	☐	

continued on the following page

continued from the previous page

Procedure 4-5	Able to Perform	Able to Perform with Assistance	Unable to Perform	Initials and Date
24. Allow client to wash hands. *Comments:*	☐	☐	☐	
25. Place call light within reach; put side rails up. *Comments:*	☐	☐	☐	
26. Wash hands. *Comments:*	☐	☐	☐	
Removing a Urinal 27. Wash hands and apply gloves. Remove the urinal. *Comments:*	☐	☐	☐	
28. Measure urine output. Empty and rinse the urinal. Place it in the client's reach. *Comments:*	☐	☐	☐	
29. Remove soiled gloves. Wash hands. *Comments:*	☐	☐	☐	
30. Allow client to wash hands. *Comments:*	☐	☐	☐	
31. Place call light in reach; put side rails up. *Comments:*	☐	☐	☐	
32. Wash hands. *Comments:*	☐	☐	☐	

Checklist for Procedure 4-6   Assisting with Feeding

Name _____ Date _____

School _____

Instructor _____

Course _____

Procedure 4-6 Assisting with Feeding	Able to Perform	Able to Perform with Assistance	Unable to Perform	Initials and Date
Assessment				
1. Assess the appropriateness of the ordered diet. *Comments:*	☐	☐	☐	
2. Assess the client's environmental needs. *Comments:*	☐	☐	☐	
3. Assess the client's immediate nutritional needs. *Comments:*	☐	☐	☐	
4. Assess the client's ability to chew and swallow. *Comments:*	☐	☐	☐	
5. Assess the client's level of understanding. *Comments:*	☐	☐	☐	
Planning/Expected Outcomes				
1. Clients will ingest calories adequate for their body requirements. *Comments:*	☐	☐	☐	
2. Clients will report being satiated and comfortable. *Comments:*	☐	☐	☐	
Implementation				
1. Wash hands. *Comments:*	☐	☐	☐	
2. Help the client wash hands and face and prepare for the meal. *Comments:*	☐	☐	☐	

continued on the following page

continued from the previous page

Procedure 4-6	Able to Perform	Able to Perform with Assistance	Unable to Perform	Initials and Date
3. Remove or move any unpleasant stimuli. *Comments:*	☐	☐	☐	
4. If possible, have the client sit upright. *Comments:*	☐	☐	☐	
5. Check that the food is the correct diet and consistency. *Comments:*	☐	☐	☐	
6. Place a napkin or protective cover over the client if needed. *Comments:*	☐	☐	☐	
7. Prepare the food in a manner that will help the client eat it. *Comments:*	☐	☐	☐	
8. If you will be feeding the client, sit at the client's eye level. *Comments:*	☐	☐	☐	
9. Allow the client to do as much as possible for him- or herself. *Comments:*	☐	☐	☐	
10. Use this time as an opportunity to connect with the client. *Comments:*	☐	☐	☐	
11. Remove the tray when the client is finished with the meal. Make sure the client is positioned properly and the call light is within reach. *Comments:*	☐	☐	☐	
12. Help the client to clean up following the meal. *Comments:*	☐	☐	☐	
13. Wash hands. *Comments:*	☐	☐	☐	

Checklist for Procedure 4-7   Bathing a Client in Bed

Name _____ Date _____

School _____

Instructor _____

Course _____

Procedure 4-7 Bathing a Client in Bed	Able to Perform	Able to Perform with Assistance	Unable to Perform	Initials and Date
Assessment				
1. Assess the client's level of ability to assist with the bath. *Comments:*	☐	☐	☐	
2. Assess the client's level of comfort with the procedure. *Comments:*	☐	☐	☐	
3. Assess the environment and equipment available. *Comments:*	☐	☐	☐	
Planning/Expected Outcomes				
1. Clients will be cleaned without damage to their skin. *Comments:*	☐	☐	☐	
2. Clients' privacy will be maintained. *Comments:*	☐	☐	☐	
3. Clients will participate in their own hygiene. *Comments:*	☐	☐	☐	
4. Clients will not experience adverse effects as a result of the bath. *Comments:*	☐	☐	☐	
Implementation				
1. Assess client's preferences about bathing. *Comments:*	☐	☐	☐	
2. Explain procedure to client. *Comments:*	☐	☐	☐	
3. Prepare environment. Provide time for elimination, and provide privacy. *Comments:*	☐	☐	☐	

continued on the following page

continued from the previous page

Procedure 4-7	Able to Perform	Able to Perform with Assistance	Unable to Perform	Initials and Date
4. Wash hands. Apply gloves. *Comments:*	☐	☐	☐	
5. Lower side rail nearest you. Position client comfortably. *Comments:*	☐	☐	☐	
6. Place bath blanket over top sheet. Remove top sheet and client's gown. *Comments:*	☐	☐	☐	
7. Fill washbasin two-thirds full with warm water. *Comments:*	☐	☐	☐	
8. Wet the washcloth and wring it out. *Comments:*	☐	☐	☐	
9. Make a bath mitten with the washcloth. *Comments:*	☐	☐	☐	
10. Wash client's face, neck, and ears. Shave client if needed. *Comments:*	☐	☐	☐	
11. Wash arms, forearms, and hands. *Comments:*	☐	☐	☐	
12. Wash chest and abdomen. *Comments:*	☐	☐	☐	
13. Wash legs and feet. *Comments:*	☐	☐	☐	
14. Wash back. *Comments:*	☐	☐	☐	
15. Assist client to supine position. Perform perineal care. *Comments:*	☐	☐	☐	
16. Apply lotion and powder as desired. Apply clean gown. *Comments:*	☐	☐	☐	

Procedure 4-7	Able to Perform	Able to Perform with Assistance	Unable to Perform	Initials and Date
17. Document skin assessment, type of bath, and client response. *Comments:*	☐	☐	☐	
18. Wash hands. *Comments:*	☐	☐	☐	

Checklist for Procedure 4-8   Oral Care

Name _____ Date _____

School _____

Instructor _____

Course _____

Procedure 4-8 Oral Care	Able to Perform	Able to Perform with Assistance	Unable to Perform	Initials and Date
Assessment				
1. Assess whether the client is able to assist with oral care. *Comments:*	☐	☐	☐	
2. Evaluate whether the client has an understanding of proper oral hygiene. *Comments:*	☐	☐	☐	
3. Check whether the client has dentures. *Comments:*	☐	☐	☐	
4. Assess the condition of the client's mouth. *Comments:*	☐	☐	☐	
5. Assess mouth for disease processes. *Comments:*	☐	☐	☐	
6. Assess what cultural practices must be considered. *Comments:*	☐	☐	☐	
7. Assess whether there are any appliances or devices present in the client's mouth. *Comments:*	☐	☐	☐	
8. Check that the proper equipment is available. *Comments:*	☐	☐	☐	
Planning/Expected Outcomes				
1. Client's mouth, teeth, gums, and lips will be clean. *Comments:*	☐	☐	☐	
2. Any disease processes present will be noted and treated. *Comments:*	☐	☐	☐	

continued on the following page

continued from the previous page

Procedure 4-8	Able to Perform	Able to Perform with Assistance	Unable to Perform	Initials and Date
3. The oral mucosa will be clean, intact, and well hydrated. *Comments:*	☐	☐	☐	
Implementation				
Self-Care Client: Flossing and Brushing 1. Assemble articles for flossing and brushing. *Comments:*	☐	☐	☐	
2. Provide privacy. *Comments:*	☐	☐	☐	
3. Place client in a high-Fowler's position. *Comments:*	☐	☐	☐	
4. Wash hands and apply gloves. *Comments:*	☐	☐	☐	
5. Arrange articles within client's reach. *Comments:*	☐	☐	☐	
6. Assist client with flossing and brushing as necessary. *Comments:*	☐	☐	☐	
7. Assist client with rinsing mouth. *Comments:*	☐	☐	☐	
8. Reposition client, raise side rails, and place call button within reach. *Comments:*	☐	☐	☐	
9. Rinse, dry, and return articles to proper place. *Comments:*	☐	☐	☐	
10. Remove gloves, wash hands, and document care. *Comments:*	☐	☐	☐	
Self-Care Client: Denture Care 11. Assemble articles for denture cleaning. *Comments:*	☐	☐	☐	

Procedure 4-8	Able to Perform	Able to Perform with Assistance	Unable to Perform	Initials and Date
12. Provide privacy. *Comments:*	☐	☐	☐	
13. Assist client to a high-Fowler's position. *Comments:*	☐	☐	☐	
14. Wash hands and apply gloves. *Comments:*	☐	☐	☐	
15. Assist client with denture removal. Place in denture cup. *Comments:*	☐	☐	☐	
16. Apply toothpaste to brush and brush dentures with cool water. *Comments:*	☐	☐	☐	
17. Rinse thoroughly. *Comments:*	☐	☐	☐	
18. Assist client with rinsing mouth and replacing dentures. *Comments:*	☐	☐	☐	
19. Reposition client, with side rails up and call button within reach. *Comments:*	☐	☐	☐	
20. Rinse, dry, and return articles to proper place. *Comments:*	☐	☐	☐	
21. Remove gloves, wash hands, and document care. *Comments:*	☐	☐	☐	
Full-Care Client: Brushing and Flossing 22. Assemble articles for flossing and brushing. *Comments:*	☐	☐	☐	
23. Provide privacy. *Comments:*	☐	☐	☐	

continued on the following page

continued from the previous page

Procedure 4-8	Able to Perform	Able to Perform with Assistance	Unable to Perform	Initials and Date
24. Wash hands and apply gloves. *Comments:*	☐	☐	☐	
25. Position client as condition allows. *Comments:*	☐	☐	☐	
26. Place towel across client's chest or under face and mouth. *Comments:*	☐	☐	☐	
27. Apply small amount of toothpaste, and brush teeth and gums. *Comments:*	☐	☐	☐	
28. Floss between all teeth. *Comments:*	☐	☐	☐	
29. Assist the client in rinsing mouth. *Comments:*	☐	☐	☐	
30. Reapply toothpaste and brush the teeth and gums. *Comments:*	☐	☐	☐	
31. Assist the client in rinsing and drying mouth. *Comments:*	☐	☐	☐	
32. Apply lip moisturizer, if appropriate. *Comments:*	☐	☐	☐	
33. Reposition client, raise side rails, and place call button within reach. *Comments:*	☐	☐	☐	
34. Rinse, dry, and return articles to proper place. *Comments:*	☐	☐	☐	
35. Remove gloves, wash hands, and document care. *Comments:*	☐	☐	☐	

Procedure 4-8	Able to Perform	Able to Perform with Assistance	Unable to Perform	Initials and Date
Clients at Risk for or with an Alteration of the Oral Cavity				
36. Assemble articles for flossing and brushing. *Comments:*	☐	☐	☐	
37. Provide privacy. *Comments:*	☐	☐	☐	
38. Wash hands and apply gloves. *Comments:*	☐	☐	☐	
39. Bleeding: a. Assess oral cavity for signs of bleeding. b. Proceed with the oral care for a full-care client, except: • Do not floss. • Use a soft toothbrush, toothette, or a padded tongue blade to swab teeth and gums. • Dispose of padded tongue blade into a biohazard bag. • Rinse with tepid water. *Comments:*	☐	☐	☐	
40. Infection: a. Assess oral cavity for signs of infection. b. Culture lesions as ordered. c. Proceed with oral care for a full-care client except: • Do not floss. • Use prescribed antiseptic solution. • Use a padded tongue blade to swab the teeth and gums. • Dispose of padded tongue blade into a biohazard bag. • Rinse mouth with tepid water. • Apply additional solution as prescribed. *Comments:*	☐	☐	☐	
41. Ulceration: a. Assess oral cavity for signs of ulceration. b. Culture lesions as ordered. c. Proceed with oral care for a full-care client except: • Do not floss. • Use prescribed antiseptic solution. • Use a padded tongue blade to swab the teeth and gums. • Dispose of padded tongue blade into a biohazard bag. • Rinse mouth with tepid water. • Apply additional solution as prescribed. *Comments:*	☐	☐	☐	

continued on the following page

continued from the previous page

Procedure 4-8	Able to Perform	Able to Perform with Assistance	Unable to Perform	Initials and Date
Unconscious (Comatose) Client:				
42. Assemble articles for flossing and brushing. *Comments:*	☐	☐	☐	
43. Provide privacy. *Comments:*	☐	☐	☐	
44. Wash hands and apply gloves. *Comments:*	☐	☐	☐	
45. Explain the procedure to the client. *Comments:*	☐	☐	☐	
46. Place the client in a lateral position, head turned toward the side. *Comments:*	☐	☐	☐	
47. Use a floss holder and floss between all teeth. *Comments:*	☐	☐	☐	
48. Moisten toothbrush, and brush the teeth and gums. Do not use toothpaste. *Comments:*	☐	☐	☐	
49. After flossing and brushing, rinse mouth and perform oral suction. *Comments:*	☐	☐	☐	
50. Dry the client's mouth. *Comments:*	☐	☐	☐	
51. Apply lip moisturizer. *Comments:*	☐	☐	☐	
52. Leave the client in a lateral position for 30–60 minutes after oral care. Suction one more time. *Comments:*	☐	☐	☐	
53. Dispose of nonreusable items appropriately. Rinse, dry, and return articles to proper place. *Comments:*	☐	☐	☐	
54. Remove gloves, wash hands, and document care. *Comments:*	☐	☐	☐	

Checklist for Procedure 4-9   Perineal and Genital Care

Name _____ Date _____

School _____

Instructor _____

Course _____

Procedure 4-9 Perineal and Genital Care	Able to Perform	Able to Perform with Assistance	Unable to Perform	Initials and Date
Assessment				
1. Evaluate client status. *Comments:*	☐	☐	☐	
2. Identify cultural preferences for perineal care. *Comments:*	☐	☐	☐	
3. Assess the client's perineal health. *Comments:*	☐	☐	☐	
4. Determine if the client is incontinent of urine or stool. *Comments:*				
5. Assess whether the client has recently had perineal/genital surgery. *Comments:*	☐	☐	☐	
Planning/Expected Outcomes				
1. Perineum and genitalia will be dry, clean, and odor free. *Comments:*	☐	☐	☐	
2. The client will report feeling comfortable and clean. *Comments:*	☐	☐	☐	
3. The client will not experience discomfort or undue embarrassment. *Comments:*	☐	☐	☐	
4. The perineum will be free of skin breakdown or irritation. *Comments:*	☐	☐	☐	

continued on the following page

continued from the previous page

Procedure 4-9	Able to Perform	Able to Perform with Assistance	Unable to Perform	Initials and Date
Implementation				
1. Wash hands and wear gloves. *Comments:*	☐	☐	☐	
2. Close privacy curtain or door. *Comments:*	☐	☐	☐	
3. Position client. *Comments:*	☐	☐	☐	
4. Place waterproof pads under the client. *Comments:*	☐	☐	☐	
5. Remove fecal debris and dispose in toilet. *Comments:*	☐	☐	☐	
6. Spray perineum with washing solution. *Comments:*	☐	☐	☐	
7. Cleanse perineum with wet washcloths. Cleanse the penis on the male. *Comments:*	☐	☐	☐	
8. Examine folds and vulva of females for debris. *Comments:*	☐	☐	☐	
9. If soap is used, spray area with clean water from the peri-bottle. *Comments:*	☐	☐	☐	
10. Change gloves. *Comments:*	☐	☐	☐	
11. Dry perineum carefully with towel. *Comments:*	☐	☐	☐	
12. If indicated, apply barrier lotion or ointment. *Comments:*	☐	☐	☐	

Procedure 4-9	Able to Perform	Able to Perform with Assistance	Unable to Perform	Initials and Date
13. Reposition or dress client as appropriate. *Comments:*	☐	☐	☐	
14. Dispose of linens and garbage appropriately. *Comments:*	☐	☐	☐	
15. Wash hands. *Comments:*	☐	☐	☐	
16. Deodorize room if appropriate. *Comments:*	☐	☐	☐	

Checklist for Procedure 4-10   Eye Care

Name _____   Date _____

School _____

Instructor _____

Course _____

Procedure 4-10 Eye Care	Able to Perform	Able to Perform with Assistance	Unable to Perform	Initials and Date
Assessment				
1. Determine if the client is wearing contact lenses or has an ocular prosthesis. Comments:	☐	☐	☐	
2. Determine availability of eye care supplies. Comments:	☐	☐	☐	
3. Assess whether the client can do his or her own eye care. Comments:	☐	☐	☐	
Planning/Expected Outcomes				
1. The client's contact lenses will be safely removed and stored. Comments:	☐	☐	☐	
2. The client's ocular prosthesis will be safely removed, cleaned, and either stored or returned to the client's eye socket. Comments:	☐	☐	☐	
3. The client's contacts or prosthesis will be cared for with a minimum of trauma to the client. Comments:	☐	☐	☐	
4. The client's eyes will be free of crusts and exudate. Comments:	☐	☐	☐	
Implementation				
Artificial Eye Removal 1. Inquire about client's care regimen and gather equipment. Comments:	☐	☐	☐	
2. Provide privacy. Comments:	☐	☐	☐	

continued on the following page

continued from the previous page

Procedure 4-10	Able to Perform	Able to Perform with Assistance	Unable to Perform	Initials and Date
3. Wash hands; apply gloves. *Comments:*	☐	☐	☐	
4. Place client in a semi-Fowler's position. *Comments:*	☐	☐	☐	
5. Place cotton balls in emesis basin filled halfway with warm water. *Comments:*	☐	☐	☐	
6. Place gauze sponges in bottom of second emesis basin filled halfway with mild soap and tepid water. *Comments:*	☐	☐	☐	
7. Squeeze excess water from a cotton ball. Cleanse the eyelid with the cotton ball. Repeat until eyelid is clean. *Comments:*	☐	☐	☐	
8. Remove the artificial eye: a. Raise the client's upper eyelid and depress the lower eyelid. b. Cup hand under the client's lower eyelid. c. Apply slight pressure between the brow and the artificial eye and remove it. Place it in the warm, soapy water. *Comments:*	☐	☐	☐	
9. Grasp a moistened cotton ball, cleanse the edge of the eye socket. *Comments:*	☐	☐	☐	
10. Inspect the eye socket for irritation, drainage, or crusting. *Comments:*	☐	☐	☐	
11. Eye socket irrigation: a. Place the client in flat, supine position. Turn head toward socket side and slightly extend neck. b. Fill the irrigation syringe with the irrigating solution. c. Separate the eyelids, resting fingers on the brow and cheekbone. d. Hold the irrigating syringe several inches above the inner canthus. Direct the flow of solution from the inner canthus along the conjunctival sac. e. Irrigate with the prescribed amount of solution.				

Procedure 4-10	Able to Perform	Able to Perform with Assistance	Unable to Perform	Initials and Date
f. Wipe the eyelids with a moistened cotton ball. g. Pat the skin dry with the towel. h. Return the client to a semi-Fowler's position. i. Remove gloves, wash hands, and apply clean gloves. *Comments:*	☐	☐	☐	
12. Rub the artificial eye between the fingers in warm, soapy water. *Comments:*	☐	☐	☐	
13. Rinse the prosthesis under running water or in the basin of tepid water. Do not dry the prosthesis. *Comments:*	☐	☐	☐	
14. Reinsert the prosthesis: a. With the thumb, raise and hold the upper eyelid open. b. Grasp the artificial eye so that the indented part is facing the client's nose and slide it under the upper eyelid. c. Depress the lower lid. d. Pull the lower lid forward to cover the edge of the prosthesis. *Comments:*	☐	☐	☐	
15. Place the cleaned eye in a labeled container with saline or tap water. *Comments:*	☐	☐	☐	
16. Grasp a moistened cotton ball, wipe the eyelid from the inner to the outer canthus. *Comments:*	☐	☐	☐	
17. Clean, dry, and replace equipment. *Comments:*	☐	☐	☐	
18. Reposition the client, raise side rails, and place call light within reach. *Comments:*	☐	☐	☐	
19. Dispose of biohazard bag appropriately. *Comments:*	☐	☐	☐	

continued on the following page

continued from the previous page

Procedure 4-10	Able to Perform	Able to Perform with Assistance	Unable to Perform	Initials and Date
20. Remove gloves and wash hands. *Comments:*	☐	☐	☐	
21. Document procedure, client's response, and client teaching. *Comments:*	☐	☐	☐	
Contact Lens Removal 22. Assemble equipment for lens removal. *Comments:*	☐	☐	☐	
23. Assess level of assistance needed, provide privacy, and explain to the client. *Comments:*	☐	☐	☐	
24. Wash hands. *Comments:*	☐	☐	☐	
25. Assist the client to a semi-Fowler's position if needed. *Comments:*	☐	☐	☐	
26. Drape a clean towel over the client's chest. *Comments:*	☐	☐	☐	
27. Prepare the lens storage case with the prescribed solution. *Comments:*	☐	☐	☐	
28. Instruct the client to look straight ahead. Assess the location of the lens. Move the lens toward the cornea. *Comments:*	☐	☐	☐	

29. Remove the lens.
  a. Hard lens:
    • Cup nondominant hand under the eye.
    • Pull outside corner of the eye toward the temple and ask client to blink. Catch the lens.
  b. Soft lens:
    • Separate the eyelid with your fingers.
    • Slide the lens downward onto the sclera and gently squeeze the lens.
    • Release the top eyelid and remove the lens.
    • If lens cannot be extracted using fingers, secure a suction cup to remove the contact lens.
Comments:
	☐	☐	☐	

Procedure 4-10	Able to Perform	Able to Perform with Assistance	Unable to Perform	Initials and Date
30. Store the lens in the correct compartment of a case labeled with the client's name. *Comments:*	☐	☐	☐	
31. Repeat Actions 29 and 30 for the second lens. *Comments:*	☐	☐	☐	
32. Assess eyes for irritation or redness. *Comments:*	☐	☐	☐	
33. Store the lens case in a safe place. *Comments:*	☐	☐	☐	
34. Dispose of soiled articles and clean and return reusable articles. *Comments:*	☐	☐	☐	
35. Reposition the client, raise side rails, and place call light within reach. *Comments:*	☐	☐	☐	
36. Remove gloves and wash hands. *Comments:*	☐	☐	☐	
37. Document procedure. *Comments:*	☐	☐	☐	

Checklist for Procedure 4-11   Hair and Scalp Care

Name _____ Date _____

School _____

Instructor _____

Course _____

Procedure 4-11 Hair and Scalp Care	Able to Perform	Able to Perform with Assistance	Unable to Perform	Initials and Date
Assessment				
1. Assess client's need for hair and scalp care. *Comments:*	☐	☐	☐	
2. Assess structure and functional integrity of the hair and scalp. *Comments:*	☐	☐	☐	
3. Assess client preferences for hair and scalp care. *Comments:*	☐	☐	☐	
4. Confirm client is not allergic to any products to be used. *Comments:*	☐	☐	☐	
5. Assess client's medical condition and health status. *Comments:*	☐	☐	☐	
6. Assess client's knowledge of the procedure. *Comments:*	☐	☐	☐	
7. Assess client's ability to perform/assist with the procedure. *Comments:*	☐	☐	☐	
Planning/Expected Outcomes				
1. The client will have healthy hair and a clean scalp. *Comments:*	☐	☐	☐	
2. The client will experience improved circulation to the scalp. *Comments:*	☐	☐	☐	

continued on the following page

continued from the previous page

Procedure 4-11	Able to Perform	Able to Perform with Assistance	Unable to Perform	Initials and Date
3. The client's comfort, self-esteem, and sense of well-being will be improved. *Comments:*	☐	☐	☐	
Implementation				
1. Inform client you will be assisting with hair care. *Comments:*	☐	☐	☐	
2. Prepare room environment and provide privacy. *Comments:*	☐	☐	☐	
3. Review client history for allergies. Confirm orders for medicated treatments. *Comments:*	☐	☐	☐	
4. Organize equipment at side of bed or chair. *Comments:*	☐	☐	☐	
5. Adjust bed to comfortable height, or position chair. *Comments:*	☐	☐	☐	
6. Wash hands and apply gloves. *Comments:*	☐	☐	☐	
7. Remove pillow or assist client to chair. *Comments:*	☐	☐	☐	
8. Place linen saver and towel under client's shoulders and head. *Comments:*	☐	☐	☐	
9. Drape client's shoulders with a second towel. *Comments:*	☐	☐	☐	
10. Gently comb client's hair, observing scalp and hair. *Comments:*	☐	☐	☐	
11. Place large pitcher(s) of warm water on bedside table. *Comments:*	☐	☐	☐	

Procedure 4-11	Able to Perform	Able to Perform with Assistance	Unable to Perform	Initials and Date
12. Place the shampoo tray under the client's neck and head. *Comments:*	☐	☐	☐	
13. Position drainage pail in line with the spout of the shampoo tray. *Comments:*	☐	☐	☐	
14. Offer washcloth for client's eyes and cotton balls for client's ears. *Comments:*	☐	☐	☐	
15. Carefully pour the warm water over the hair, moistening thoroughly. *Comments:*	☐	☐	☐	
16. Massage a small amount of shampoo into the hair. Gently massage the shampoo into the scalp. *Comments:*	☐	☐	☐	
17. Rinse the hair by using the small pitcher to pour warm water over the hair and scalp. *Comments:*	☐	☐	☐	
18. Repeat application of shampoo and massage scalp and hair for a longer period of time. *Comments:*	☐	☐	☐	
19. Rinse again until hair and scalp are free of shampoo. *Comments:*	☐	☐	☐	
20. Apply conditioner or rinse as per product directions. *Comments:*	☐	☐	☐	
21. Support client's head while you remove the shampoo tray. *Comments:*	☐	☐	☐	
22. Wrap client's hair/head with the towel drape. Dry the scalp and hair with the towel. *Comments:*	☐	☐	☐	

continued on the following page

continued from the previous page

Procedure 4-11	Able to Perform	Able to Perform with Assistance	Unable to Perform	Initials and Date
23. Remove the linen saver and towel from the bed. *Comments:*	☐	☐	☐	
24. Elevate the head of bed to desired angle. *Comments:*	☐	☐	☐	
25. Thoroughly dry your hands and/or change gloves. *Comments:*	☐	☐	☐	
26. Turn hair dryer on to warm setting and check the temperature. *Comments:*	☐	☐	☐	
27. Dry hair. *Comments:*	☐	☐	☐	
28. Gently comb/brush the hair. *Comments:*	☐	☐	☐	
29. Style hair per client preference. *Comments:*	☐	☐	☐	
30. Reposition the client comfortably and provide for client safety. *Comments:*	☐	☐	☐	
31. Empty the water. Remove, clean, and return equipment. *Comments:*	☐	☐	☐	
32. Remove gloves and wash your hands. *Comments:*	☐	☐	☐	

Checklist for Procedure 4-12   Hand and Foot Care

Name _____ Date _____

School _____

Instructor _____

Course _____

Procedure 4-12 Hand and Foot Care	Able to Perform	Able to Perform with Assistance	Unable to Perform	Initials and Date
Assessment				
1. Assess skin integrity. *Comments:*	☐	☐	☐	
2. Assess nail integrity. *Comments:*	☐	☐	☐	
3. Assess structural integrity of hands and feet. *Comments:*	☐	☐	☐	
4. Assess functional status of hands and feet. *Comments:*	☐	☐	☐	
5. Identify allergies. *Comments:*	☐	☐	☐	
6. Assess client's ability to perform basic hand and foot care. *Comments:*	☐	☐	☐	
7. Assess client's preferences for equipment to be used in the procedure. *Comments:*	☐	☐	☐	
Planning/Expected Outcomes				
1. The client's hands and feet will be clean, odor free, soft, and hydrated. *Comments:*	☐	☐	☐	
2. The client will experience maximized function of hands and feet. *Comments:*	☐	☐	☐	
3. The client will be comfortable and relaxed. *Comments:*	☐	☐	☐	

continued on the following page

continued from the previous page

Procedure 4-12	Able to Perform	Able to Perform with Assistance	Unable to Perform	Initials and Date
Implementation				
1. Explain planned procedure and confirm allergy status. *Comments:*	☐	☐	☐	
2. Assemble equipment. *Comments:*	☐	☐	☐	
3. For feet, seat client in stable, comfortable chair or pull bedding out at the foot of the bed. *Comments:*	☐	☐	☐	
4. Place linen saver under client's hands/feet. *Comments:*	☐	☐	☐	
5. Wash hands; apply gloves. *Comments:*	☐	☐	☐	
6. Fill basin halfway with warm water. Place basin on the linen saver. *Comments:*	☐	☐	☐	
7. Immerse client's hand/foot in the basin. *Comments:*	☐	☐	☐	
8. Soak hand/foot 2–10 minutes. *Comments:*	☐	☐	☐	
9. Wash hand/foot with scant amount of a mild antibacterial soap. *Comments:*	☐	☐	☐	
10. Rinse well to be sure all soap is removed. *Comments:*	☐	☐	☐	
11. Remove hand/foot from the basin and place onto clean towel. *Comments:*	☐	☐	☐	
12. Pat and then gently rub dry. *Comments:*	☐	☐	☐	
13. Gently push the cuticle and subungual skin back. *Comments:*	☐	☐	☐	

Procedure 4-12	Able to Perform	Able to Perform with Assistance	Unable to Perform	Initials and Date
14. Use a towel or stone pumice on any thickened, dry skin areas. *Comments:*	☐	☐	☐	
15. Lightly powder between and under fingers/toes. *Comments:*	☐	☐	☐	
16. Concurrently assess skin and function. *Comments:*	☐	☐	☐	
17. Check pulses, turgor, and capillary refill. *Comments:*	☐	☐	☐	
18. Empty basin and refill. Repeat with other hand/foot. *Comments:*	☐	☐	☐	
19. While other hand/foot soaks, perform nail care on the first hand/foot. *Comments:*	☐	☐	☐	
20. Lightly apply cream, massaging into the hand/foot. *Comments:*	☐	☐	☐	
21. Towel off any excess cream. *Comments:*	☐	☐	☐	
22. Perform range of motion (ROM) exercises. *Comments:*	☐	☐	☐	
23. Place lamb's wool or cotton in areas that are rubbing. Put on clean socks after foot care. *Comments:*	☐	☐	☐	
24. Check the interior of shoes for foreign objects or scratchy edges prior to putting them on. *Comments:*	☐	☐	☐	
25. Remove, clean, and/or replace equipment/supplies. *Comments:*	☐	☐	☐	
26. Dispose of gloves and wash hands. *Comments:*	☐	☐	☐	

Checklist for Procedure 4-13 Shaving a Client

Name _____ Date _____

School _____

Instructor _____

Course _____

Procedure 4-13 Shaving a Client	Able to Perform	Able to Perform with Assistance	Unable to Perform	Initials and Date
Assessment				
1. Assess whether the client is able to perform self-care. Comments:	☐	☐	☐	
2. Assess the client's skin. Comments:	☐	☐	☐	
3. Assess whether the client is at increased risk of bleeding. Comments:	☐	☐	☐	
4. Assess the client's ability to manipulate the razor. Comments:	☐	☐	☐	
5. Assess the client's shaving preferences. Comments:	☐	☐	☐	
Planning/Expected Outcomes				
1. The client will be neat and well-groomed. Comments:	☐	☐	☐	
2. The client's skin integrity will remain intact. Comments:	☐	☐	☐	
3. The client will attain a sense of independence. Comments:	☐	☐	☐	
4. The client will be comfortable following the procedure. Comments:	☐	☐	☐	
Implementation				
1. Wash hands and apply gloves. Comments:	☐	☐	☐	
2. If the client can shave himself, set up the equipment. Comments:	☐	☐	☐	

continued on the following page

continued from the previous page

Procedure 4-13	Able to Perform	Able to Perform with Assistance	Unable to Perform	Initials and Date
3. Place a towel over the client's chest and shoulder. *Comments:*	☐	☐	☐	
4. Position the client. *Comments:*	☐	☐	☐	
5. Fill a washbasin with warm water. *Comments:*	☐	☐	☐	
6. Wet and wring out washcloth. Apply cloth over the client's face. Remove washcloth. *Comments:*	☐	☐	☐	
7. Apply shaving cream. *Comments:*	☐	☐	☐	
8. Holding the razor at a 45° angle, start shaving the client's face. *Comments:*	☐	☐	☐	
9. Dip the razor in water as cream accumulates. *Comments:*	☐	☐	☐	
10. Check the face to see if all the facial hair is removed. *Comments:*	☐	☐	☐	
11. Rinse the face thoroughly with a moistened washcloth. *Comments:*	☐	☐	☐	
12. Dry the face and apply after-shave lotion if desired. *Comments:*	☐	☐	☐	
13. Allow client to inspect the results of your shave. *Comments:*	☐	☐	☐	
14. Dispose of equipment in proper receptacle. *Comments:*	☐	☐	☐	
15. Wash hands. *Comments:*	☐	☐	☐	

Checklist for Procedure 4-14   Giving a Back Rub

Name _____ Date _____

School _____

Instructor _____

Course _____

Procedure 4-14 Giving a Back Rub	Able to Perform	Able to Perform with Assistance	Unable to Perform	Initials and Date
Assessment				
1. Assess the client's willingness to have a massage. *Comments:*	☐	☐	☐	
2. Assess the client for contraindications of a back rub. *Comments:*	☐	☐	☐	
3. Assess any limitations the client has in positioning. *Comments:*	☐	☐	☐	
4. Assess the client for fatigue, stiffness, or soreness. *Comments:*	☐	☐	☐	
5. Assess the client for anxiety or emotional disturbances. *Comments:*	☐	☐	☐	
6. Have the client quantify the degree of discomfort. *Comments:*	☐	☐	☐	
Planning/Expected Outcomes				
1. The client will experience a reduction in stress symptoms. *Comments:*	☐	☐	☐	
2. The nurse will establish a better rapport with the client. *Comments:*	☐	☐	☐	
Implementation				
1. Wash your hands and apply gloves if necessary. *Comments:*	☐	☐	☐	
2. Help client to a prone or side-lying position. *Comments:*	☐	☐	☐	

continued on the following page

continued from the previous page

Procedure 4-14	Able to Perform	Able to Perform with Assistance	Unable to Perform	Initials and Date
3. Expose client's back, shoulder, and sacral area. *Comments:*	☐	☐	☐	
4. Warm a small amount of lotion between your palms. *Comments:*	☐	☐	☐	
5. Begin in the sacral area moving upward toward the shoulders. *Comments:*	☐	☐	☐	
6. Assess client's back during the massage. *Comments:*	☐	☐	☐	
7. Provide petrissage to areas of increased tension. *Comments:*	☐	☐	☐	
8. Complete the massage with long, light brush strokes. *Comments:*	☐	☐	☐	
9. Wipe off excess lubricant and cover the client up. *Comments:*	☐	☐	☐	
10. Wash your hands. *Comments:*	☐	☐	☐	

Checklist for Procedure 4-15   Changing the IV Gown

Name _____ Date _____

School _____

Instructor _____

Course _____

Procedure 4-15 Changing the IV Gown	Able to Perform	Able to Perform with Assistance	Unable to Perform	Initials and Date
Assessment				
1. Assess the client for the presence of an IV line or lines. *Comments:*	☐	☐	☐	
2. Assess the client's current gown. *Comments:*	☐	☐	☐	
3. Determine whether the infusion can be turned off briefly. *Comments:*	☐	☐	☐	
4. Assess availability of gowns made for clients with IVs. *Comments:*	☐	☐	☐	
Planning/Expected Outcomes				
1. The IV line will remain intact during the change. *Comments:*	☐	☐	☐	
2. The privacy of the client will be preserved. *Comments:*	☐	☐	☐	
3. The IV gown will not become tangled in the IV line. *Comments:*	☐	☐	☐	
4. The gown will be changed without compromising the client's health. *Comments:*	☐	☐	☐	
Implementation				
1. Wash hands. *Comments:*	☐	☐	☐	
2. Untie or unsnap the back fasteners on the old gown. *Comments:*	☐	☐	☐	

continued on the following page

continued from the previous page

Procedure 4-15	Able to Perform	Able to Perform with Assistance	Unable to Perform	Initials and Date
Gown with Shoulder Snaps				
3. Unsnap the gown sleeves. *Comments:*	☐	☐	☐	
4. Cover the client with the clean gown. *Comments:*	☐	☐	☐	
5. Pull the old gown out from underneath the clean gown. *Comments:*	☐	☐	☐	
6. Snap the sleeves of the clean gown around the client's arms. *Comments:*	☐	☐	☐	
Gown with Solid Sleeves 1				
7. Place the clean gown over the client in the proper orientation. *Comments:*	☐	☐	☐	
8. Remove the old gown from the arm without IV access. *Comments:*	☐	☐	☐	
9. Determine if the client will tolerate a brief interruption in the IV infusion. *Comments:*	☐	☐	☐	
10. Clamp the IV tubing or shut off the IV pump and remove the tubing from the pump. *Comments:*	☐	☐	☐	
11. Remove the IV bottle from the IV stand. *Comments:*	☐	☐	☐	
12. Hold the IV bottle in nondominant hand, and use the other hand to slide the old gown off the arm with IV access onto the hand holding the IV bottle. *Comments:*	☐	☐	☐	
13. Take the IV bottle in the free hand and remove the client gown from your hand. *Comments:*	☐	☐	☐	

Procedure 4-15	Able to Perform	Able to Perform with Assistance	Unable to Perform	Initials and Date
14. With the IV bottle in dominant hand, place the other hand into the clean gown, from the distal end toward the proximal end of the sleeve. *Comments:*	☐	☐	☐	
15. Place the IV bottle in the hand with the clean gown on it. Use the free hand to slide the sleeve of the clean gown over the IV equipment and over the client's arm. *Comments:*	☐	☐	☐	
16. Replace the IV bottle on the IV stand. Restart the IV flow. *Comments:*	☐	☐	☐	
17. Check the IV flow rate and the IV access site. *Comments:*	☐	☐	☐	
18. Slide the gown sleeve over the client's other arm. *Comments:*	☐	☐	☐	
Gown with Solid Sleeves 2 19. Check the IV flow rate and the IV access site. *Comments:*	☐	☐	☐	
20. Fasten the client's gown and provide for the client's comfort. *Comments:*	☐	☐	☐	
21. Wash hands. *Comments:*	☐	☐	☐	

Checklist for Procedure 4-16   Assisting from Bed to Stretcher

Name _____ Date _____

School _____

Instructor _____

Course _____

Procedure 4-16 Assisting from Bed to Stretcher	Able to Perform	Able to Perform with Assistance	Unable to Perform	Initials and Date
Assessment				
1. Assess the client's current level of mobility. *Comments:*	☐	☐	☐	
2. Assess for injury. *Comments:*	☐	☐	☐	
3. Assess for any impediments to mobility. *Comments:*	☐	☐	☐	
4. Assess the client's level of understanding. *Comments:*	☐	☐	☐	
5. Assess the client's environment. *Comments:*	☐	☐	☐	
6. Make sure the stretcher is safe to use. *Comments:*	☐	☐	☐	
Planning/Expected Outcomes				
1. The client will be transferred without pain or injury. *Comments:*	☐	☐	☐	
2. Drainage tubes, IVs, or other devices will remain intact. *Comments:*	☐	☐	☐	
3. The client's skin will be intact and undamaged. *Comments:*	☐	☐	☐	
Implementation				
Transferring a Client with Minimum Assistance 1. Inform client about desired purpose and destination. *Comments:*	☐	☐	☐	

continued on the following page

continued from the previous page

Procedure 4-16	Able to Perform	Able to Perform with Assistance	Unable to Perform	Initials and Date
2. Raise the bed 1 inch higher than the stretcher, and lock brakes of bed and stretcher. *Comments:*	☐	☐	☐	
3. Instruct client to move close to stretcher. Lower side rails of bed and stretcher. *Comments:*	☐	☐	☐	
4. Stand at outer side of stretcher and push it toward bed. *Comments:*	☐	☐	☐	
5. Instruct client to move onto stretcher. Assist as needed. *Comments:*	☐	☐	☐	
6. Cover client with sheet or bath blanket. *Comments:*	☐	☐	☐	
7. Elevate side rails on stretcher and secure safety belts. Release brakes of stretcher. *Comments:*	☐	☐	☐	
8. Stand at head of stretcher to guide it when pushing. *Comments:*	☐	☐	☐	
9. Wash hands. *Comments:*	☐	☐	☐	
Transferring a Client with Maximum Assistance 10. Repeat Actions 1 and 2. *Comments:*	☐	☐	☐	
11. Assess amount of assistance required for transfer. *Comments:*	☐	☐	☐	
12. Lock wheels of bed and stretcher. *Comments:*	☐	☐	☐	
13. Have one nurse stand close to client's head. *Comments:*	☐	☐	☐	

Procedure 4-16	Able to Perform	Able to Perform with Assistance	Unable to Perform	Initials and Date
14. Log roll the client and place a lift sheet under the client. *Comments:*	☐	☐	☐	
15. Empty all drainage bags. Record amounts. Secure drainage system to client's gown. *Comments:*	☐	☐	☐	
16. Move client to edge of bed near stretcher. *Comments:*	☐	☐	☐	
17. The nurse on nonstretcher side of bed holds the stretcher side of the lift sheet up to prevent the client from falling. *Comments:*	☐	☐	☐	
18. Place pillow or slider board overlapping the bed and stretcher. *Comments:*	☐	☐	☐	
19. Have staff members grasp edges of lift sheet. *Comments:*	☐	☐	☐	
20. On the count of three, staff members pull lift sheet and the client onto the stretcher. *Comments:*	☐	☐	☐	
21. Position client on stretcher. Cover with a sheet or bath blanket. *Comments:*	☐	☐	☐	
22. Secure safety belts and elevate side rails of stretcher. *Comments:*	☐	☐	☐	
23. Move IV from bed pole to stretcher IV pole after client transfer. *Comments:*	☐	☐	☐	
24. Wash hands. *Comments:*	☐	☐	☐	

Checklist for Procedure 4-17   Assisting from Bed to Wheelchair, Commode, or Chair

Name _____ Date _____

School _____

Instructor _____

Course _____

Procedure 4-17 Assisting from Bed to Wheelchair, Commode, or Chair	Able to Perform	Able to Perform with Assistance	Unable to Perform	Initials and Date
Assessment				
1. Assess the client's current level of mobility. *Comments:*	☐	☐	☐	
2. Assess for any impediments to mobility. *Comments:*	☐	☐	☐	
3. Assess the client's level of understanding and anxiety regarding the procedure. *Comments:*	☐	☐	☐	
4. Assess the client's environment. *Comments:*	☐	☐	☐	
5. Assess the equipment. *Comments:*	☐	☐	☐	
Planning/Expected Outcomes				
1. The client will be transferred without pain or injury. *Comments:*	☐	☐	☐	
2. Drainage tubes, IVs, or other devices will be intact. *Comments:*	☐	☐	☐	
3. The client's skin will be intact and undamaged. *Comments:*	☐	☐	☐	
Implementation				
1. Inform client about desired purpose and destination. *Comments:*	☐	☐	☐	

continued on the following page

continued from the previous page

Procedure 4-17	Able to Perform	Able to Perform with Assistance	Unable to Perform	Initials and Date
2. Assess client for ability to assist with and understand the transfer. *Comments:*	☐	☐	☐	
3. Lock the bed in position. *Comments:*	☐	☐	☐	
4. Place any splints, braces, or other devices on the client. *Comments:*	☐	☐	☐	
5. Place shoes or slippers on the client's feet. *Comments:*	☐	☐	☐	
6. Lower the height of the bed to lowest possible position. *Comments:*	☐	☐	☐	
7. Slowly raise the head of the bed if this is not contraindicated. *Comments:*	☐	☐	☐	
8. Place an arm under the client's legs and behind the client's back. Pivot the client so he or she is sitting on the edge of the bed. *Comments:*	☐	☐	☐	
9. Allow client to dangle for 2–5 minutes. *Comments:*	☐	☐	☐	
10. Place the chair or wheelchair at a 45° angle close to the bed. *Comments:*	☐	☐	☐	
11. Lock wheelchair brakes and elevate the foot pedals. *Comments:*	☐	☐	☐	
12. Place gait belt around the client's waist, if needed. *Comments:*	☐	☐	☐	

Procedure 4-17	Able to Perform	Able to Perform with Assistance	Unable to Perform	Initials and Date
13. Assist client to side of bed until feet are firmly on the floor and slightly apart. *Comments:*	☐	☐	☐	
14. Grasp the sides of the gait belt or place your hands just below the client's axilla. Bend your knees and assist the client to a standing position. *Comments:*	☐	☐	☐	
15. Standing close to the client, pivot until the client's back is toward the chair. *Comments:*	☐	☐	☐	
16. Have client place hands on the arm supports. *Comments:*	☐	☐	☐	
17. Bend at the knees, easing the client into a sitting position. *Comments:*	☐	☐	☐	
18. Assist client to maintain proper posture. *Comments:*	☐	☐	☐	
19. Secure the safety belt, place client's feet on foot pedals, and release brakes to move client. If the client is sitting in a chair, offer a footstool. *Comments:*	☐	☐	☐	
20. Wash hands. *Comments:*	☐	☐	☐	

Checklist for Procedure 4-18 Assisting from Bed to Walking

Name _____ Date _____

School _____

Instructor _____

Course _____

Procedure 4-18 Assisting from Bed to Walking	Able to Perform	Able to Perform with Assistance	Unable to Perform	Initials and Date
Assessment				
1. Assess the client's ambulating potential. *Comments:*	☐	☐	☐	
2. Assess client's limitations to mobility and ability to perform activities of daily living. *Comments:*	☐	☐	☐	
Planning/Expected Outcomes				
1. The client's functional abilities will improve. *Comments:*	☐	☐	☐	
2. The client's strength and endurance will improve. *Comments:*	☐	☐	☐	
3. The effects of immobility will be minimized or avoided. *Comments:*	☐	☐	☐	
Implementation				
1. Wash hands. *Comments:*	☐	☐	☐	
2. Explain procedure to the client to elicit client cooperation. *Comments:*	☐	☐	☐	
3. Provide for client privacy. *Comments:*	☐	☐	☐	
4. Adjust bed to a comfortable working height. Lower side rail. *Comments:*	☐	☐	☐	
5. Gather all necessary equipment. Adjust client equipment to accommodate the new position. *Comments:*	☐	☐	☐	

continued on the following page

continued from the previous page

Procedure 4-18	Able to Perform	Able to Perform with Assistance	Unable to Perform	Initials and Date
6. Flatten bed and assist client in rolling toward you. *Comments:*	☐	☐	☐	
7. While client is in the side-lying position, assist him or her into the sitting position with feet on the floor. *Comments:*	☐	☐	☐	
8. Monitor vital signs while client is sitting, as appropriate. *Comments:*	☐	☐	☐	
9. Secure gait belt around client's waist. Place ambulation device within client's reach. Assist client to stand. *Comments:*	☐	☐	☐	
10. Monitor vital signs while client is standing, as appropriate. *Comments:*	☐	☐	☐	
11. If client is able to proceed, assume a position beside the client and assist the client, as necessary, using the gait belt. *Comments:*	☐	☐	☐	
12. During ambulation, monitor client vital signs, as necessary. *Comments:*	☐	☐	☐	
13. Following ambulation, return client to bed, remove gait belt, and monitor vital signs, as necessary. *Comments:*	☐	☐	☐	
14. Replace side rails to upright position. *Comments:*	☐	☐	☐	
15. Place the call light within reach of the client. *Comments:*	☐	☐	☐	
16. Place items of frequent use within reach of the client. *Comments:*	☐	☐	☐	
17. Wash hands. *Comments:*	☐	☐	☐	

Checklist for Procedure 4-19   Using a Hydraulic Lift

Name _____ Date _____

School _____

Instructor _____

Course _____

Procedure 4-19 **Using a Hydraulic Lift**	Able to Perform	Able to Perform with Assistance	Unable to Perform	Initials and Date
Assessment				
1. Identify clients with any injuries of the vertebrae. *Comments:*	☐	☐	☐	
2. Identify any equipment that is connected to the client. *Comments:*	☐	☐	☐	
3. Assess client's need for transfer and physical and mental condition. *Comments:*	☐	☐	☐	
4. Assess client's ability to understand and assist in transfer. *Comments:*	☐	☐	☐	
5. Assess number of staff needed for transfer. *Comments:*	☐	☐	☐	
6. Determine whether client is in appropriate clothes and ready for transfer. *Comments:*	☐	☐	☐	
Planning/Expected Outcomes				
1. Client will be transferred safely. *Comments:*	☐	☐	☐	
2. Client will not experience anxiety during the transfer. *Comments:*	☐	☐	☐	
3. Client will incur no injuries. *Comments:*	☐	☐	☐	
4. Privacy will be maintained. *Comments:*	☐	☐	☐	

continued on the following page

continued from the previous page

Procedure 4-19	Able to Perform	Able to Perform with Assistance	Unable to Perform	Initials and Date
Implementation				
1. Wash hands. *Comments:*	☐	☐	☐	
2. Check the orders to determine the length of time the client may sit. *Comments:*	☐	☐	☐	
3. Check the client's medical diagnosis and any other problems. *Comments:*	☐	☐	☐	
4. Ask the client how long ago he or she last sat. *Comments:*	☐	☐	☐	
5. Lock the wheels of the bed. *Comments:*	☐	☐	☐	
6. Position the chair close to the bed. *Comments:*	☐	☐	☐	
7. Position drainage bags and tubing on the chair side of the bed. *Comments:*	☐	☐	☐	
8. Clamp and disconnect any tubing, if permitted. *Comments:*	☐	☐	☐	
9. Roll the client on his or her side and position the sling beside the client. *Comments:*	☐	☐	☐	
10. Roll the client on the other side, pull the sling through, and position the sling on the bed. *Comments:*	☐	☐	☐	
11. Roll the client back onto the sling and fold the arms over the chest. *Comments:*	☐	☐	☐	
12. Make sure the sling is centered. *Comments:*	☐	☐	☐	

Procedure 4-19	Able to Perform	Able to Perform with Assistance	Unable to Perform	Initials and Date
13. Lower the side rail. Position the lift on the chair side of the bed. Spread the base of the hydraulic lift. *Comments:*	☐	☐	☐	
14. Lift the frame and pass it over the client. Lower the frame and attach the hooks to the sling. *Comments:*	☐	☐	☐	
15. Raise the client from the bed by pumping the handle. *Comments:*	☐	☐	☐	
16. Secure the client with a safety belt and cover with a blanket. *Comments:*	☐	☐	☐	
17. Steer the client away from the bed and slide a chair through the base of the lift. *Comments:*	☐	☐	☐	
18. Lower the client into the chair and disconnect the sling from the lift. *Comments:*	☐	☐	☐	
19. Reposition and reconnect any tubing necessary. *Comments:*	☐	☐	☐	
20. Assess how well the client tolerated the move. *Comments:*	☐	☐	☐	
21. Place call light within reach, cover appropriately, and apply restraints if needed. *Comments:*	☐	☐	☐	
22. Reverse the procedure to return the client to the bed. *Comments:*	☐	☐	☐	
23. Wash hands. *Comments:*	☐	☐	☐	

Checklist for Procedure 4-20   Administering Preoperative Care

Name _____ Date _____

School _____

Instructor _____

Course _____

Procedure 4-20 Administering Preoperative Care	Able to Perform	Able to Perform with Assistance	Unable to Perform	Initials and Date
Assessment				
1. Assess the client's diagnosis and the planned surgery. *Comments:*	☐	☐	☐	
2. Assess the client's surgical history. *Comments:*	☐	☐	☐	
3. Assess for complicating factors. *Comments:*	☐	☐	☐	
4. Assess for any allergies. *Comments:*	☐	☐	☐	
5. Assess the client for prostheses. *Comments:*	☐	☐	☐	
6. Determine when client last ate or drank. *Comments:*	☐	☐	☐	
7. Assess the client's level of understanding regarding the plan of care. *Comments:*	☐	☐	☐	
8. Make sure signed surgical consent has been obtained. *Comments:*	☐	☐	☐	
Planning/Expected Outcomes				
1. The client will experience decreased anxiety. *Comments:*	☐	☐	☐	
2. The client will not experience any adverse reactions. *Comments:*	☐	☐	☐	

continued on the following page

continued from the previous page

Procedure 4-20	Able to Perform	Able to Perform with Assistance	Unable to Perform	Initials and Date
3. The client will not experience any loss of belongings. *Comments:*	☐	☐	☐	
4. The client will not experience any disruption or delay of the surgery. *Comments:*	☐	☐	☐	
Implementation				
1. Wash hands. *Comments:*	☐	☐	☐	
2. Verify admission orders. *Comments:*	☐	☐	☐	
3. Verify the client by checking name tag and asking name. *Comments:*	☐	☐	☐	
4. Check the client's understanding of the procedure. *Comments:*	☐	☐	☐	
5. Complete the preoperative checklist. *Comments:*	☐	☐	☐	
6. Perform neurological assessment. *Comments:*	☐	☐	☐	
7. Perform vascular assessment. *Comments:*	☐	☐	☐	
8. Auscultate the lungs bilaterally front and back. *Comments:*	☐	☐	☐	
9. Assess the gastrointestinal system. *Comments:*	☐	☐	☐	
10. Assess the genital/urinary system. *Comments:*	☐	☐	☐	
11. Assess skin integrity and muscle tone. *Comments:*	☐	☐	☐	

Procedure 4-20	Able to Perform	Able to Perform with Assistance	Unable to Perform	Initials and Date
12. Ascertain any allergies or adverse reactions during previous surgeries. *Comments:*	☐	☐	☐	
13. Obtain medication history. *Comments:*	☐	☐	☐	
14. Ascertain any history of drug/alcohol use. *Comments:*	☐	☐	☐	
15. Check weight. *Comments:*	☐	☐	☐	
16. Check if family is available and who is present. *Comments:*	☐	☐	☐	
17. Ascertain if client has signed the surgical consent. *Comments:*	☐	☐	☐	
18. Remove all valuables. Tape rings in place. Document valuable disposition. *Comments:*	☐	☐	☐	
19. Check if eyeglasses and dentures are removed. *Comments:*	☐	☐	☐	
20. Administer intravenous fluids according to orders. *Comments:*	☐	☐	☐	
21. Administer medications according to orders. *Comments:*	☐	☐	☐	
22. Ascertain that preoperative checklist is complete. *Comments:*	☐	☐	☐	
23. Transport the client to appropriate area. *Comments:*	☐	☐	☐	
24. Inform family members where surgical waiting area is. *Comments:*	☐	☐	☐	

Checklist for Procedure 4-21   Preparing a Surgical Site

Name _____ Date _____

School _____

Instructor _____

Course _____

Procedure 4-21 Preparing a Surgical Site	Able to Perform	Able to Perform with Assistance	Unable to Perform	Initials and Date
Assessment				
1. Assess the client for sensitivity or allergies to the scrub solution. *Comments:*	☐	☐	☐	
2. Assess skin integrity. *Comments:*	☐	☐	☐	
3. Assess the client's knowledge of the surgical preparation procedure. *Comments:*	☐	☐	☐	
4. Assess for existing appliances or other instrumentation. *Comments:*	☐	☐	☐	
5. Assess the client's level of mobility at the surgical site. *Comments:*	☐	☐	☐	
Planning/Expected Outcomes				
1. The surgical preparation will be performed without injury or trauma to the client. *Comments:*	☐	☐	☐	
2. The client will understand the procedure. *Comments:*	☐	☐	☐	
3. The client will not experience any allergic reaction or skin sensitivity. *Comments:*	☐	☐	☐	
4. The client will not experience infection secondary to site preparation. *Comments:*	☐	☐	☐	

continued on the following page

continued from the previous page

Procedure 4-21	Able to Perform	Able to Perform with Assistance	Unable to Perform	Initials and Date
5. The client will not experience disruption to any existing instrumentation. *Comments:*	☐	☐	☐	
6. The client will not experience any injury secondary to perioperative positioning. *Comments:*	☐	☐	☐	
Implementation				
1. Review chart to determine the exact area to be prepped. *Comments:*	☐	☐	☐	
2. Wash hands. *Comments:*	☐	☐	☐	
3. Assess client's level of consciousness and mobility. *Comments:*	☐	☐	☐	
4. Explain the procedure to client. *Comments:*	☐	☐	☐	
5. Be sure that hairpins, jewelry, and prostheses were removed during the preoperative preparation. *Comments:*	☐	☐	☐	
6. Assist client with transfer to the surgical table. *Comments:*	☐	☐	☐	
7. Position the client for optimal access to the surgical site. *Comments:*	☐	☐	☐	
8. Cover with blanket. Provide privacy. *Comments:*	☐	☐	☐	
9. Cover hair if required. *Comments:*	☐	☐	☐	
10. Assemble equipment needed. *Comments:*	☐	☐	☐	

Procedure 4-21	Able to Perform	Able to Perform with Assistance	Unable to Perform	Initials and Date
11. Remove your ring(s) and watch. Wash your hands and apply clean gloves. *Comments:*	☐	☐	☐	
12. The surgical prep site depends on the type of surgery to be performed. *Comments:*	☐	☐	☐	
13. Arrange for adequate light on the area to be prepared. *Comments:*	☐	☐	☐	
14. Using warm water, hold the skin taut with the razor at a 45° angle. Stroke in the direction of hair growth. Rinse the razor to remove accumulated hair. *Comments:*	☐	☐	☐	
15. Dry the client's skin with a sterile towel. *Comments:*	☐	☐	☐	
16. Clear the shaving supplies from the preparation area. *Comments:*	☐	☐	☐	
17. Apply sterile gloves and gown. *Comments:*	☐	☐	☐	
18. Scrub the surgical site with an antibacterial cleaner. *Comments:*	☐	☐	☐	
19. Continue this process for 3–10 minutes. *Comments:*	☐	☐	☐	
20. Clean any hidden areas in the surgical site using cotton swabs. *Comments:*	☐	☐	☐	
21. Rinse the area with sterile water. Wait for the site to dry or pat dry with a sterile towel. *Comments:*	☐	☐	☐	
22. Cover the area with sterile drapes leaving the surgical site exposed. *Comments:*	☐	☐	☐	

Checklist for Procedure 4-22   Administering Immediate Postoperative Care

Name _____ Date _____

School _____

Instructor _____

Course _____

Procedure 4-22 **Administering Immediate Postoperative Care**	Able to Perform	Able to Perform with Assistance	Unable to Perform	Initials and Date
Assessment				
1. Assess the client's sedation level and mental status. *Comments:*	☐	☐	☐	
2. Assess the client's cardiovascular status. *Comments:*	☐	☐	☐	
3. Assess the client's respiratory status. *Comments:*	☐	☐	☐	
4. Assess the client's level of pain. *Comments:*	☐	☐	☐	
5. Assess the surgical site and surgical appliances. *Comments:*	☐	☐	☐	
6. Assess the client's fluid status. *Comments:*	☐	☐	☐	
7. Assess the neurovascular status of the client's extremities. *Comments:*	☐	☐	☐	
Planning/Expected Outcomes				
1. The client's airway will be patent. *Comments:*	☐	☐	☐	
2. The client's vital signs will be stable for at least one hour. *Comments:*	☐	☐	☐	
3. The client will be alert and oriented when stimulated. *Comments:*	☐	☐	☐	
4. The client's respiratory status will be adequate. *Comments:*	☐	☐	☐	

continued on the following page

continued from the previous page

Procedure 4-22	Able to Perform	Able to Perform with Assistance	Unable to Perform	Initials and Date
5. The client's pain control will be adequate. *Comments:*	☐	☐	☐	
6. With regional anesthesia, motor and sensory function will be at an adequate level. *Comments:*	☐	☐	☐	
7. The client's surgical site will be intact with an appropriate dressing. *Comments:*	☐	☐	☐	
8. The client's intravenous access will be intact and patent. *Comments:*	☐	☐	☐	
9. The client's output will be within normal limits. *Comments:*	☐	☐	☐	
10. The client's temperature will be within normal limits. *Comments:*	☐	☐	☐	
Implementation				
1. Wash hands; apply gloves. *Comments:*	☐	☐	☐	
2. Check the client's vital signs upon the client's arrival in the unit. *Comments:*	☐	☐	☐	
3. Identify client via armband and verify the client's identity with the chart. *Comments:*	☐	☐	☐	
4. Inform the client that he is out of the operating room and in the recovery room. *Comments:*	☐	☐	☐	
5. Attach bedside electrocardiogram (EKG) leads to the client and run a baseline EKG strip. *Comments:*	☐	☐	☐	

Procedure 4-22	Able to Perform	Able to Perform with Assistance	Unable to Perform	Initials and Date
6. Attach the oximeter to the client. *Comments:*	☐	☐	☐	
7. Check intravenous (IV) site, solution, and flow rate. *Comments:*	☐	☐	☐	
8. Check surgical dressing and site. *Comments:*	☐	☐	☐	
9. Complete a total head to toe assessment. Airway: • Check the patency of the client's airway. • Assess for the presence of equal breath sounds. • Note the presence of adventitious sounds. Respiratory: • Note the presence of any supplemental oxygen. • Assess the client's blood oxygen saturation and respirations. Cardiovascular: • Check pulses, especially those distal to the surgical site. • Note the color, temperature, and capillary refill of extremities. • Note cardiac rate, rhythm, blood pressure, and any indications of bleeding. Temperature: • Check the client's core temperature. Neurological: • Assess the client's level of awareness, equality of pupils, verbal response, and equality of movement and feeling. Gastrointestinal: • Evaluate for the presence of nausea or vomiting. Observe function and patency of nasogastric (NG) tube, if present. • Assess gastric secretions for color and amount. Genitourinary: • Evaluate the amount and color of the client's urinary output. • Assess that the catheter is draining appropriately. Pain: • Assess the client's level of pain and treat as appropriate. • Assess other means of controlling pain, such as repositioning. Fluid balance: • Evaluate the client's fluid status. • Check for peripheral edema or jugular venous distention. Vital signs: • Reevaluate the client's vital signs and status as needed, at least every 15 minutes. *Comments:*	☐	☐	☐	

continued on the following page

continued from the previous page

Procedure 4-22	Able to Perform	Able to Perform with Assistance	Unable to Perform	Initials and Date
10. Encourage the client to deep breathe, cough, and use the incentive spirometer. *Comments:*	☐	☐	☐	
11. Check and implement postoperative orders. *Comments:*	☐	☐	☐	
12. Inform the client's family or significant other that the client is in the recovery room. *Comments:*	☐	☐	☐	
13. Turn the client every hour, maintaining proper alignment. *Comments:*	☐	☐	☐	
14. Upon discharge by the postanesthesia caregiver, a full report should be given to the nurse assuming care of the client. *Comments:*	☐	☐	☐	
15. Remove gloves and wash hands. *Comments:*	☐	☐	☐	

Checklist for Procedure 4-23   Postoperative Exercise Instruction

Name _____ Date _____

School _____

Instructor _____

Course _____

Procedure 4-23 **Postoperative Exercise Instruction**	Able to Perform	Able to Perform with Assistance	Unable to Perform	Initials and Date
Assessment				
1. Assess the client's current understanding of postoperative procedures. *Comments:*	☐	☐	☐	
2. Assess the client's ability to understand the postoperative exercise instructions. *Comments:*	☐	☐	☐	
3. Assess client limitations that would prevent or impair the performance of postoperative exercises. *Comments:*	☐	☐	☐	
Planning/Expected Outcomes				
1. The client will be able to successfully demonstrate postoperative exercises and out-of-bed transfers. *Comments:*	☐	☐	☐	
2. The client will be able to successfully demonstrate proper use of the incentive spirometer. *Comments:*	☐	☐	☐	
Implementation				
1. Wash hands and organize equipment. *Comments:*	☐	☐	☐	
2. Check the client's identification band. *Comments:*	☐	☐	☐	
3. Apply gloves. *Comments:*	☐	☐	☐	
4. Place client in a sitting position. *Comments:*	☐	☐	☐	

continued on the following page

continued from the previous page

Procedure 4-23	Able to Perform	Able to Perform with Assistance	Unable to Perform	Initials and Date
5. Demonstrate deep breathing exercises. • Place one hand on abdomen during inhalation. • Expand the abdomen and rib cage on inspiration. • Inhale slowly and evenly through your nose. • Hold breath for 2–3 seconds. • Slowly exhale through your mouth. *Comments:*	☐	☐	☐	
6. Have the client return demonstrate the deep breathing exercises. *Comments:*	☐	☐	☐	
7. Have the client repeat the exercise 3–4 times. *Comments:*	☐	☐	☐	
8. Instruct the client on the use of an incentive spirometer. • Hold the volume-oriented spirometer upright. • Exhale, seal lips tightly around the mouthpiece; take a slow deep breath to elevate the balls in the plastic tube, hold the inspiration for at least 3 seconds. • The client measures the amount of inspired air volume. • Remove the mouthpiece and exhale normally. • Take several normal breaths. *Comments:*	☐	☐	☐	
9. Have the client repeat the procedure 4–5 times. *Comments:*	☐	☐	☐	
10. Have the client cough after the incentive effort. *Comments:*	☐	☐	☐	
11. Demonstrate splinting and coughing. • Have the client slowly raise head and sniff the air. • Have the client bend forward and exhale slowly through pursed lips. • Repeat breathing 2–3 times. • When the client is ready to cough, place a folded pillow against the abdomen held with clasped hands. • Have client take a deep breath and begin coughing immediately after inspiration is completed. • Have a tissue ready. *Comments:*	☐	☐	☐	
12. Have the client return demonstrate splinting and coughing. *Comments:*	☐	☐	☐	

Procedure 4-23	Able to Perform	Able to Perform with Assistance	Unable to Perform	Initials and Date
13. Wash the incentive spirometer mouthpiece and store in a clean container. Change disposable mouthpieces every 24 hours. *Comments:*	☐	☐	☐	
14. Teach the client leg and foot exercises. • With heels on bed, push toes of both feet toward the foot of the bed until the calf muscles tighten, then relax feet. Pull the toes toward the chin until calf muscles tighten; then relax feet. • With heels on bed, lift and circle both ankles, first to the right and then to the left; repeat three times, relax. • Flex and extend each knee alternately, sliding foot up along the bed; relax. *Comments:*	☐	☐	☐	
15. Have the client return demonstrate the leg and foot exercises. *Comments:*	☐	☐	☐	
16. Explain how to turn in bed and get out of bed. *Comments:*	☐	☐	☐	
17. Clients with a left-sided abdominal or chest incision should turn to the right side of bed and sit up as follows: • Flex the knees. • With the right hand, splint the incision with hand or small pillow. • Turn toward right side by pushing with the left foot and grasping the nurse or side rail of the bed with the left hand. • Sit up on the side of the bed using the left arm and hand to push down against the mattress or side rail. *Comments:*	☐	☐	☐	
18. Reverse instructions in Action 17 for the client with a right-sided incision. *Comments:*	☐	☐	☐	
19. Instruct clients who have had orthopedic surgery how to use an overhead trapeze. *Comments:*	☐	☐	☐	
20. Wash hands. *Comments:*	☐	☐	☐	

Checklist for Procedure 4-24   Administering Passive Range of Motion (ROM) Exercises

Name _____ Date _____

School _____

Instructor _____

Course _____

Procedure 4-24 Administering Passive Range of Motion (ROM) Exercises	Able to Perform	Able to Perform with Assistance	Unable to Perform	Initials and Date
Assessment				
1. Be aware of the client's medical diagnosis. *Comments:*	☐	☐	☐	
2. Familiarize yourself with the client's current range of motion. *Comments:*	☐	☐	☐	
3. Assess client consciousness and cognitive function. *Comments:*	☐	☐	☐	
Planning/Expected Outcomes				
1. Client will maintain or improve current functional mobility. *Comments:*	☐	☐	☐	
2. Client will regain or improve strength and movement in involved areas. *Comments:*	☐	☐	☐	
3. Client will avoid complications of immobility. *Comments:*	☐	☐	☐	
Implementation				
1. Wash hands and wear gloves. *Comments:*	☐	☐	☐	
2. Explain procedure to client. *Comments:*	☐	☐	☐	
3. Provide for privacy, exposing only the extremity to be exercised. *Comments:*	☐	☐	☐	

continued on the following page

continued from the previous page

Procedure 4-24	Able to Perform	Able to Perform with Assistance	Unable to Perform	Initials and Date
4. Adjust bed to comfortable height for performing ROM. *Comments:*	☐	☐	☐	
5. Lower bed rail only on the side you are working. *Comments:*	☐	☐	☐	
6. Start at the client's head and perform ROM exercises down each side of the body. *Comments:*	☐	☐	☐	
7. Repeat each ROM exercise as the client tolerates to a maximum of five times. *Comments:*	☐	☐	☐	
8. Describe the passive ROM exercises you are performing. *Comments:*	☐	☐	☐	
9. Head With the client in a sitting position, if possible. • Rotation: Turn the head from side to side. • Flexion and extension: Tilt the head toward the chest and then slightly upward. • Lateral flexion: Tilt the head on each side so as to almost touch the ear to the shoulder. *Comments:*	☐	☐	☐	
10. Neck With the client in a sitting position, if possible. • Rotation: Rotate the neck in a semicircle while supporting the head. *Comments:*	☐	☐	☐	
11. Trunk With the client in a sitting position, if possible. • Flexion and extension: Bend the trunk forward, straighten, and then extend slightly backward. • Rotation: Turn the shoulders forward and return to normal position. • Lateral flexion: Tip trunk to the left side, straighten, tip to the right side. *Comments:*	☐	☐	☐	

Procedure 4-24	Able to Perform	Able to Perform with Assistance	Unable to Perform	Initials and Date
12. Arm • Flexion and extension: Extend a straight arm upward toward the head, then downward along the side. • Adduction and abduction: Extend a straight arm toward the midline and away from the midline. *Comments:*	☐	☐	☐	
13. Shoulder • Internal and external rotation: Bend the elbow at a 90° angle with upper arm parallel to the shoulder. Move the lower arm upward and downward. *Comments:*	☐	☐	☐	
14. Elbow • Flexion and extension: Supporting the arm, flex and extend the elbow. • Pronation and supination: Flex elbow, move the hand in a palm-up and palm-down position. *Comments:*	☐	☐	☐	
15. Wrist • Flexion and extension: Supporting the wrist, flex and extend the wrist. • Adduction and abduction: Supporting the lower arm, turn wrist right to left, left to right, then rotate the wrist in a circular motion. *Comments:*	☐	☐	☐	
16. Hand • Flexion and extension: Support the wrist, flex and extend the fingers. • Adduction and abduction: Support the wrist, spread fingers apart and then bring them close together. • Opposition: Supporting the wrist, touch each finger with the tip of the thumb. • Thumb rotation: Support the wrist, rotate the thumb in a circular manner. *Comments:*	☐	☐	☐	
17. Hip and leg With the client in a supine position, if possible. • Flexion and extension: Support the lower leg, flex the leg toward the chest and then extend the leg. • Internal and external rotation: Support the lower leg, angle the foot inward and outward. • Adduction and abduction: Slide the leg away from the client's midline and then back to the midline. *Comments:*	☐	☐	☐	

continued on the following page

continued from the previous page

Procedure 4-24	Able to Perform	Able to Perform with Assistance	Unable to Perform	Initials and Date
18. Knee • Flexion and extension: Support the lower leg, flex and extend the knee. *Comments:*	☐	☐	☐	
19. Ankle • Flexion and extension: Support the lower leg, flex and extend the ankle. *Comments:*	☐	☐	☐	
20. Foot • Adduction and abduction: Support the ankle, spread the toes apart and then bring them close together. • Flexion and extension: Support the ankle, extend the toes upward and then flex the toes downward. *Comments:*	☐	☐	☐	
21. Observe client for signs of exertion, pain, or fatigue. *Comments:*	☐	☐	☐	
22. Replace covers and position client in proper body alignment. *Comments:*	☐	☐	☐	
23. Place side rails in original position. *Comments:*	☐	☐	☐	
24. Place call light within reach. *Comments:*	☐	☐	☐	
25. Wash hands. *Comments:*	☐	☐	☐	

Checklist for Procedure 4-25 Postmortem Care

Name _____ Date _____

School _____

Instructor _____

Course _____

Procedure 4-25 Postmortem Care	Able to Perform	Able to Perform with Assistance	Unable to Perform	Initials and Date
Assessment				
1. Verify that respiration and heart activity have ceased and that the physician has pronounced death. *Comments:*	☐	☐	☐	
2. Assess the family's response to the news of the client's death. *Comments:*	☐	☐	☐	
3. If not already known or required, ask the family's preference for an autopsy. *Comments:*	☐	☐	☐	
4. Follow hospital policy regarding seeking permission for organ donation. *Comments:*	☐	☐	☐	
Planning/Expected Outcomes				
1. Next of kin will be informed of the client's death and offered the option to visit the deceased. *Comments:*	☐	☐	☐	
2. The client will be bathed and prepared for the morgue. *Comments:*	☐	☐	☐	
3. The client's body alignment will be maintained during family visitation. *Comments:*	☐	☐	☐	
4. The family will experience no undue emotional shock or trauma from debris, blood, or tubes protruding from the body. *Comments:*	☐	☐	☐	

continued on the following page

continued from the previous page

Procedure 4-25	Able to Perform	Able to Perform with Assistance	Unable to Perform	Initials and Date
Implementation				
1. Close the drapes and/or door. Allow the family to stay if desired. *Comments:*	☐	☐	☐	
2. Have physician and/or other qualified person pronounce the client's death. *Comments:*	☐	☐	☐	
3. Notify all departments that need to know of the client's death. *Comments:*	☐	☐	☐	
4. Wash hands and apply gloves and other protective equipment. *Comments:*	☐	☐	☐	
5. Bathe the body. Put a gown on the client, and clean the immediate environment. *Comments:*	☐	☐	☐	
6. Follow the institution's policy about removing or inserting prostheses. *Comments:*	☐	☐	☐	
7. Gently close the client's eyes, if open. *Comments:*	☐	☐	☐	
8. Allow family and friends of the deceased time to view the body, if desired. *Comments:*	☐	☐	☐	
9. Inventory the client's belongings. *Comments:*	☐	☐	☐	
10. Send the client's belongings home with the family if possible. Document the name of the person who received the items. *Comments:*	☐	☐	☐	

Procedure 4-25	Able to Perform	Able to Perform with Assistance	Unable to Perform	Initials and Date
11. Place identifying tags on the deceased. *Comments:*	☐	☐	☐	
12. Wrap the body in a sheet or shroud. *Comments:*	☐	☐	☐	
13. Transfer the body to the stretcher or morgue cart. *Comments:*	☐	☐	☐	
14. Arrange for transportation to the morgue. *Comments:*	☐	☐	☐	
15. Leave the morgue cart in the room until ready to transport. *Comments:*	☐	☐	☐	
16. Document the time of death and disposition of the body and personal effects. *Comments:*	☐	☐	☐	
17. Wash hands. *Comments:*	☐	☐	☐	

Checklist for Procedure 5-1   Administering Oral, Sublingual, and Buccal Medications

Name _____ Date _____

School _____

Instructor _____

Course _____

Procedure 5-1 Administering Oral, Sublingual, and Buccal Medications	Able to Perform	Able to Perform with Assistance	Unable to Perform	Initials and Date
Assessment				
1. Assess five rights: right client, right medication, right route, right dose, and right time. *Comments:*	☐	☐	☐	
2. Review the action, purpose, normal dosage and route, common side effects, time of onset and peak action, and nursing implications of each drug. *Comments:*	☐	☐	☐	
3. Assess the client's condition and the written order. *Comments:*	☐	☐	☐	
4. Assess the client's ability to swallow food and fluid. *Comments:*	☐	☐	☐	
5. Assess for any contraindications for oral medication. *Comments:*	☐	☐	☐	
6. Assess the client's medical record for allergies. *Comments:*	☐	☐	☐	
7. Assess the client's knowledge about the use of medications. *Comments:*	☐	☐	☐	
8. Assess the client's age. *Comments:*	☐	☐	☐	
9. Assess the client's need for fluids. *Comments:*	☐	☐	☐	
10. Assess the client's ability to sit or turn to the side. *Comments:*	☐	☐	☐	

continued on the following page

continued from the previous page

Procedure 5-1	Able to Perform	Able to Perform with Assistance	Unable to Perform	Initials and Date
Planning/Expected Outcomes				
1. The client will swallow the prescribed medication. *Comments:*	☐	☐	☐	
2. The client will understand the medication's purpose and schedule. *Comments:*	☐	☐	☐	
3. The client will have no discomfort or alterations in function. *Comments:*	☐	☐	☐	
4. The client will show the desired response to the medication. *Comments:*	☐	☐	☐	
Implementation				
1. Wash hands and put on clean gloves. *Comments:*	☐	☐	☐	
2. Arrange the medication tray and cups. *Comments:*	☐	☐	☐	
3. Unlock the medication cart or log on to the computer. *Comments:*	☐	☐	☐	
4. Prepare medication for one client at a time using the five rights. *Comments:*	☐	☐	☐	
5. To prepare a tablet or capsule: • Pour into the medication cup without touching it. • Scored tablets may be broken or crushed. • Do not open unit-dose tablets. *Comments:*	☐	☐	☐	
6. To prepare a liquid medication: • Remove the bottle cap and place cap upside down. • Pour medication at eye level to the desired dose. *Comments:*	☐	☐	☐	
7. To prepare a narcotic, obtain the key and sign out the dose. *Comments:*	☐	☐	☐	

Procedure 5-1	Able to Perform	Able to Perform with Assistance	Unable to Perform	Initials and Date
8. Check expiration date on all medications. • Double-check the medication administration record (MAR) with the prepared drugs and place with the client's medications. • Return stock medications to their shelf or drawer. *Comments:*	☐	☐	☐	
9. Administer medications to client: • Observe the correct time to give the medication. • Identify the client. • Check to ensure that this is the correct medication type and dosage. • Assess suitability of the form of the medication. • Perform any assessment required for specific medications. • Explain the purpose of the drug and answer any questions. • Assist the client to a sitting or lateral position. • Allow client to hold the tablet or medication cup. • Give a glass of liquid, and straw if needed. • For *sublingual* medications, instruct client to dissolve medication under the tongue. • For *buccal* medications, instruct the client to dissolve medication in the mouth against the cheek. • For medications given through a *nasogastric tube,* crush tablets or open capsules and dissolve with warm water. • Remain with the client until each medication has been swallowed or dissolved. • Assist the client into a comfortable position. *Comments:*	☐	☐	☐	
10. Dispose of soiled supplies and wash hands. *Comments:*	☐	☐	☐	
11. Record the time and route on the MAR. *Comments:*	☐	☐	☐	
12. Return the cart; clean and restock as needed. *Comments:*	☐	☐	☐	

Checklist for Procedure 5-2   Administering Eye and Ear Medications

Name _____ Date _____

School _____

Instructor _____

Course _____

Procedure 5-2 Administering Eye and Ear Medications	Able to Perform	Able to Perform with Assistance	Unable to Perform	Initials and Date
Assessment				
1. Assess the five rights: right client, right medication, right route, right dose, and right time. *Comments:*	☐	☐	☐	
2. Assess the condition of the client's eyes and/or ears. *Comments:*	☐	☐	☐	
3. Assess the medication order. *Comments:*	☐	☐	☐	
Planning/Expected Outcomes				
1. The client will receive the medication according to the five rights. *Comments:*	☐	☐	☐	
2. The client will encounter the minimum of discomfort. *Comments:*	☐	☐	☐	
3. The client will receive maximum benefit from the medication. *Comments:*	☐	☐	☐	
Implementation				
Eye Medication 1. Check for allergies or other contraindications. *Comments:*	☐	☐	☐	
2. Gather the necessary equipment. *Comments:*	☐	☐	☐	
3. Follow the five rights of drug administration. *Comments:*	☐	☐	☐	

continued on the following page

continued from the previous page

Procedure 5-2	Able to Perform	Able to Perform with Assistance	Unable to Perform	Initials and Date
4. Place the medication on a clean surface in the client's room. *Comments:*	☐	☐	☐	
5. Check client's identification armband. *Comments:*	☐	☐	☐	
6. Explain the procedure; assist the client as needed. *Comments:*	☐	☐	☐	
7. Wash hands. Apply nonsterile gloves if needed. *Comments:*	☐	☐	☐	
8. Place client in a supine position with the head slightly hyperextended. *Comments:*	☐	☐	☐	
Instilling Eyedrops 9. Remove cap from bottle and place cap on its side. *Comments:*	☐	☐	☐	
10. Squeeze the prescribed dose of medication into the eyedropper. *Comments:*	☐	☐	☐	
11. Place a tissue below the lower lid. *Comments:*	☐	☐	☐	
12. With dominant hand, hold eyedropper one-half to three-quarters of an inch above the eyeball; rest hand on client's forehead to stabilize. *Comments:*	☐	☐	☐	
13. Place hand on cheekbone and expose lower conjunctival sac by pulling down on cheek. *Comments:*	☐	☐	☐	
14. Instruct the client to look up and drop the prescribed number of drops into center of conjuctival sac. *Comments:*	☐	☐	☐	

Procedure 5-2	Able to Perform	Able to Perform with Assistance	Unable to Perform	Initials and Date
15. While client closes and moves eyes, place fingers on either side of the client's nose. *Comments:*	☐	☐	☐	
16. Remove gloves; wash hands. *Comments:*	☐	☐	☐	
17. Record route, site, and time on the MAR. *Comments:*	☐	☐	☐	
Eye Ointment Application 18. Repeat Actions 1–8. *Comments:*	☐	☐	☐	
Lower Lid 19. • With nondominant hand, gently separate client's eyelids with thumb and finger and grasp lower lid near margin immediately below the lashes; exert pressure downward over the bony prominence of the cheek. • Instruct the client to look up. • Apply eye ointment along inside edge of the lower eyelid. *Comments:*	☐	☐	☐	
Upper Lid 20. • Instruct client to look down. • Grasp lashes near center of upper lid and draw lid up and away from eyeball. • Squeeze ointment along upper lid starting at inner canthus. *Comments:*	☐	☐	☐	
21. Repeat Actions 16 and 17. *Comments:*	☐	☐	☐	
Medication Disk 22. Repeat Actions 1–8. *Comments:*	☐	☐	☐	
23. Open package and press sterile gloved finger against the disk. *Comments:*	☐	☐	☐	

continued on the following page

continued from the previous page

Procedure 5-2	Able to Perform	Able to Perform with Assistance	Unable to Perform	Initials and Date
24. Instruct the client to look up. *Comments:*	☐	☐	☐	
25. Pull the client's lower eyelid down and place the disk horizontally in the conjunctival sac. • Pull the lower eyelid out, up, and over the disk. • Instruct the client to blink several times. • If disk is still visible, repeat steps. • Instruct the client to press the fingers against the closed lids. • If the disk falls out, rinse it under cool water and reinsert. *Comments:*	☐	☐	☐	
26. If the disk is prescribed for both eyes, repeat Actions 23–25. *Comments:*	☐	☐	☐	
27. Repeat Actions 16 and 17. *Comments:*	☐	☐	☐	
Removing an Eye Medication Disk 28. Repeat Actions 3 and 5–8. *Comments:*	☐	☐	☐	
29. Remove the disk: • Invert the lower eyelid and identify the disk. • If in the upper eye, stroke the client's closed eyelid to move the disk to the corner of eye. • Slide the disk onto the lower eyelid and out of the client's eye. *Comments:*	☐	☐	☐	
30. Remove gloves; wash hands. *Comments:*	☐	☐	☐	
31. Record on the MAR the removal of the disk. *Comments:*	☐	☐	☐	
Ear Medication 1. Check with client and chart for any known allergies. *Comments:*	☐	☐	☐	

Procedure 5-2	Able to Perform	Able to Perform with Assistance	Unable to Perform	Initials and Date
2. Check the MAR against the written orders. *Comments:*	☐	☐	☐	
3. Wash hands. *Comments:*	☐	☐	☐	
4. Calculate the dose. *Comments:*	☐	☐	☐	
5. Use the identification armband to properly identify the client. *Comments:*	☐	☐	☐	
6. Explain the procedure to the client. *Comments:*	☐	☐	☐	
7. Place the client in a side-lying position with the affected ear facing up. *Comments:*	☐	☐	☐	
8. Straighten the ear canal by pulling the pinna down and back for children less than 3 years of age or upward and outward in adults and older children. *Comments:*	☐	☐	☐	
9. Instill the drops into the ear canal by holding the dropper at least one-half inch above the ear canal. *Comments:*	☐	☐	☐	
10. Ask the client to maintain the position for 2–3 minutes. *Comments:*	☐	☐	☐	
11. Place a cotton ball on the outermost part of the canal. *Comments:*	☐	☐	☐	
12. Wash hands. *Comments:*	☐	☐	☐	
13. Document the drug, amount, time, and ear medicated. *Comments:*	☐	☐	☐	

Checklist for Procedure 5-3 Administering Skin/Topical Medications

Name _____ Date _____

School _____

Instructor _____

Course _____

Procedure 5-3 Administering Skin/Topical Medications	Able to Perform	Able to Perform with Assistance	Unable to Perform	Initials and Date
Assessment				
1. Assess the five rights: right client, right medication, right route, right dose, and right time. *Comments:*	☐	☐	☐	
2. Assess the baseline condition of the area of application. *Comments:*	☐	☐	☐	
3. If drug is for systemic effect, assess area for skin aberrations. *Comments:*	☐	☐	☐	
Planning/Expected Outcomes				
1. Good skin integrity. *Comments:*	☐	☐	☐	
2. Relief of itching, irritation, or pain. *Comments:*	☐	☐	☐	
3. Improved circulation. *Comments:*	☐	☐	☐	
Implementation				
1. Wash hands. *Comments:*	☐	☐	☐	
2. Obtain order for medication. *Comments:*	☐	☐	☐	
3. Ascertain client's allergic status. *Comments:*	☐	☐	☐	
4. If unfamiliar with medication, seek appropriate information. *Comments:*	☐	☐	☐	

continued on the following page

continued from the previous page

Procedure 5-3	Able to Perform	Able to Perform with Assistance	Unable to Perform	Initials and Date
5. Select and verify medication with orders. *Comments:*	☐	☐	☐	
6. Check expiration date. *Comments:*	☐	☐	☐	
7. Read medication label again. *Comments:*	☐	☐	☐	
8. Take medication to client's room and introduce yourself. *Comments:*	☐	☐	☐	
9. Ask if the client has any drug allergies or had any previous reactions. *Comments:*	☐	☐	☐	
10. Explain the purpose of the medication. *Comments:*	☐	☐	☐	
11. Read the label for the third time and check the client's identification band. *Comments:*	☐	☐	☐	
12. Position the client appropriately for administration of medication. *Comments:*	☐	☐	☐	
13. Put on gloves. *Comments:*	☐	☐	☐	
14. Clean the skin surface thoroughly and pat skin dry. *Comments:*	☐	☐	☐	
15. Assess the client's skin condition. *Comments:*	☐	☐	☐	
16. Change gloves. *Comments:*	☐	☐	☐	

Procedure 5-3	Able to Perform	Able to Perform with Assistance	Unable to Perform	Initials and Date
17. Apply medication according to label or orders. *Comments:*	☐	☐	☐	
18. If an aerosol spray is used, shake the container and administer according to directions. *Comments:*	☐	☐	☐	
19. If gels or pastes are used, applicators may be needed. Apply evenly. *Comments:*	☐	☐	☐	
20. If powders are used, dust lightly and avoid inhalation. *Comments:*	☐	☐	☐	
21. If nitroglycerin ointment or paste is used: • Remove the old ointment strip and clean the old site. • Cleanse the new site. • Squeeze the dose out onto the enclosed measuring strip. • Flatten the roll of ointment to spread it over a wider area. • Apply the measuring paper, ointment side down, to a nonhairy portion of the client's body. • Tape the paper in place. *Comments:*	☐	☐	☐	
22. If a transdermal patch is used: • Remove the old patch and wash the site of the old patch. • Wash and prepare the skin at a new site. • Remove the protective covering and apply. *Comments:*	☐	☐	☐	
23. Remove gloves; wash hands. *Comments:*	☐	☐	☐	
24. Chart the medication, site, and the client's response. *Comments:*	☐	☐	☐	

Checklist for Procedure 5-4   Administering Nasal Medications

Name _____ Date _____

School _____

Instructor _____

Course _____

Procedure 5-4 **Administering Nasal Medications**	Able to Perform	Able to Perform with Assistance	Unable to Perform	Initials and Date
Assessment				
1. Assess the five rights: right client, right medication, right route, right dose, and right time. *Comments:*	☐	☐	☐	
2. Assess the client's nasal congestion and nasal obstruction. *Comments:*	☐	☐	☐	
3. Assess the client's discharge and nasal mucosa. *Comments:*	☐	☐	☐	
4. Assess the client's pain and/or discomfort level in the sinuses. *Comments:*	☐	☐	☐	
5. Assess the client for adverse systemic conditions. *Comments:*	☐	☐	☐	
Planning/Expected Outcomes				
1. The client will be free of nasal congestion. *Comments:*	☐	☐	☐	
2. The client will be free of nasal discharge and odor. *Comments:*	☐	☐	☐	
3. The client will breathe freely through the nasal passages. *Comments:*	☐	☐	☐	
4. The client will be free of sinus pain and nasal pain. *Comments:*	☐	☐	☐	
5. The client's nasal passages will be moist and pink. *Comments:*	☐	☐	☐	

continued on the following page

continued from the previous page

Procedure 5-4	Able to Perform	Able to Perform with Assistance	Unable to Perform	Initials and Date
Implementation				
1. Wash hands. Wear a mask if needed. *Comments:*	☐	☐	☐	
2. Explain the purpose of the medication and the desired head position. *Comments:*	☐	☐	☐	
3. Explain the sensation of the medications. *Comments:*	☐	☐	☐	
4. If a nasal inhaler is used, explain how inhalers work. Follow the five rights. *Comments:*	☐	☐	☐	
5. Have the client blow nose and assume desired position. Squeeze nose drops into dropper. *Comments:*	☐	☐	☐	
6. Have the client exhale and close one nostril. *Comments:*	☐	☐	☐	
7. Have client inhale while medication is sprayed into the first nostril. If drops are used, insert dropper and instill the prescribed dosage. *Comments:*	☐	☐	☐	
8. Ask client to blot excess drainage; do not blow nose. *Comments:*	☐	☐	☐	
9. Repeat the procedure on the other nostril. *Comments:*	☐	☐	☐	
10. Help the client resume a comfortable position. If nose drops are used, have client maintain a therapeutic position. *Comments:*	☐	☐	☐	
11. Dispose of soiled articles appropriately. Wash hands. *Comments:*	☐	☐	☐	
12. Evaluate the effect of the medication in 15–20 minutes. *Comments:*	☐	☐	☐	

Checklist for Procedure 5-5   Administering Rectal Medications

Name _____ Date _____

School _____

Instructor _____

Course _____

Procedure 5-5 **Administering Rectal Medications**	Able to Perform	Able to Perform with Assistance	Unable to Perform	Initials and Date
Assessment				
1. Assess the five rights: right client, right medication, right route, right dose, and right time. *Comments:*	☐	☐	☐	
2. Review the order and identify the medication to be delivered. *Comments:*	☐	☐	☐	
3. Assess the client's need for rectal medication administration. *Comments:*	☐	☐	☐	
4. Consider any adjustments needed due to the age of the client. *Comments:*	☐	☐	☐	
5. Observe for the desired effects or any adverse reactions. *Comments:*	☐	☐	☐	
6. Assess the client's understanding of the procedure. *Comments:*	☐	☐	☐	
Planning/Expected Outcomes				
1. The medication will be delivered appropriately and safely. *Comments:*	☐	☐	☐	
2. The desired outcome will be verbalized by the client and documented by the nurse. *Comments:*	☐	☐	☐	
3. The treatment will be completed quickly and efficiently. *Comments:*	☐	☐	☐	

continued on the following page

continued from the previous page

Procedure 5-5	Able to Perform	Able to Perform with Assistance	Unable to Perform	Initials and Date
4. Client will state relief of complaint. *Comments:*	☐	☐	☐	

Implementation

	Able to Perform	Able to Perform with Assistance	Unable to Perform	Initials and Date
1. Assess the client's need for the medication. *Comments:*	☐	☐	☐	
2. Check physician or qualified practitioner's written order. *Comments:*	☐	☐	☐	
3. Check the MAR against the medication order. *Comments:*	☐	☐	☐	
4. Check for any drug allergies. *Comments:*	☐	☐	☐	
5. Review the client's history for surgeries or bleeding. *Comments:*	☐	☐	☐	
6. Gather the equipment needed before entering the room. *Comments:*	☐	☐	☐	
7. Assess the client's readiness. Provide privacy. *Comments:*	☐	☐	☐	
8. Wash hands. *Comments:*	☐	☐	☐	
9. Apply disposable gloves. *Comments:*	☐	☐	☐	
10. Ask the client's name and check identification band. *Comments:*	☐	☐	☐	
11. Assist client into correct position. *Comments:*	☐	☐	☐	
12. Visually assess the client's external anus. *Comments:*	☐	☐	☐	

Procedure 5-5	Able to Perform	Able to Perform with Assistance	Unable to Perform	Initials and Date
13. Lubricate the enema tip or remove suppository from wrapper and lubricate. *Comments:*	☐	☐	☐	
14. Explain that client will experience a cool sensation and pressure. *Comments:*	☐	☐	☐	
15. Retract buttocks, visualizing the anus. • Gently insert the suppository through the anus. • Insert the enema tip and instill the contents. *Comments:*	☐	☐	☐	
16. Remove finger or enema tip and clean client's anal area. *Comments:*	☐	☐	☐	
17. Discard gloves. *Comments:*	☐	☐	☐	
18. Wash hands. *Comments:*	☐	☐	☐	
19. Have client remain in bed or on side for 10 minutes. *Comments:*	☐	☐	☐	
20. Place call light within reach. *Comments:*	☐	☐	☐	
21. Record administration of medication. *Comments:*	☐	☐	☐	
22. Document effectiveness or any side effects of treatment. *Comments:*	☐	☐	☐	

Checklist for Procedure 5-6 Administering Vaginal Medications

Name _____ Date _____

School _____

Instructor _____

Course _____

Procedure 5-6 Administering Vaginal Medications	Able to Perform	Able to Perform with Assistance	Unable to Perform	Initials and Date
Assessment				
1. Assess the client's comfort level and symptoms. *Comments:*	☐	☐	☐	
2. Assess the client's knowledge of the purpose of the treatment. *Comments:*	☐	☐	☐	
3. Assess the client's ability to self-administer the medication. *Comments:*	☐	☐	☐	
Planning/Expected Outcomes				
1. Client will experience an absence of infection. *Comments:*	☐	☐	☐	
2. Client will experience an absence of symptoms. *Comments:*	☐	☐	☐	
3. Client will understand the need to perform the entire course of treatment. *Comments:*	☐	☐	☐	
4. Client will understand the importance of personal hygiene. *Comments:*	☐	☐	☐	
5. Client will understand the need to clean and store equipment. *Comments:*	☐	☐	☐	
Implementation				
1. Verify orders. *Comments:*	☐	☐	☐	

continued on the following page

continued from the previous page

Procedure 5-6	Able to Perform	Able to Perform with Assistance	Unable to Perform	Initials and Date
2. Ascertain that the client understands the procedure. *Comments:*	☐	☐	☐	
3. Ask the client to void. *Comments:*	☐	☐	☐	
4. Wash hands. *Comments:*	☐	☐	☐	
5. Arrange equipment at client's bedside. *Comments:*	☐	☐	☐	
6. Provide privacy. *Comments:*	☐	☐	☐	
7. Assist the client into a dorsal-recumbent or Sim's position. *Comments:*	☐	☐	☐	
8. Drape the client as appropriate. *Comments:*	☐	☐	☐	
9. Position lighting to illuminate vaginal orifice. *Comments:*	☐	☐	☐	
10. Assess the perineal area. *Comments:*	☐	☐	☐	
11. • If using an applicator, fill with medication. • If using a suppository, remove the suppository from the foil and position in the applicator. • Apply water-soluble lubricant to suppository or applicator. *Comments:*	☐	☐	☐	
12. For suppository, retract the labia. *Comments:*	☐	☐	☐	
13. Insert applicator 2–3 inches into the vagina. Push the plunger to administer the medication. Insert the suppository, tapered end first, along the posterior wall of the vagina. *Comments:*	☐	☐	☐	

Procedure 5-6	Able to Perform	Able to Perform with Assistance	Unable to Perform	Initials and Date
14. Withdraw the applicator and place on a towel. *Comments:*	☐	☐	☐	
15. If administering a douche or irrigation: • Warm solution to slightly above body temperature. • Position the client on a bedpan, toilet seat, or in a tub. • Apply lubricant to the irrigation nozzle and insert into the vagina. • Hang the irrigant container approximately 2 feet above the vaginal area. • Open the clamp and allow a small amount of solution to flow into the vagina. • Move the nozzle and rotate around the entire vaginal area. *Comments:*	☐	☐	☐	
16. Wipe and clean the client's perineal area. *Comments:*	☐	☐	☐	
17. Apply a perineal pad. *Comments:*	☐	☐	☐	
18. Wash and store the applicator. *Comments:*	☐	☐	☐	
19. Remove gloves and wash hands. *Comments:*	☐	☐	☐	
20. Instruct the client to remain flat for at least 30 minutes. *Comments:*	☐	☐	☐	
21. Raise side rails and place the call light within reach. *Comments:*	☐	☐	☐	

Checklist for Procedure 5-7   Administering Nebulized Medications

Name _____ Date _____

School _____

Instructor _____

Course _____

Procedure 5-7 **Administering Nebulized Medications**	Able to Perform	Able to Perform with Assistance	Unable to Perform	Initials and Date
Assessment				
1. Assess the five rights: right client, right medication, right route, right dose, and right time. *Comments:*	☐	☐	☐	
2. Assess the client's respiratory status. *Comments:*	☐	☐	☐	
3. Evaluate the history of this episode of the client's distress. *Comments:*	☐	☐	☐	
4. Assess the client's ability to use the nebulizer or metered dose inhaler. *Comments:*	☐	☐	☐	
5. Assess the medication(s) currently ordered. *Comments:*	☐	☐	☐	
6. Assess the medications the client is currently taking. *Comments:*	☐	☐	☐	
7. Assess the client's knowledge of the medications and the delivery method. *Comments:*	☐	☐	☐	
Planning/Expected Outcomes				
1. The client will experience improved gas exchange. *Comments:*	☐	☐	☐	
2. The client's breathing pattern will become effective. *Comments:*	☐	☐	☐	
3. The client will understand the need for the medication and the delivery system. *Comments:*	☐	☐	☐	

continued on the following page

continued from the previous page

Procedure 5-7	Able to Perform	Able to Perform with Assistance	Unable to Perform	Initials and Date
4. The client will not experience any adverse effects. *Comments:*	☐	☐	☐	
5. The client's anxiety level will decrease following treatment. *Comments:*	☐	☐	☐	

Implementation

Hand-Held Nebulizer

	Able to Perform	Able to Perform with Assistance	Unable to Perform	Initials and Date
1. Assess client's ability to use the nebulizer. *Comments:*	☐	☐	☐	
2. Check the MAR against the orders. *Comments:*	☐	☐	☐	
3. Check for drug allergies and hypersensitivity. *Comments:*	☐	☐	☐	
4. Wash your hands before setting up the nebulizer. *Comments:*	☐	☐	☐	
5. Set up the medication(s) for one client at a time. *Comments:*	☐	☐	☐	
6. Look at the medication at eye level if using droppers. *Comments:*	☐	☐	☐	
7. Pour the entire amount of the drug(s) into the nebulizer cup. *Comments:*	☐	☐	☐	
8. Cover the cup with the cap and fasten. *Comments:*	☐	☐	☐	
9. Fasten the T-piece to the top of the cap. *Comments:*	☐	☐	☐	
10. Fasten a short length of tubing to one end of the T-piece. *Comments:*	☐	☐	☐	

Procedure 5-7	Able to Perform	Able to Perform with Assistance	Unable to Perform	Initials and Date
11. Fasten the mouthpiece or mask to the other end of the T-piece. *Comments:*	☐	☐	☐	
12. Identify the client prior to administration of medication(s). *Comments:*	☐	☐	☐	
13. Identify the medication(s) to the client and explain purpose(s) of the medication(s). *Comments:*	☐	☐	☐	
14. Advise the client to sit in an upright position. *Comments:*	☐	☐	☐	
15. Attach tubing to the bottom of the nebulizer cup. Attach the other end to the air outlet. • Adjust the air valve to 6 liters/min. • Leave the air on until the medication is used up. *Comments:*	☐	☐	☐	
16. Instruct the client to breathe in and out slowly and deeply with his lips sealed around the mouthpiece. *Comments:*	☐	☐	☐	
17. Observe that client is using proper technique. *Comments:*	☐	☐	☐	
18. Wash your hands with soap and water. *Comments:*	☐	☐	☐	
19. Record the date, time, medication, and dosage on the chart. *Comments:*	☐	☐	☐	
20. When the nebulizer cup is empty: • Turn off the compressor or wall air. • Detach tubing from the air and the nebulizer cup. • If disposable, dispose of the nebulizer appropriately. • If reusable, wash, rinse, and dry the nebulizer components. *Comments:*	☐	☐	☐	

continued on the following page

continued from the previous page

Procedure 5-7	Able to Perform	Able to Perform with Assistance	Unable to Perform	Initials and Date
21. Immediately following the treatment, assess for results or adverse effects. Comments:	☐	☐	☐	
22. Reassess the client 5–10 minutes following the treatment. Comments:	☐	☐	☐	
23. Wash your hands. Comments:	☐	☐	☐	
Metered-Dose Nebulizer 24. Assess the client's ability to use the metered-dose nebulizer. Comments:	☐	☐	☐	
25. Check the MAR against the orders. Comments:	☐	☐	☐	
26. Check for drug allergies and hypersensitivity. Comments:	☐	☐	☐	
27. Wash your hands. Comments:	☐	☐	☐	
28. Shake the prepackaged nebulizer. Comments:	☐	☐	☐	
29. Place the nebulizer into the applicator. Comments:	☐	☐	☐	
30. Place the aerochamber onto the nebulizer if needed. Comments:	☐	☐	☐	
31. Have the client place the mouthpiece in his or her mouth. Comments:	☐	☐	☐	
32. Have client press down on the dispenser and inhale simultaneously. Comments:	☐	☐	☐	

continued from the previous page

Procedure 5-7	Able to Perform	Able to Perform with Assistance	Unable to Perform	Initials and Date
33. If an aerochamber is used, have the client inhale slowly and deeply. *Comments:*	☐	☐	☐	
34. Observe client to assess for possible adverse effects. *Comments:*	☐	☐	☐	
35. Wash your hands. *Comments:*	☐	☐	☐	
36. Record the medication administration and your observations. *Comments:*	☐	☐	☐	

Checklist for Procedure 5-8 Administering an Intradermal Injection

Name _____ Date _____

School _____

Instructor _____

Course _____

Procedure 5-8 **Administering an Intradermal Injection**	Able to Perform	Able to Perform with Assistance	Unable to Perform	Initials and Date
Assessment				
1. Assess the five rights: right client, right medication, right route, right dose, and right time. *Comments:*	☐	☐	☐	
2. Review physician's or qualified practitioner's order. *Comments:*	☐	☐	☐	
3. Review information regarding the expected outcomes. *Comments:*	☐	☐	☐	
4. Assess for the indications for intradermal injection. *Comments:*	☐	☐	☐	
5. Check the expiration date of the medication vial. *Comments:*	☐	☐	☐	
6. Assess client's knowledge regarding the medication to be received. *Comments:*	☐	☐	☐	
7. Assess the client's response to discussion about an injection. *Comments:*	☐	☐	☐	
Planning/Expected Outcomes				
1. The client will experience minimal pain at the injection site. *Comments:*	☐	☐	☐	
2. The client will experience no allergic reaction or side effects. *Comments:*	☐	☐	☐	
3. The client will be able to explain the significance of a skin reaction. *Comments:*	☐	☐	☐	

continued on the following page

continued from the previous page

Procedure 5-8	Able to Perform	Able to Perform with Assistance	Unable to Perform	Initials and Date
4. The client will keep follow-up appointments. *Comments:*	☐	☐	☐	
Implementation				
1. Wash hands and put on clean gloves. *Comments:*	☐	☐	☐	
2. Provide privacy. Identify client. *Comments:*	☐	☐	☐	
3. Select injection site. *Comments:*	☐	☐	☐	
4. Select one-quarter- to five-eighths-inch 25- to 27-gauge needle. *Comments:*	☐	☐	☐	
5. Assist client into a comfortable position. • Relax the arm with forearm extended on a flat surface. • Distract client by talking about an interesting subject. *Comments:*	☐	☐	☐	
6. Use antiseptic swab in a circular motion to clean skin at site. *Comments:*	☐	☐	☐	
7. Pull cap from needle. *Comments:*	☐	☐	☐	
8. Administer injection: • Stretch skin over site with forefinger and thumb. • Insert needle slowly until resistance is felt; then advance to no more than an eighth of an inch. • Slowly inject the medication. • Note a small bleb forming under the skin surface *Comments:*	☐	☐	☐	
9. Withdraw the needle, applying gentle pressure with the swab. *Comments:*	☐	☐	☐	

continued from the previous page

Procedure 5-8	Able to Perform	Able to Perform with Assistance	Unable to Perform	Initials and Date
10. Do not massage the site. *Comments:*	☐	☐	☐	
11. Assist the client to a comfortable position. *Comments:*	☐	☐	☐	
12. Discard the uncapped needle and syringe safely. *Comments:*	☐	☐	☐	
13. Remove gloves and wash hands. *Comments:*	☐	☐	☐	

Checklist for Procedure 5-9 Administering a Subcutaneous Injection

Name _____ Date _____

School _____

Instructor _____

Course _____

Procedure 5-9 Administering a Subcutaneous Injection	Able to Perform	Able to Perform with Assistance	Unable to Perform	Initials and Date
Assessment				
1. Assess the five rights: right client, right medication, right route, right dose, and right time. *Comments:*	☐	☐	☐	
2. Review physician's or qualified practitioner's order. *Comments:*	☐	☐	☐	
3. Review information regarding the drug ordered. *Comments:*	☐	☐	☐	
4. Assess client for factors that may influence an injection. *Comments:*	☐	☐	☐	
5. Assess for previous subcutaneous injections. *Comments:*	☐	☐	☐	
6. Assess for the indications for subcutaneous injection. *Comments:*	☐	☐	☐	
7. Assess the client's age. *Comments:*	☐	☐	☐	
8. Assess client's knowledge regarding the medication. *Comments:*	☐	☐	☐	
9. Assess the client's response to discussion about an injection. *Comments:*	☐	☐	☐	
Planning/Expected Outcomes				
1. The client will experience minimal pain or burning at the injection site. *Comments:*	☐	☐	☐	

continued on the following page

continued from the previous page

Procedure 5-9	Able to Perform	Able to Perform with Assistance	Unable to Perform	Initials and Date
2. The client will experience no allergic reaction or other side effects. *Comments:*	☐	☐	☐	
3. The client will be able to explain the purpose, action, schedule, and side effects of the medication. *Comments:*	☐	☐	☐	
Implementation				
1. Wash hands and put on clean gloves. *Comments:*	☐	☐	☐	
2. Identify client. Provide privacy. *Comments:*	☐	☐	☐	
3. Select injection site. *Comments:*	☐	☐	☐	
4. Select needle size. *Comments:*	☐	☐	☐	
5. Assist client into a comfortable position. Distract client. *Comments:*	☐	☐	☐	
6. Use antiseptic swab to clean skin at site. *Comments:*	☐	☐	☐	
7. While holding swab between fingers, pull cap from needle. *Comments:*	☐	☐	☐	
8. Administer injection: • Hold syringe like a dart. • Pinch skin with nondominant hand. • Inject needle quickly and firmly. • Release the skin. • Grasp the lower end of the syringe with one hand, and position other hand at the end of the plunger. • Pull back on the plunger. If no blood appears, slowly inject the medication. *Comments:*	☐	☐	☐	

Procedure 5-9	Able to Perform	Able to Perform with Assistance	Unable to Perform	Initials and Date
9. Withdraw the needle while applying pressure with the swab. *Comments:*	☐	☐	☐	
10. Apply pressure. Massaging the site is contraindicated for some medications. *Comments:*	☐	☐	☐	
11. Assist the client to a comfortable position. *Comments:*	☐	☐	☐	
12. Discard the uncapped needle and syringe appropriately. *Comments:*	☐	☐	☐	
13. Remove gloves and wash hands. *Comments:*	☐	☐	☐	

Checklist for Procedure 5-10   Administering an Intramuscular Injection

Name _____ Date _____

School _____

Instructor _____

Course _____

Procedure 5-10 **Administering an Intramuscular Injection**	Able to Perform	Able to Perform with Assistance	Unable to Perform	Initials and Date
Assessment				
1. Assess the five rights: right client, right medication, right route, right dose, and right time. *Comments:*	☐	☐	☐	
2. Review physician's or qualified practitioner's order. *Comments:*	☐	☐	☐	
3. Review information regarding the drug ordered. *Comments:*	☐	☐	☐	
4. Assess client for factors that may influence an injection. *Comments:*	☐	☐	☐	
5. Assess for previous intramuscular injections. *Comments:*	☐	☐	☐	
6. Assess for the indications for intramuscular injections. *Comments:*	☐	☐	☐	
7. Assess the client's age. *Comments:*	☐	☐	☐	
8. Assess client's knowledge regarding the medication to be received. *Comments:*	☐	☐	☐	
9. Assess the client's response to discussion about an injection. *Comments:*	☐	☐	☐	
10. Assess the client's size and muscle development. *Comments:*	☐	☐	☐	

continued on the following page

continued from the previous page

Procedure 5-10	Able to Perform	Able to Perform with Assistance	Unable to Perform	Initials and Date
Planning/Expected Outcomes				
1. The client will experience minimal pain at the injection site. *Comments:*	☐	☐	☐	
2. The client will experience no allergic reaction or other side effects. *Comments:*	☐	☐	☐	
3. The client will be able to explain the action, side effects, dosage, and schedule of the medication. *Comments:*	☐	☐	☐	
Implementation				
1. Wash hands and put on clean gloves. *Comments:*	☐	☐	☐	
2. Identify client. Provide privacy. *Comments:*	☐	☐	☐	
3. Select injection site. *Comments:*	☐	☐	☐	
4. Select needle size. *Comments:*	☐	☐	☐	
5. Assist client into a comfortable position. *Comments:*	☐	☐	☐	
6. Use antiseptic swab to clean skin at site. *Comments:*	☐	☐	☐	
7. While holding swab between fingers, pull cap from needle. *Comments:*	☐	☐	☐	
8. Administer injection: • Hold syringe between thumb and forefinger, like a dart. • Spread skin tightly. • Inject needle quickly and firmly. • Release the skin. • Grasp the lower end of the syringe with one hand and position other hand at the end of the plunger. • Pull back on the plunger. If no blood appears, inject the medication. *Comments:*	☐	☐	☐	

Procedure 5-10	Able to Perform	Able to Perform with Assistance	Unable to Perform	Initials and Date
9. Withdraw the needle while applying pressure with the swab. *Comments:*	☐	☐	☐	
10. Gently massage the site. *Comments:*	☐	☐	☐	
11. Assist the client to a comfortable position. *Comments:*	☐	☐	☐	
12. Discard the uncapped needle and syringe appropriately. *Comments:*	☐	☐	☐	
13. Remove gloves and wash hands. *Comments:*	☐	☐	☐	

Checklist for Procedure 5-11   Administering Medication via Z-Track Injection

Name _____ Date _____

School _____

Instructor _____

Course _____

Procedure 5-11 **Administering Medication via Z-Track Injection**	Able to Perform	Able to Perform with Assistance	Unable to Perform	Initials and Date
Assessment				
1. Assess the five rights: right client, right medication, right route, right dose, and right time. *Comments:*	☐	☐	☐	
2. Assess the client's understanding of the proposed injection. *Comments:*	☐	☐	☐	
3. Verify the physician's or qualified practitioner's order. *Comments:*	☐	☐	☐	
4. Consider the appropriateness of the therapy. *Comments:*	☐	☐	☐	
5. Replace any missing or faded identification bracelets. *Comments:*	☐	☐	☐	
6. Check the client's drug allergy history. *Comments:*	☐	☐	☐	
Planning/Expected Outcomes				
1. The correct client will receive the correct medication. *Comments:*	☐	☐	☐	
2. The client will not experience pain or skin staining secondary to the medication. *Comments:*	☐	☐	☐	
3. The client will obtain the expected benefit from the medication. *Comments:*	☐	☐	☐	

continued on the following page

continued from the previous page

Procedure 5-11	Able to Perform	Able to Perform with Assistance	Unable to Perform	Initials and Date
Implementation				
1. Wash hands. *Comments:*	☐	☐	☐	
2. Assess the client for knowledge of planned injection. *Comments:*	☐	☐	☐	
3. Check the MAR against the order. *Comments:*	☐	☐	☐	
4. Check for drug allergies. *Comments:*	☐	☐	☐	
5. Prepare the medication for only one client at a time. *Comments:*	☐	☐	☐	
6. Select the correct medication and double-check against the MAR. *Comments:*	☐	☐	☐	
7. Calculate the medication dose, if necessary. *Comments:*	☐	☐	☐	
8. Draw up the medication with a large-bore needle. Replace it with an appropriate size needle. *Comments:*	☐	☐	☐	
9. Add 0.1–0.2 ml of air to the dose in the syringe. *Comments:*	☐	☐	☐	
10. Identify client. Locate the appropriate injection site. *Comments:*	☐	☐	☐	
11. Wash your hands using an antibacterial soap. *Comments:*	☐	☐	☐	
12. Clean the injection site thoroughly and allow to dry. *Comments:*	☐	☐	☐	

Procedure 5-11	Able to Perform	Able to Perform with Assistance	Unable to Perform	Initials and Date
13. Pull the skin and subcutaneous tissue to the side or downward. *Comments:*	☐	☐	☐	
14. Remove the needle guard. *Comments:*	☐	☐	☐	
15. While maintaining traction on the skin, dart the needle into the skin. *Comments:*	☐	☐	☐	
16. Aspirate for a minimum of 5 seconds. Observe for a blood return. *Comments:*	☐	☐	☐	
17. If no blood return is present, slowly inject the medication. *Comments:*	☐	☐	☐	
18. If injecting an irritating substance, allow the needle to stay in place for 10 seconds after the injection. *Comments:*	☐	☐	☐	
19. While maintaining traction on the skin, remove the needle and allow the skin to slide over the injection track. *Comments:*	☐	☐	☐	
20. Do not rub or wipe the skin after removal of the needle. *Comments:*	☐	☐	☐	
21. Dispose of needle in a nonpenetrable container. *Comments:*	☐	☐	☐	
22. Wash hands. *Comments:*	☐	☐	☐	

Checklist for Procedure 5-12   Withdrawing Medication from a Vial

Name _____ Date _____

School _____

Instructor _____

Course _____

Procedure 5-12 **Withdrawing Medication from a Vial**	Able to Perform	Able to Perform with Assistance	Unable to Perform	Initials and Date
Assessment				
1. Assess the expiration date on the vial to be sure it is current. *Comments:*	☐	☐	☐	
2. Assess the contents of the vial for the correct medication and dosage. *Comments:*	☐	☐	☐	
3. Assess the contents of the vial for color, consistency, and debris. *Comments:*	☐	☐	☐	
4. Assess the integrity of the vial and the stopper. *Comments:*	☐	☐	☐	
5. Assess the integrity of the syringe and needle that will be used. *Comments:*	☐	☐	☐	
Planning/Expected Outcomes				
1. The correct medication will be drawn from the vial using sterile technique. *Comments:*	☐	☐	☐	
2. The correct dose will be drawn from the vial. *Comments:*	☐	☐	☐	
3. The remaining contents of multiuse vials will not be contaminated. *Comments:*	☐	☐	☐	
4. The date the vial was opened will be marked on the vial in ink. *Comments:*	☐	☐	☐	

continued on the following page

continued from the previous page

Procedure 5-12	Able to Perform	Able to Perform with Assistance	Unable to Perform	Initials and Date
Implementation				
1. Wash hands. Apply gloves if desired. *Comments:*	☐	☐	☐	
2. Select the appropriate vial. *Comments:*	☐	☐	☐	
3. Verify physician's or qualified practitioner's orders. *Comments:*	☐	☐	☐	
4. Check expiration date. *Comments:*	☐	☐	☐	
5. Determine the medication route and select the appropriate size syringe and needle. *Comments:*	☐	☐	☐	
6. Withdraw the plunger to the desired volume of medication. *Comments:*	☐	☐	☐	
7. Clean the rubber top of the vial with an alcohol pad. *Comments:*	☐	☐	☐	
8. Remove the cap from the needle. *Comments:*	☐	☐	☐	
9. Lay the needle cap on a clean surface. *Comments:*	☐	☐	☐	
10. Placing the needle in the center of the vial, inject air slowly. *Comments:*	☐	☐	☐	
11. Invert the vial and withdraw the medication. *Comments:*	☐	☐	☐	
12. Determine that the appropriate dose/volume has been reached. *Comments:*	☐	☐	☐	

Procedure 5-12	Able to Perform	Able to Perform with Assistance	Unable to Perform	Initials and Date
13. Slowly withdraw the needle from the vial. *Comments:*	☐	☐	☐	
14. Using ink, mark the current date, time, and initials on the vial. *Comments:*	☐	☐	☐	
15. Label the syringe with drug, dose, date, and time. *Comments:*	☐	☐	☐	
16. Wash hands. *Comments:*	☐	☐	☐	

Checklist for Procedure 5-13   Withdrawing Medication from an Ampule

Name _____ Date _____

School _____

Instructor _____

Course _____

Procedure 5-13 **Withdrawing Medication from an Ampule**	Able to Perform	Able to Perform with Assistance	Unable to Perform	Initials and Date
Assessment				
1. Identify the correct ampule. *Comments:*	☐	☐	☐	
2. Assess the syringe, filter needle, and injection needle. *Comments:*	☐	☐	☐	
3. Assess the fluid in the ampule. *Comments:*	☐	☐	☐	
4. Identify the medication's intended action, purpose, and nursing implications. *Comments:*	☐	☐	☐	
Planning/Expected Outcomes				
1. The correct medication ampule will be selected. *Comments:*	☐	☐	☐	
2. The medication will be drawn into an appropriate syringe. *Comments:*	☐	☐	☐	
3. Microorganisms will not be introduced into the sterile system. *Comments:*	☐	☐	☐	
4. Foreign objects will not be introduced into the sterile system. *Comments:*	☐	☐	☐	
Implementation				
1. Wash hands. *Comments:*	☐	☐	☐	

continued on the following page

continued from the previous page

Procedure 5-13	Able to Perform	Able to Perform with Assistance	Unable to Perform	Initials and Date
2. Select appropriate ampule. *Comments:*	☐	☐	☐	
3. Select syringe with filter needle. *Comments:*	☐	☐	☐	
4. Obtain a sterile gauze pad. *Comments:*	☐	☐	☐	
5. Select and set aside the appropriate length of needle for planned injection. *Comments:*	☐	☐	☐	
6. Clear a work space. *Comments:*	☐	☐	☐	
7. Observe ampule for location of the fluid. *Comments:*	☐	☐	☐	
8. If fluid is trapped in the top, flick the neck of the ampule. *Comments:*	☐	☐	☐	
9. Wrap the sterile gauze pad around the neck and snap off the top in an outward motion. *Comments:*	☐	☐	☐	
10. Invert ampule, place the needle into the liquid, and withdraw fluid into the syringe. *Comments:*	☐	☐	☐	
11. Alternately, place the ampule on the counter, hold and tilt slightly. Insert the needle into liquid and draw liquid into the syringe. *Comments:*	☐	☐	☐	
12. Remove the filter needle and replace with the injection needle. *Comments:*	☐	☐	☐	

Procedure 5-13	Able to Perform	Able to Perform with Assistance	Unable to Perform	Initials and Date
13. Dispose of filter needle and glass ampule appropriately. *Comments:*	☐	☐	☐	
14. Label the syringe with drug, dose, date, and time. *Comments:*	☐	☐	☐	
15. Wash hands. *Comments:*	☐	☐	☐	

Checklist for Procedure 5-14 Mixing Medications from Two Vials into One Syringe

Name _____ Date _____

School _____

Instructor _____

Course _____

Procedure 5-14 Mixing Medications from Two Vials into One Syringe	Able to Perform	Able to Perform with Assistance	Unable to Perform	Initials and Date
Assessment				
1. Identify the medications, dosage, and route ordered and the normal dosage and route. *Comments:*	☐	☐	☐	
2. Consider whether the order of drawing up medications makes a difference. *Comments:*	☐	☐	☐	
3. Assess client's knowledge regarding this skill if the client will be doing this at home. *Comments:*	☐	☐	☐	
Planning/Expected Outcomes				
1. The ordered medications will be drawn up using sterile technique. *Comments:*	☐	☐	☐	
2. The correct dose of medication will be drawn from the vials. *Comments:*	☐	☐	☐	
3. The remaining contents of multiuse vials will not be contaminated. *Comments:*	☐	☐	☐	
4. If needed, client will be instructed in performing this skill. *Comments:*	☐	☐	☐	
Implementation				
1. Check MAR against the written orders. *Comments:*	☐	☐	☐	
2. Check for drug allergies. *Comments:*	☐	☐	☐	

continued on the following page

continued from the previous page

Procedure 5-14	Able to Perform	Able to Perform with Assistance	Unable to Perform	Initials and Date
3. Wash your hands. *Comments:*	☐	☐	☐	
4. Gather the equipment needed. Prepare the medication for one client at a time. *Comments:*	☐	☐	☐	
5. Check the need for one medication to be drawn up before the other. *Comments:*	☐	☐	☐	
6. Determine the total volume of the combined medications. *Comments:*	☐	☐	☐	
7. Swab the top of each vial with alcohol. *Comments:*	☐	☐	☐	
8. Draw air into the syringe equal to the volume to be drawn up from the second vial. Inject the air into the second vial and remove the syringe and needle from the vial. *Comments:*	☐	☐	☐	
9. Draw air into the syringe equal to the volume to be drawn up from the first vial. Inject air into the first vial. Keep the needle and syringe in the vial. *Comments:*	☐	☐	☐	
10. Withdraw the correct amount of medication from the first vial. *Comments:*	☐	☐	☐	
11. Remove the syringe from the first vial and insert it into the second vial. Withdraw medication from second vial to the volume total of both medications summed together. *Comments:*	☐	☐	☐	
12. Follow the institutional policy regarding recapping needles. *Comments:*	☐	☐	☐	
13. Wash hands. *Comments:*	☐	☐	☐	

Procedure 5-14	Able to Perform	Able to Perform with Assistance	Unable to Perform	Initials and Date
Mixing Insulin 14. • Check client's most recent blood-glucose level, dietary intake, oral intake status (i.e., is NPO), and signs and symptoms related to glucose level. • Repeat Actions 1–4. • Remove caps from insulin vials (if necessary). Gently rotate (never shake) the suspension insulin, such as NPH, intermediate, or long-acting insulin, until no sediment is at the bottom of the vial. • Wipe off tops on insulin vials with alcohol sponge. • Draw back the amount of air into the syringe that equals the total dose of both insulin solutions. Insert the needle and syringe into the vial with the cloudy suspension (intermediate or long-acting insulin) and inject air equal to the amount to be given of that insulin. Do no touch solution with needle. • Insert needle and syringe into vial of short-acting or regular insulin and inject air equal to the amount to be given. • Keep needle and syringe in solution. Invert vial and withdraw medication slowly and accurately. • Withdraw needle and expel any air bubbles. Check dose with another nurse. • Invert the vial with longer-acting insulin, holding plunger carefully, and withdraw long-acting insulin, being careful not to inject any regular insulin into vial. • Store insulin properly. • Wash hands and prepare to administer injection. *Comments:*	☐	☐	☐	

Checklist for Procedure 5-15   Preparing an IV Solution

Name _____ Date _____

School _____

Instructor _____

Course _____

Procedure 5-15 Preparing an IV Solution	Able to Perform	Able to Perform with Assistance	Unable to Perform	Initials and Date
Assessment				
1. Check the order for the IV solution and infusion rate. *Comments:*	☐	☐	☐	
2. Review information regarding the solution and nursing implications. *Comments:*	☐	☐	☐	
3. Check all additives in the solution and other medications. *Comments:*	☐	☐	☐	
4. Assess the client's understanding of the purpose of the IV infusion. *Comments:*	☐	☐	☐	
Planning/Expected Outcomes				
1. The appropriate fluids at the ordered dosages will be available. *Comments:*	☐	☐	☐	
2. The IV infusion will be sterile, without precipitate or contamination. *Comments:*	☐	☐	☐	
3. The caregiver preparing the IV solution will not be endangered. *Comments:*	☐	☐	☐	
Implementation				
1. Check the order for the IV solution. *Comments:*	☐	☐	☐	

continued on the following page

continued from the previous page

Procedure 5-15	Able to Perform	Able to Perform with Assistance	Unable to Perform	Initials and Date
2. Wash hands. Apply gloves if needed. *Comments:*	☐	☐	☐	
3. Remove protective cover from bag or bottle. *Comments:*	☐	☐	☐	
4. Inspect the bag or bottle. Inspect the fluid. Check expiration date. *Comments:*	☐	☐	☐	
5. Prepare a label for the IV bag or bottle: • Note date, time, and your initials. • Note the rate at which the solution is to infuse. • Mark approximate infusion intervals on the label. • Attach the label to the bag or bottle upside-down. *Comments:*	☐	☐	☐	
6. Store the prepared IV solution in the assigned area. *Comments:*	☐	☐	☐	
7. Remove gloves and dispose with all used materials. *Comments:*	☐	☐	☐	
8. Wash hands. *Comments:*	☐	☐	☐	
9. Document the preparation of the IV solution. *Comments:*	☐	☐	☐	
Hanging the Prepared IV 10. Wash hands. *Comments:*	☐	☐	☐	
11. Obtain the ordered IV solution. Check to be sure it matches the order. *Comments:*	☐	☐	☐	
12. Inspect the bag or bottle. Inspect the fluid. *Comments:*	☐	☐	☐	

Procedure 5-15	Able to Perform	Able to Perform with Assistance	Unable to Perform	Initials and Date
13. Check client's identification bracelet. *Comments:*	☐	☐	☐	
14. Prepare an IV time tape noting the IV rate and approximate infusion intervals. Attach tape to solution upside-down. *Comments:*	☐	☐	☐	
15. With the tubing clamp closed, remove the plastic covering the infusion port and insert the tubing spike into the port. *Comments:*	☐	☐	☐	
16. Compress the drip chamber to fill halfway. *Comments:*	☐	☐	☐	
17. Loosen protective cap from end of tubing, open the roller clamp, and flush tubing with IV solution. *Comments:*	☐	☐	☐	
18. Close the roller clamp and tighten the cap protector. *Comments:*	☐	☐	☐	
19. When ready to initiate the infusion, remove the cap protector and attach the tubing to the IV catheter. *Comments:*	☐	☐	☐	
20. Open the clamp and regulate the flow of solution. *Comments:*	☐	☐	☐	
21. Wash hands. *Comments:*	☐	☐	☐	

Checklist for Procedure 5-16   Adding Medications to an IV Solution

Name _____ Date _____

School _____

Instructor _____

Course _____

Procedure 5-16 Adding Medications to an IV Solution	Able to Perform	Able to Perform with Assistance	Unable to Perform	Initials and Date
Assessment				
1. Assess the five rights: right client, right medication, right route, right dose, and right time. *Comments:*	☐	☐	☐	
2. Review information regarding the drug. *Comments:*	☐	☐	☐	
3. Determine the additives in the solution of an existing IV line. *Comments:*	☐	☐	☐	
4. Assess the patency of the IV. *Comments:*	☐	☐	☐	
5. Assess the skin at the IV site. *Comments:*	☐	☐	☐	
6. Check the client's drug allergy history. *Comments:*	☐	☐	☐	
7. Assess the client's understanding of the purpose of the medication. *Comments:*	☐	☐	☐	
Planning/Expected Outcomes				
1. The appropriate fluids and medications at the ordered dosages will be mixed for IV infusion. *Comments:*	☐	☐	☐	
2. The IV infusion will not be contaminated during the procedure. *Comments:*	☐	☐	☐	

continued on the following page

continued from the previous page

Procedure 5-16	Able to Perform	Able to Perform with Assistance	Unable to Perform	Initials and Date
3. The caregiver mixing the IV will not be endangered. *Comments:*	☐	☐	☐	
4. The medication will be infused without trauma to the client. *Comments:*	☐	☐	☐	
Implementation				
1. Check order for the IV solution and additives ordered. *Comments:*	☐	☐	☐	
2. Determine whether the ordered additives are compatible with the IV solution and with each other. *Comments:*	☐	☐	☐	
3. Wash hands; apply gloves, if needed. *Comments:*	☐	☐	☐	
4. Using the appropriate technique, draw up ordered additives. *Comments:*	☐	☐	☐	
Adding Medication to a New Solution 5. Remove protective cover from new bag or bottle. *Comments:*	☐	☐	☐	
6. Inspect the bag or bottle. Inspect the fluid. Check expiration date. *Comments:*	☐	☐	☐	
7. Add medication to IV solution: • For plastic IV bag, locate port with rubber stopper. • For IV bottle, locate the X, circle, or triangle over the IV injection site. • Wipe off port or site with antiseptic swab. • Insert needle into center of port or site. • Inject medication into bag. • Remove needle from bag. *Comments:*	☐	☐	☐	
8. Mix medication into IV solution. *Comments:*	☐	☐	☐	

Procedure 5-16	Able to Perform	Able to Perform with Assistance	Unable to Perform	Initials and Date
9. Label the bag: • Write the name and dose of medication, date, time, and nurse's initials. • Apply to bag upside-down. *Comments:*	☐	☐	☐	
10. Store the prepared IV solution in the assigned area. *Comments:*	☐	☐	☐	
Adding Medication to an Existing Solution 11. Identify client using armband and calling name. *Comments:*	☐	☐	☐	
12. Explain the purpose and route of the medication. *Comments:*	☐	☐	☐	
13. Clamp the IV tubing and remove bag from IV pole. *Comments:*	☐	☐	☐	
14. Add medication to IV solution: • For plastic IV bag, locate port with rubber stopper. • For IV bottle, locate the X, circle, or triangle over the IV injection site. • Wipe off port or site with antiseptic swab. • Insert needle into center of port or site. • Inject medication into bag. • Remove needle from bag. *Comments:*	☐	☐	☐	
15. Mix medication into IV solution. *Comments:*	☐	☐	☐	
16. Apply a new label: • Write the name and dose of medication, date, time, and nurse's initials. • Apply to bag upside-down. *Comments:*	☐	☐	☐	
17. Unclamp the tubing and regulate the flow. *Comments:*	☐	☐	☐	
18. Remove gloves and dispose of all used materials appropriately. *Comments:*	☐	☐	☐	

continued on the following page

continued from the previous page

Procedure 5-16	Able to Perform	Able to Perform with Assistance	Unable to Perform	Initials and Date
19. Wash hands. *Comments:*	☐	☐	☐	
20. Document the preparation of the IV solution. *Comments:*	☐	☐	☐	

Checklist for Procedure 5-17   Administering Medications via Secondary Administration Sets (Piggyback)

Name _____ Date _____

School _____

Instructor _____

Course _____

Procedure 5-17 Administering Medications via Secondary Administration Sets (Piggyback)	Able to Perform	Able to Perform with Assistance	Unable to Perform	Initials and Date
Assessment				
1. Assess the five rights: right client, right medication, right route, right dose, and right time. *Comments:*	☐	☐	☐	
2. Review information regarding the drug. *Comments:*	☐	☐	☐	
3. Determine the additives in the solution of an existing IV line. *Comments:*	☐	☐	☐	
4. Assess the placement of the IV catheter in the vein. *Comments:*	☐	☐	☐	
5. Assess the skin at the IV site. *Comments:*	☐	☐	☐	
6. Check the client's drug allergy history. *Comments:*	☐	☐	☐	
7. Assess the client's understanding of the purpose of the medication. *Comments:*	☐	☐	☐	
8. Assess the compatibility of the piggyback IV medication with the primary IV solution. *Comments:*	☐	☐	☐	
Planning/Expected Outcomes				
1. The drug is infused into the vein without complications. *Comments:*	☐	☐	☐	
2. The IV site remains free of swelling and inflammation. *Comments:*	☐	☐	☐	

continued on the following page

continued from the previous page

Procedure 5-17	Able to Perform	Able to Perform with Assistance	Unable to Perform	Initials and Date
3. The client will be able to discuss the purpose of the drug. *Comments:*	☐	☐	☐	
Implementation				
1. Check physician's or qualified practitioner's order. *Comments:*	☐	☐	☐	
2. Wash hands and put on clean gloves. *Comments:*	☐	☐	☐	
3. Check client's identification bracelet. *Comments:*	☐	☐	☐	
4. Explain procedure and reason drug is being given. *Comments:*	☐	☐	☐	
5. Prepare medication bag: • Close clamp on tubing of secondary infusion set. • Spike medication bag with secondary infusion tubing. • Open clamp. • Allow tubing to fill with solution. *Comments:*	☐	☐	☐	
6. Hang piggyback medication bag above level of primary IV bag. *Comments:*	☐	☐	☐	
7. Connect piggyback tubing to primary tubing at Y-port: • For needleless system, remove port cap and connect tubing. • If a needle is used, clean port with antiseptic swab and insert small-gauge needle into center of port. • Secure tubing with adhesive tape. *Comments:*	☐	☐	☐	
8. Administer the medication: • Check the prescribed length of time for the infusion. • Regulate the flow rate of the piggyback. • Observe that primary infusion has stopped during drug administration. *Comments:*	☐	☐	☐	

Procedure 5-17	Able to Perform	Able to Perform with Assistance	Unable to Perform	Initials and Date
9. Check primary infusion line when medication is finished: • Regulate primary infusion rate. • Leave secondary bag and tubing in place. *Comments:*	☐	☐	☐	
10. Remove gloves and dispose of contaminated materials appropriately. *Comments:*	☐	☐	☐	
11. Wash hands. *Comments:*	☐	☐	☐	

Checklist for Procedure 5-18   Administering Medications via IV Bolus or IV Push

Name _____ Date _____

School _____

Instructor _____

Course _____

Procedure 5-18 **Administering Medications via IV Bolus or IV Push**	Able to Perform	Able to Perform with Assistance	Unable to Perform	Initials and Date
Assessment				
1. Assess the five rights: right client, right medication, right route, right dose, and right time. *Comments:*	☐	☐	☐	
2. Review information regarding the drug. *Comments:*	☐	☐	☐	
3. Determine the additives in the solution of an existing IV line. *Comments:*	☐	☐	☐	
4. Assess the placement of the IV needle. *Comments:*	☐	☐	☐	
5. Assess the skin at the IV site. *Comments:*	☐	☐	☐	
6. Check the client's drug allergy history. *Comments:*	☐	☐	☐	
7. Assess the client's understanding of the purpose of the medication. *Comments:*	☐	☐	☐	
8. Assess the medication to be given. *Comments:*	☐	☐	☐	
Planning/Expected Outcomes				
1. The drug will be infused into the vein without complications. *Comments:*	☐	☐	☐	
2. The IV site will remain free of swelling and inflammation. *Comments:*	☐	☐	☐	

continued on the following page

continued from the previous page

Procedure 5-18	Able to Perform	Able to Perform with Assistance	Unable to Perform	Initials and Date
3. The client will be able to discuss the purpose of the drug. *Comments:*	☐	☐	☐	
4. Any adverse reactions to the drug will be identified and treated. *Comments:*	☐	☐	☐	
Implementation				
1. Check order to give drug. *Comments:*	☐	☐	☐	
2. Wash hands and put on clean gloves. *Comments:*	☐	☐	☐	
3. Using the appropriate technique, draw the medication up into a syringe. *Comments:*	☐	☐	☐	
4. Check client's identification bracelet. *Comments:*	☐	☐	☐	
5. Explain procedure and reason drug is being given. *Comments:*	☐	☐	☐	
6. Using an injection port on an existing primary IV: • Select an injection port close to the IV insertion site. • Check for a blood return. • Administer the medication. • After the bolus is infused, clear the tubing of medication. *Comments:*	☐	☐	☐	
7. Using a saline lock: • Clean the lock with antiseptic swab and insert saline-filled syringe into center of diaphragm. • Check for blood return and then flush the lock with saline. • Remove the saline syringe. • Clean the injection port again with an antiseptic swab. • Insert the medication syringe into the injection port and slowly inject the medication over the prescribed time. • Remove the syringe. • Clean the injection port with an antiseptic swab. • Insert another saline-filled syringe into the injection port and slowly flush. *Comments:*	☐	☐	☐	

Procedure 5-18	Able to Perform	Able to Perform with Assistance	Unable to Perform	Initials and Date
8. Using a three-way stopcock: • Turn off the stopcock to the port that will be used. • For stopcocks without an injection port, remove the port cap and attach the needleless syringe. • For stopcocks with an injection port, clean with an antiseptic swab and insert a small-gauge needle into the port. • If the infusion catheter is only used intermittently, attach a syringe of saline prior to the syringe containing medication. • Open the stopcock so the fluid will flow from the syringe to the client. • Check for blood return. • If flushing with saline, turn the stopcock off, remove the syringe, clean the cap (if present), insert the syringe filled with medication, and turn the stopcock on. • Slowly inject the medication over the prescribed time period. • Turn off the stopcock to the injection port. • Reinitiate the flow of IV fluid, if applicable. • Flush the tubing or catheter with saline and heparinized solution if there is no continuous IV flow. *Comments:*	☐	☐	☐	
9. Remove the needle from the port and clean with an antiseptic swab. *Comments:*	☐	☐	☐	
10. Remove gloves and dispose of material appropriately. *Comments:*	☐	☐	☐	
11. Wash hands. *Comments:*	☐	☐	☐	

Checklist for Procedure 5-19   Administering Medications via Volume-Control Sets

Name _____ Date _____

School _____

Instructor _____

Course _____

Procedure 5-19 **Administering Medications via Volume-Control Sets**	Able to Perform	Able to Perform with Assistance	Unable to Perform	Initials and Date
Assessment				
1. Identify and review the drug(s) ordered. *Comments:*	☐	☐	☐	
2. Check allergies and replace identification bracelets if needed. *Comments:*	☐	☐	☐	
3. Assess client's knowledge regarding medications. *Comments:*	☐	☐	☐	
4. Assess client's IV access. *Comments:*	☐	☐	☐	
Planning/Expected Outcomes				
1. Correct dose of medication will be administered over correct time period. *Comments:*	☐	☐	☐	
2. Client will be instructed, if needed, on use of intermittent infusion or additive set. *Comments:*	☐	☐	☐	
3. The client will not suffer any adverse effects. *Comments:*	☐	☐	☐	
Implementation				
1. Wash hands. *Comments:*	☐	☐	☐	
2. Check MAR against the written orders. *Comments:*	☐	☐	☐	
3. Check for drug allergies. *Comments:*	☐	☐	☐	

continued on the following page

continued from the previous page

Procedure 5-19	Able to Perform	Able to Perform with Assistance	Unable to Perform	Initials and Date
4. Prepare the medication for one client at a time. *Comments:*	☐	☐	☐	
5. Decide what type of infusion set is needed. Assemble equipment. *Comments:*	☐	☐	☐	
6. Familiarize yourself with the equipment prior to using it. *Comments:*	☐	☐	☐	
7. Close clamps and open air vent on chamber. Connect the primary IV bag to the volume-control set. If needed, connect a primary IV tubing set to the volume-control set. *Comments:*	☐	☐	☐	
8. Open the upper clamp and let IV solution partially fill the chamber. Close the clamp. *Comments:*	☐	☐	☐	
9. Open the lower clamp and allow the solution to fill the tubing. *Comments:*	☐	☐	☐	
10. Draw up the medication into a syringe. *Comments:*	☐	☐	☐	
11. Check the client's armband. *Comments:*	☐	☐	☐	
12. Identify the drug for the client and its therapeutic purpose. *Comments:*	☐	☐	☐	
13. Clean the volume-control set injection port with alcohol. *Comments:*	☐	☐	☐	
14. Inject the medication into the chamber and gently mix. *Comments:*	☐	☐	☐	

Procedure 5-19	Able to Perform	Able to Perform with Assistance	Unable to Perform	Initials and Date
15. Open upper clamp and add IV solution until diluent is at the prescribed amount. Close clamp. *Comments:*	☐	☐	☐	
16. Adjust the flow rate to infuse the medication at the prescribed rate. *Comments:*	☐	☐	☐	
17. Label the chamber with medication, date, time, and initials. *Comments:*	☐	☐	☐	
18. Observe the client for side effects or adverse reactions. *Comments:*	☐	☐	☐	
19. When the volume in the chamber has infused, close the air vent and reset the IV flow rate. *Comments:*	☐	☐	☐	
20. Wash hands. *Comments:*	☐	☐	☐	

Checklist for Procedure 5-20   Administering Medication via a Cartridge System

Name _____ Date _____

School _____

Instructor _____

Course _____

Procedure 5-20 Administering Medication via a Cartridge System	Able to Perform	Able to Perform with Assistance	Unable to Perform	Initials and Date
Assessment				
1. Assess the five rights: right client, right medication, right route, right dose, and right time. *Comments:*	☐	☐	☐	
2. Identify and review the drug ordered. *Comments:*	☐	☐	☐	
3. Check allergies and replace any missing or faded identification bracelets. *Comments:*	☐	☐	☐	
4. Assess client's knowledge regarding medications. *Comments:*	☐	☐	☐	
5. Assess IV or SQ access. *Comments:*	☐	☐	☐	
6. Assess rate of infusion. *Comments:*	☐	☐	☐	
Planning/Expected Outcomes				
1. Correct dose of medication will be administered over a set time period. *Comments:*	☐	☐	☐	
2. Client will demonstrate knowledge regarding the use and programming of the cartridge system. *Comments:*	☐	☐	☐	
3. Client will not suffer any adverse effects secondary to the cartridge system. *Comments:*	☐	☐	☐	

continued on the following page

continued from the previous page

Procedure 5-20	Able to Perform	Able to Perform with Assistance	Unable to Perform	Initials and Date
Implementation				
1. Wash hands. *Comments:*	☐	☐	☐	
2. Check MAR against the written orders. *Comments:*	☐	☐	☐	
3. Check for drug allergies. *Comments:*	☐	☐	☐	
4. Prepare the medication for one client at a time. • Decide if a cartridge infusion replacement set is needed. • Assemble needed equipment (check battery). • Ensure air is completely expelled from tubing. *Comments:*	☐	☐	☐	
5. Check the client's identification bracelet before administering the medication. *Comments:*	☐	☐	☐	
6. Review the drug information with the client. *Comments:*	☐	☐	☐	
7. Administer the medication using the cartridge set through the ordered site. *Comments:*	☐	☐	☐	
8. Observe the client for side effects or adverse reactions. *Comments:*	☐	☐	☐	
9. Wash hands. *Comments:*	☐	☐	☐	

Checklist for Procedure 5-21 Administering Patient-Controlled Analgesia (PCA)

Name _____ Date _____

School _____

Instructor _____

Course _____

Procedure 5-21 Administering Patient-Controlled Analgesia (PCA)	Able to Perform	Able to Perform with Assistance	Unable to Perform	Initials and Date
Assessment				
1. Assess the five rights: right client, right medication, right route, right dose, and right time. *Comments:*	☐	☐	☐	
2. Assess client consciousness level and cognitive function. *Comments:*	☐	☐	☐	
3. Identify the PCA ordered. *Comments:*	☐	☐	☐	
4. Assess client pain. *Comments:*	☐	☐	☐	
5. Measure client blood pressure and respiratory rate if opioid is prescribed. *Comments:*	☐	☐	☐	
Planning/Expected Outcomes				
1. Client reports lessening or absence of pain. *Comments:*	☐	☐	☐	
2. Client can correctly press the PCA button to self-administer analgesic. *Comments:*	☐	☐	☐	
3. Client experiences no unwanted physical changes. *Comments:*	☐	☐	☐	
4. Client experiences no uncontrollable side effects. *Comments:*	☐	☐	☐	
Implementation				
1. Wash hands. *Comments:*	☐	☐	☐	

continued on the following page

continued from the previous page

Procedure 5-21	Able to Perform	Able to Perform with Assistance	Unable to Perform	Initials and Date
2. Assess the client's comfort level. *Comments:*	☐	☐	☐	
3. Assess the client's consciousness level and ability to understand the instruction. *Comments:*	☐	☐	☐	
4. Check the PCA order. *Comments:*	☐	☐	☐	
5. Check the PCA medication label against the written order, and follow the five rights principle. *Comments:*	☐	☐	☐	
6. Read the instructions before assembling and programming the PCA pump. *Comments:*	☐	☐	☐	
7. Place the filled PCA syringe into the chamber in the PCA pump. *Comments:*	☐	☐	☐	
8. Program the pump according to the prescribed parameters. *Comments:*	☐	☐	☐	
9. Apply gloves. *Comments:*	☐	☐	☐	
10. Inspect the existing IV line and site. *Comments:*	☐	☐	☐	
11. Prime the PCA pump tubing and connect tubing to the primary IV line. *Comments:*	☐	☐	☐	
12. Give the client the control button and instruct how and when to press the button. *Comments:*	☐	☐	☐	
13. Record the procedure. *Comments:*	☐	☐	☐	
14. Wash hands. *Comments:*	☐	☐	☐	

Checklist for Procedure 5-22   Administering Epidural Analgesia

Name _____   Date _____

School _____

Instructor _____

Course _____

Procedure 5-22 **Administering Epidural Analgesia**	Able to Perform	Able to Perform with Assistance	Unable to Perform	Initials and Date
Assessment				
1. Assess the five rights: right client, right medication, right route, right dose, and right time. *Comments:*	☐	☐	☐	
2. Assess client's pain level. *Comments:*	☐	☐	☐	
3. Assess the catheter site for symptoms of infection. *Comments:*	☐	☐	☐	
4. Assess catheter intactness. *Comments:*	☐	☐	☐	
5. Assess vital signs. *Comments:*	☐	☐	☐	
Planning/Expected Outcomes				
1. Client's pain will be relieved. *Comments:*	☐	☐	☐	
2. Client's mobility will be improved due to relief from pain. *Comments:*	☐	☐	☐	
3. Catheter and tubing will be taped securely in place. *Comments:*	☐	☐	☐	
4. There will be no signs or symptoms of infection. *Comments:*	☐	☐	☐	
5. The client will be able to void without difficulty. *Comments:*	☐	☐	☐	

continued on the following page

continued from the previous page

Procedure 5-22	Able to Perform	Able to Perform with Assistance	Unable to Perform	Initials and Date
Implementation				
1. Wash hands. *Comments:*	☐	☐	☐	
2. Verify medication with order. *Comments:*	☐	☐	☐	
3. Gather equipment needed and verify client. *Comments:*	☐	☐	☐	
4. Set up sterile field. *Comments:*	☐	☐	☐	
For Bolus Injection				
5. Draw up solution, using a filter needle, into a 10-cc syringe. *Comments:*	☐	☐	☐	
6. Remove the filter needle and replace with 20-gauge needle or needleless system. *Comments:*	☐	☐	☐	
7. Clean injection cap with povidone-iodine. *Comments:*	☐	☐	☐	
8. Insert needle into injection cap and aspirate. *Comments:*	☐	☐	☐	
9. If 0.5 cc or less clear fluid is aspirated, inject drug slowly. *Comments:*	☐	☐	☐	
10. Remove needle from injection cap and dispose of properly. *Comments:*	☐	☐	☐	
For Continuous Infusion				
11. Attach preservative-free opioid to infusion pump tubing and prime tubing. *Comments:*	☐	☐	☐	

Procedure 5-22	Able to Perform	Able to Perform with Assistance	Unable to Perform	Initials and Date
12. Attach the distal end of the tubing to the catheter. Luer-Lok all connections. Tape a tension loop of tubing to client. Start pump. *Comments:*	☐	☐	☐	
13. Ensure pump is infusing at desired rate. *Comments:*	☐	☐	☐	
14. Label tubing as epidural catheter tubing, with name of drug, date, and time. *Comments:*	☐	☐	☐	
15. Dispose of gloves and wash hands. *Comments:*	☐	☐	☐	
16. Document in client's chart. *Comments:*	☐	☐	☐	

Checklist for Procedure 5-23   Managing Controlled Substances

Name _____ Date _____

School _____

Instructor _____

Course _____

Procedure 5-23 Managing Controlled Substances	Able to Perform	Able to Perform with Assistance	Unable to Perform	Initials and Date
Assessment				
1. Assess the security of the controlled substance storage safe. Comments:	☐	☐	☐	
2. Assess the contents of the safe for any evidence of tampering. Comments:	☐	☐	☐	
3. Assess the controlled substance record for integrity of records. Comments:	☐	☐	☐	
4. Assess the method used for the storage and safeguarding of the safe keys. Comments:	☐	☐	☐	
5. Assess the method used for signing out controlled substances. Comments:	☐	☐	☐	
6. Assess the method used for wasting unused controlled substances. Comments:	☐	☐	☐	
7. Assess the method used to document controlled substances received from and returned to the pharmacy. Comments:	☐	☐	☐	
Planning/Expected Outcomes				
1. The controlled substances will be stored in a legal, safe, and secure manner. Comments:	☐	☐	☐	

continued on the following page

continued from the previous page

Procedure 5-23	Able to Perform	Able to Perform with Assistance	Unable to Perform	Initials and Date
2. The controlled substance packaging will be intact. *Comments:*	☐	☐	☐	
3. The controlled substance record will be accurate. *Comments:*	☐	☐	☐	
4. The keys to the safe will be maintained in a secure place and manner. *Comments:*	☐	☐	☐	
5. When removed from the safe, controlled substances will be recorded and dispensed safely and legally. *Comments:*	☐	☐	☐	
6. Unused portions of controlled substances will be disposed of safely and legally. *Comments:*	☐	☐	☐	
7. Controlled substances will be received from and returned to the pharmacy using a secure and legal method. *Comments:*	☐	☐	☐	

Implementation

Dispensing a Controlled Substance to a Client

	Able to Perform	Able to Perform with Assistance	Unable to Perform	Initials and Date
1. Wash hands. *Comments:*	☐	☐	☐	
2. Check the client's MAR for the type and dosage of the controlled substance. *Comments:*	☐	☐	☐	
3. Obtain the keys to the controlled substance safe. *Comments:*	☐	☐	☐	
4. Open both locks on the controlled substance safe. *Comments:*	☐	☐	☐	
5. Remove the ordered medication and check it against the client's MAR. *Comments:*	☐	☐	☐	

Procedure 5-23	Able to Perform	Able to Perform with Assistance	Unable to Perform	Initials and Date
6. Remove the ordered dosage from the safe and relock the safe. *Comments:*	☐	☐	☐	
7. Record the removal of the medication on the sign-out record. Sign the record. *Comments:*	☐	☐	☐	
8. Secure the controlled substance safe keys. *Comments:*	☐	☐	☐	
9. Dispense the controlled substance using the appropriate method. *Comments:*	☐	☐	☐	
Disposing of Unused Portions of Controlled Substances 10. Obtain the assistance of a second registered nurse. *Comments:*	☐	☐	☐	
11. With the second nurse as a witness, safely dispose of the unused controlled substance. *Comments:*	☐	☐	☐	
12. On the controlled substance record, note the amount of substance wasted. Both nurses sign the wastage record. *Comments:*	☐	☐	☐	
13. Dispose of any needles or biohazardous substances appropriately. *Comments:*	☐	☐	☐	
14. Wash hands. *Comments:*	☐	☐	☐	
Inventorying Controlled Substances 15. Obtain the assistance of a registered nurse from the next or previous shift. *Comments:*	☐	☐	☐	
16. Obtain the keys to the controlled substance safe. *Comments:*	☐	☐	☐	

continued on the following page

continued from the previous page

Procedure 5-23	Able to Perform	Able to Perform with Assistance	Unable to Perform	Initials and Date
17. One nurse physically counts the controlled substances in the safe, informing the second nurse of each total. *Comments:*	☐	☐	☐	
18. The second nurse records the counted totals in the appropriate space in the controlled substance record. *Comments:*	☐	☐	☐	
19. Any discrepancies must be accounted for before the administering nurses can be dismissed. *Comments:*	☐	☐	☐	
20. All sets of keys must be accounted for and collected before the administering nurses can be dismissed. *Comments:*	☐	☐	☐	
21. Relock the controlled substance safe and secure the keys. *Comments:*	☐	☐	☐	

Checklist for Procedure 6-1   Inserting and Maintaining a Nasogastric Tube

Name _____ Date _____

School _____

Instructor _____

Course _____

Procedure 6-1 Inserting and Maintaining a Nasogastric Tube	Able to Perform	Able to Perform with Assistance	Unable to Perform	Initials and Date
Assessment				
1. Assess client's consciousness level. *Comments:*	☐	☐	☐	
2. Check the client's chart for any history of nostril surgery or unusual nostril bleeding. *Comments:*	☐	☐	☐	
3. Use a penlight to assess nostrils for a deviated septum. *Comments:*	☐	☐	☐	
4. Ask the client to breathe, occluding one nostril at a time. *Comments:*	☐	☐	☐	
5. Assess for latex allergy. Prevents reaction to latex and determines if there is a need to use latex-free tubes and gloves. *Comments:*	☐	☐	☐	
Planning/Expected Outcomes				
1. Client's nutritional status will improve. *Comments:*	☐	☐	☐	
2. Client's nutritional needs will be met. *Comments:*	☐	☐	☐	
3. Client will maintain a patent airway. *Comments:*	☐	☐	☐	
4. Client will not have diarrhea due to nasogastric (NG) feeding. *Comments:*	☐	☐	☐	
5. Mouth mucous membranes will remain moist and intact. *Comments:*	☐	☐	☐	

continued on the following page

continued from the previous page

Procedure 6-1	Able to Perform	Able to Perform with Assistance	Unable to Perform	Initials and Date
6. Client will maintain a normal fluid volume. *Comments:*	☐	☐	☐	
7. Client's comfort level will increase. *Comments:*	☐	☐	☐	
8. Skin around the tube will remain intact. *Comments:*	☐	☐	☐	
Implementation				
1. Review client's medical history. *Comments:*	☐	☐	☐	
2. Explain the procedure and develop a hand signal. *Comments:*	☐	☐	☐	
3. Prepare the equipment. *Comments:*	☐	☐	☐	
4. Prepare the environment. Place the bed in a high-Fowler's position and cover the client's chest with a towel. *Comments:*	☐	☐	☐	
5. Wash hands, and then apply gloves. *Comments:*	☐	☐	☐	
6. Assess the client's nostrils. Have the client blow his or her nose, one nostril at a time. *Comments:*	☐	☐	☐	
7. Measure the NG tube against the client. Mark this distance with a piece of tape. *Comments:*	☐	☐	☐	
8. Lubricate first 4 inches of the tube with water-soluble lubricant. *Comments:*	☐	☐	☐	
9. Ask the client to slightly flex the neck backward. *Comments:*	☐	☐	☐	

Procedure 6-1	Able to Perform	Able to Perform with Assistance	Unable to Perform	Initials and Date
10. Gently insert the tube into a naris. *Comments:*	☐	☐	☐	
11. Tip the client's head forward once the tube reaches the nasopharynx. If the client continues to gag, stop for a moment. *Comments:*	☐	☐	☐	
12. Advance the tube several inches at a time as the client swallows. *Comments:*	☐	☐	☐	
13. Withdraw the tube immediately if there are signs of respiratory distress. *Comments:*	☐	☐	☐	
14. Advance the tube until the taped mark is reached. *Comments:*	☐	☐	☐	
15. Split a 4-inch strip of tape lengthwise 2 inches. Secure the tube with the tape. Tape to cheek as well if desired. *Comments:*	☐	☐	☐	
16. Check the placement of the tube: • Inject 30 cc of air and auscultate. • Aspirate gastric content and measure pH. • Prepare the client for x-ray check-up, if prescribed. *Comments:*	☐	☐	☐	
17. Connect the distal end of the tube to suction, draining bag, or adapter. *Comments:*	☐	☐	☐	
18. Secure the tube with a rubber band and safety pin to client's gown or bed sheet. *Comments:*	☐	☐	☐	
19. Remove gloves, dispose of used materials appropriately, and wash hands. *Comments:*	☐	☐	☐	
20. Position client comfortably with the call light in reach. *Comments:*	☐	☐	☐	

continued on the following page

continued from the previous page

Procedure 6-1	Able to Perform	Able to Perform with Assistance	Unable to Perform	Initials and Date
21. Document procedure. *Comments:*	☐	☐	☐	
Maintaining a Nasogastric Tube 22. Wash hands, and then apply gloves. *Comments:*	☐	☐	☐	
23. Check tube placement (following the steps in Action 16) before instilling anything per NG tube or at least every 8 hours. *Comments:*	☐	☐	☐	
24. Assess for signs that the tube has become blocked. *Comments:*	☐	☐	☐	
25. Do not irrigate or rotate a tube that has been placed during gastric or esophageal surgery. *Comments:*	☐	☐	☐	
26. Provide oral hygiene and assist client to clean nares daily. *Comments:*	☐	☐	☐	
27. Remove gloves, dispose of used materials appropriately, and wash hands. *Comments:*	☐	☐	☐	

Checklist for Procedure 6-2   Assessing Placement of a Large-Bore Feeding Tube

Name _____ Date _____

School _____

Instructor _____

Course _____

Procedure 6-2 Assessing Placement of a Large-Bore Feeding Tube	Able to Perform	Able to Perform with Assistance	Unable to Perform	Initials and Date
Assessment				
1. Check the written order for the type and size of feeding tube to place. *Comments:*	☐	☐	☐	
2. Review the client's medical record for a history of prior tube use or displacement. *Comments:*	☐	☐	☐	
3. Assess the client for signs of inadvertent respiratory placement. *Comments:*	☐	☐	☐	
4. Assess the client for symptoms that increase the risk of tube dislocation. *Comments:*	☐	☐	☐	
Planning/Expected Outcomes				
1. The tube will remain in place and intact. *Comments:*	☐	☐	☐	
2. The tube feeding or medication will infuse into the client's gastrointestinal tract. *Comments:*	☐	☐	☐	
3. The client will not experience any respiratory distress. *Comments:*	☐	☐	☐	
4. The client will not experience any pain. *Comments:*	☐	☐	☐	
5. The client will understand the reason for checking the tube's placement. *Comments:*	☐	☐	☐	

continued on the following page

continued from the previous page

Procedure 6-2	Able to Perform	Able to Perform with Assistance	Unable to Perform	Initials and Date
Implementation				
1. Check the written order for the feeding tube. *Comments:*	☐	☐	☐	
2. Wash hands. Put on gloves. *Comments:*	☐	☐	☐	
3. Assess placement of the tube by auscultation: • Place stethoscope over left upper quadrant of the abdomen. • Quickly inject 10–20 ml air. • Assess for resistance. • Listen for sound. *Comments:*	☐	☐	☐	
4. Measure pH of gastrointestinal (GI) contents: • Aspirate 10 cc GI contents with 60-cc syringe. • If unable to aspirate, reposition client and try again. • Measure pH of GI contents with pH indicator strip. *Comments:*	☐	☐	☐	
5. Proceed with feeding and medication. Continue to monitor the client. *Comments:*	☐	☐	☐	
6. Recheck tube placement following the tube feeding: • Flush tube with 30 cc warm water after medication or tube feeding. • Wait 1 hour before testing pH. • Inject 30 cc air and auscultate for sound. • Aspirate 10 cc of GI contents and check for pH. *Comments:*	☐	☐	☐	
7. Remove gloves and wash hands. *Comments:*	☐	☐	☐	

Checklist for Procedure 6-3   Assessing Placement of a Small-Bore Feeding Tube

Name _____ Date _____

School _____

Instructor _____

Course _____

Procedure 6-3 Assessing Placement of a Small-Bore Feeding Tube	Able to Perform	Able to Perform with Assistance	Unable to Perform	Initials and Date
Assessment				
1. Assess client for any signs of respiratory distress. *Comments:*	☐	☐	☐	
2. Check for a tape marker on the tube, near the nose. *Comments:*	☐	☐	☐	
3. Assess sputum for features that would indicate aspiration. *Comments:*	☐	☐	☐	
4. Assess for latex allergy. *Comments:*	☐	☐	☐	
Planning/Expected Outcomes				
1. The client's feeding tube will be intact. *Comments:*	☐	☐	☐	
2. The client will not experience aspiration. *Comments:*	☐	☐	☐	
Implementation				
1. Wash hands and apply clean gloves. *Comments:*	☐	☐	☐	
2. Prepare equipment. *Comments:*	☐	☐	☐	
3. Clamp the tube feeding infusion if it has been running. *Comments:*	☐	☐	☐	
4. Locate the connection between the feeding tube and feeding bag tubing. *Comments:*	☐	☐	☐	

continued on the following page

continued from the previous page

Procedure 6-3	Able to Perform	Able to Perform with Assistance	Unable to Perform	Initials and Date
5. Disconnect infusion tubing and attach a cap to tubing and feeding tube. *Comments:*	☐	☐	☐	
6. Draw 10–20 ml of air into syringe. *Comments:*	☐	☐	☐	
7. Attach syringe to proximal end of feeding tube. *Comments:*	☐	☐	☐	
8. Place diaphragm of stethoscope in epigastric area. *Comments:*	☐	☐	☐	
9. Inject air quickly into feeding tube and listen for air rush. *Comments:*	☐	☐	☐	
10. If unsuccessful in hearing rush of air, repeat Actions 6–9. *Comments:*	☐	☐	☐	
11. Aspirate approximately 20 ml of gastric contents. *Comments:*	☐	☐	☐	
12. Check the contents and obtain pH level. • pH below 4 means tube is in stomach. • pH range of 6–7 means tube is in intestine. *Comments:*	☐	☐	☐	
13. Assess the color of aspirate. *Comments:*	☐	☐	☐	
14. If unable to aspirate contents or unsure of results, call qualified practitioner and consider x-ray confirmation. *Comments:*	☐	☐	☐	
15. Record method of verification and results. *Comments:*	☐	☐	☐	
16. If placement in stomach is verified, resume tube feedings. Recheck placement every 4 hours if feeding is continuous. *Comments:*	☐	☐	☐	
17. Wash hands. *Comments:*	☐	☐	☐	

Checklist for Procedure 6-4 Removing a Nasogastric Tube

Name _____ Date _____

School _____

Instructor _____

Course _____

Procedure 6-4 Removing a Nasogastric Tube	Able to Perform	Able to Perform with Assistance	Unable to Perform	Initials and Date
Assessment				
1. Assess client's consciousness level. Comments:	☐	☐	☐	
2. Check the client's chart for orders to remove the tube. Comments:	☐	☐	☐	
3. Use a penlight to assess nostrils for irritation and dryness. Comments:	☐	☐	☐	
Planning/Expected Outcomes				
1. Client will be able to tolerate the removal of the tube. Comments:	☐	☐	☐	
2. Client will understand the reasons for tube removal. Comments:	☐	☐	☐	
3. Skin around the tube will remain intact. Comments:	☐	☐	☐	
4. Client will understand signs and symptoms to report. Comments:	☐	☐	☐	
Implementation				
1. Wash hands. Comments:	☐	☐	☐	
2. Check the written order for tube removal. Comments:	☐	☐	☐	
3. Assess client's ability to understand. Explain the procedure. Comments:	☐	☐	☐	

continued on the following page

continued from the previous page

Procedure 6-4	Able to Perform	Able to Perform with Assistance	Unable to Perform	Initials and Date
4. Prepare the equipment. *Comments:*	☐	☐	☐	
5. Provide privacy and place the client in a high-Fowler's position. *Comments:*	☐	☐	☐	
6. Apply gloves. *Comments:*	☐	☐	☐	
7. Place a clean towel over client's chest. *Comments:*	☐	☐	☐	
8. Have the client hold emesis basin and a towel or tissue during removal. *Comments:*	☐	☐	☐	
9. Disconnect suction or feeding pump, if any. Remove the tape and safety pin. *Comments:*	☐	☐	☐	
10. Check placement of the tube. *Comments:*	☐	☐	☐	
11. Flush tube with 30–50 cc normal saline followed by 10 cc air. *Comments:*	☐	☐	☐	
12. Ask the client to take a deep breath and hold still. Remove the tube over the course of 3–6 seconds. *Comments:*	☐	☐	☐	
13. Cover or wrap the tube in a towel and remove from the client's bedside. *Comments:*	☐	☐	☐	
14. Provide oral hygiene and assist the client to clean nares. *Comments:*	☐	☐	☐	

continued from the previous page

Procedure 6-4	Able to Perform	Able to Perform with Assistance	Unable to Perform	Initials and Date
15. Remove gloves, dispose of used materials appropriately, and wash hands. *Comments:*	☐	☐	☐	
16. Document the NG tube removal and client's responses. *Comments:*	☐	☐	☐	
17. Wash hands. *Comments:*	☐	☐	☐	
18. Review the original purpose of the tube. Assess for signs that the tube may need to be reinserted. *Comments:*	☐	☐	☐	

Checklist for Procedure 6-5   Feeding and Medicating via a Gastrostomy Tube

Name _____ Date _____

School _____

Instructor _____

Course _____

Procedure 6-5 Feeding and Medicating via a Gastrostomy Tube	Able to Perform	Able to Perform with Assistance	Unable to Perform	Initials and Date
Assessment				
1. Assess the client for signs of gastric distress. *Comments:*	☐	☐	☐	
2. Assess the feeding tube placement every 4 hours. *Comments:*	☐	☐	☐	
3. Assess the client's respiratory status. *Comments:*	☐	☐	☐	
4. Assess the client's ongoing nutritional status. *Comments:*	☐	☐	☐	
5. Assess the client's intake and output. *Comments:*	☐	☐	☐	
Planning/Expected Outcomes				
1. The client will receive the correct volume and formula over the correct time period. *Comments:*	☐	☐	☐	
2. The client will not experience any undesirable effects. *Comments:*	☐	☐	☐	
3. The client's weight and nutritional status will remain stable or improve. *Comments:*	☐	☐	☐	
4. The client will not experience any adverse skin or gastrointestinal effects. *Comments:*	☐	☐	☐	

continued on the following page

continued from the previous page

Procedure 6-5	Able to Perform	Able to Perform with Assistance	Unable to Perform	Initials and Date
Implementation				
1. Review client's medical record for formula, amount, and time. *Comments:*	☐	☐	☐	
2. Gather equipment and formula. *Comments:*	☐	☐	☐	
3. Check client's armband. *Comments:*	☐	☐	☐	
4. Explain procedure to client. *Comments:*	☐	☐	☐	
5. Assemble equipment. Add color to formula if used. Fill bag with prescribed amount of formula. *Comments:*	☐	☐	☐	
6. Place client on right side in a high-Fowler's position. *Comments:*	☐	☐	☐	
7. Wash hands and apply nonsterile gloves. *Comments:*	☐	☐	☐	
8. Provide for privacy. *Comments:*	☐	☐	☐	
9. Check for abdominal distention; auscultate for bowel sounds. *Comments:*	☐	☐	☐	
10. Aspirate stomach contents. If residual contents are greater than 50–100 ml, hold feeding. Instill aspirated contents back into stomach. *Comments:*	☐	☐	☐	
11. Administer tube feeding. *Comments:*	☐	☐	☐	
Intermittent Bolus 12. Pinch the tubing. *Comments:*	☐	☐	☐	

Procedure 6-5	Able to Perform	Able to Perform with Assistance	Unable to Perform	Initials and Date
13. Remove plunger from barrel of syringe and attach to adapter. *Comments:*	☐	☐	☐	
14. Fill syringe with formula. *Comments:*	☐	☐	☐	
15. Infuse slowly; add to syringe until prescribed amount has been administered. *Comments:*	☐	☐	☐	
16. Flush tubing with 30–60 ml or prescribed amount of water. *Comments:*	☐	☐	☐	
Intermittent Gavage Feeding 17. Hang bag on IV pole 18 inches above the client's head. *Comments:*	☐	☐	☐	
18. Remove air from bag's tubing. *Comments:*	☐	☐	☐	
19. Attach tubing to feeding tube adapter and adjust drip rate. *Comments:*	☐	☐	☐	
20. When bag empties of formula, infuse 30–60 ml of water; close clamp. *Comments:*	☐	☐	☐	
21. Change bags every 24 hours. *Comments:*	☐	☐	☐	
Continuous Gavage 22. Check tube placement at least every 4 hours. *Comments:*	☐	☐	☐	
23. Check residual at least every 8 hours. *Comments:*	☐	☐	☐	
24. If residual is above 100 ml, stop feeding. *Comments:*	☐	☐	☐	

continued on the following page

continued from the previous page

Procedure 6-5	Able to Perform	Able to Perform with Assistance	Unable to Perform	Initials and Date
25. Add formula to bag for a 4-hour period; dilute with water if prescribed. *Comments:*	☐	☐	☐	
26. Hang gavage bag on IV pole. Prime tubing. *Comments:*	☐	☐	☐	
27. Thread tubing through feeding pump and attach tubing to feeding tube adapter. *Comments:*	☐	☐	☐	
28. Adjust drip rate. *Comments:*	☐	☐	☐	
29. Monitor infusion rate and watch for signs of respiratory distress or diarrhea. *Comments:*	☐	☐	☐	
30. Flush tube with water every 4 hours or following administration of medications. *Comments:*	☐	☐	☐	
31. Replace disposable feeding bag at least every 24 hours. *Comments:*	☐	☐	☐	
32. Turn client every 2 hours. *Comments:*	☐	☐	☐	
33. Provide oral hygiene every 2–4 hours. *Comments:*	☐	☐	☐	
34. Administer water as prescribed, with and between feedings. *Comments:*	☐	☐	☐	
35. Remove gloves and wash hands. *Comments:*	☐	☐	☐	
36. Document tube feeding. *Comments:*	☐	☐	☐	

Checklist for Procedure 6-6   Maintaining Gastrointestinal Suction Devices

Name _____ Date _____

School _____

Instructor _____

Course _____

Procedure 6-6 **Maintaining Gastrointestinal Suction Devices**	Able to Perform	Able to Perform with Assistance	Unable to Perform	Initials and Date
Assessment				
1. Review the chart. *Comments:*	☐	☐	☐	
2. Assess the client's ability to cooperate. *Comments:*	☐	☐	☐	
3. Assess for proper placement of the NG tube. *Comments:*	☐	☐	☐	
4. Assess for patency of the NG tube. *Comments:*	☐	☐	☐	
5. Monitor gastric contents. *Comments:*	☐	☐	☐	
6. Assess the client's understanding of the suctioning procedure. *Comments:*	☐	☐	☐	
Planning/Expected Outcomes				
1. The client will have a patent NG tube with effective suction. *Comments:*	☐	☐	☐	
2. The client will understand the need for suctioning. *Comments:*	☐	☐	☐	
3. The client will not experience pain or discomfort from the suction or the NG tube. *Comments:*	☐	☐	☐	
4. The client will not experience trauma. *Comments:*	☐	☐	☐	

continued on the following page

continued from the previous page

Procedure 6-6	Able to Perform	Able to Perform with Assistance	Unable to Perform	Initials and Date
Implementation				
1. Assess the physician's or qualified practitioner's order. *Comments:*	☐	☐	☐	
2. Gather the equipment needed at the client's bedside. *Comments:*	☐	☐	☐	
3. Explain the procedure and reassure the client. *Comments:*	☐	☐	☐	
4. Set up the suction source. *Comments:*	☐	☐	☐	
5. Attach the tubing and canister to the suction head. Test the equipment. Turn the suction off. *Comments:*	☐	☐	☐	
6. Wash hands and apply gloves. *Comments:*	☐	☐	☐	
7. Connect the NG tube to the suction tubing; set the suction control as prescribed. *Comments:*	☐	☐	☐	
8. Upon instituting suction and at least every four hours thereafter: • Observe gastric drainage. Empty drainage container regularly. • Assess client for abdominal distress. • Assess the nares and the skin for signs of breakdown. *Comments:*	☐	☐	☐	
9. Remove gloves, dispose of contaminated materials appropriately, and wash hands. *Comments:*	☐	☐	☐	
10. Position client for comfort and place the call light within reach. *Comments:*	☐	☐	☐	
11. Document the procedure. *Comments:*	☐	☐	☐	

Checklist for Procedure 6-7   Applying a Condom Catheter

Name _____ Date _____

School _____

Instructor _____

Course _____

Procedure 6-7 **Applying a Condom Catheter**	Able to Perform	Able to Perform with Assistance	Unable to Perform	Initials and Date
Assessment				
1. Assess skin integrity around the penis and perineal area. *Comments:*	☐	☐	☐	
2. Assess the client for ability to cooperate. *Comments:*	☐	☐	☐	
3. Assess the amount and pattern of urinary incontinence. *Comments:*	☐	☐	☐	
4. Assess for latex allergy. *Comments:*	☐	☐	☐	
Planning/Expected Outcomes				
1. The client will have a condom catheter in place. *Comments:*	☐	☐	☐	
2. The client will have no skin irritation. *Comments:*	☐	☐	☐	
3. The client will understand and cooperate with placement and retention of the condom catheter. *Comments:*	☐	☐	☐	
4. Assess for latex allergy. *Comments:*	☐	☐	☐	
Implementation				
1. Wash hands. *Comments:*	☐	☐	☐	
2. Provide privacy. *Comments:*	☐	☐	☐	

continued on the following page

continued from the previous page

Procedure 6-7	Able to Perform	Able to Perform with Assistance	Unable to Perform	Initials and Date
3. Position the client comfortably. Raise the bed to a comfortable height for the nurse. *Comments:*	☐	☐	☐	
4. Apply gloves. *Comments:*	☐	☐	☐	
5. Fold the client's gown across the abdomen and pull the sheet up over the client's legs. *Comments:*	☐	☐	☐	
6. Assess the client's penis. *Comments:*	☐	☐	☐	
7. Clean the client's penis with warm soapy water. *Comments:*	☐	☐	☐	
8. Return the client's foreskin to its normal position. *Comments:*	☐	☐	☐	
9. Shave any excess hair around the base of the penis. *Comments:*	☐	☐	☐	
10. Rinse and dry the area. *Comments:*	☐	☐	☐	
11. If a condom kit is used, apply skin preparation solution to the shaft of the penis. *Comments:*	☐	☐	☐	
12. Apply the double-sided adhesive strip around the base of the client's penis in a spiral fashion. *Comments:*	☐	☐	☐	
13. Position the rolled condom at the distal portion of the penis and unroll it, covering the penis and the double-sided strip of adhesive. *Comments:*	☐	☐	☐	
14. Gently press the condom to the adhesive strip. *Comments:*	☐	☐	☐	

Procedure 6-7	Able to Perform	Able to Perform with Assistance	Unable to Perform	Initials and Date
15. Attach the drainage bag tubing to the catheter tubing. Secure the drainage bag. *Comments:*	☐	☐	☐	
16. Determine that the condom and tubing are not twisted. *Comments:*	☐	☐	☐	
17. Cover the client. *Comments:*	☐	☐	☐	
18. Dispose of the used equipment appropriately and wash hands. *Comments:*	☐	☐	☐	
19. Return the client's bed to the lowest position and reposition client comfortably. *Comments:*	☐	☐	☐	
20. Empty the bag, measure the urinary output, and record every 4 hours. *Comments:*	☐	☐	☐	
21. Remove the condom once a day to clean the area and assess the skin. *Comments:*	☐	☐	☐	

Checklist for Procedure 6-8 Inserting an Indwelling Catheter: Male

Name _____ Date _____

School _____

Instructor _____

Course _____

Procedure 6-8 **Inserting an Indwelling Catheter: Male**	Able to Perform	Able to Perform with Assistance	Unable to Perform	Initials and Date
Assessment				
1. Assess the need for catheterization and the type of catheterization ordered. *Comments:*	☐	☐	☐	
2. Assess the need for peritoneal care prior to catheterization. *Comments:*	☐	☐	☐	
3. Assess the urinary meatus. Ask the client for any history of difficulty with prior catheterizations. *Comments:*	☐	☐	☐	
4. Assess the client's ability to assist with the procedure. *Comments:*	☐	☐	☐	
5. Assess the light. *Comments:*	☐	☐	☐	
6. Assess for an allergy to povidone-iodine. *Comments:*	☐	☐	☐	
7. Watch for indications of distress or embarrassment. *Comments:*	☐	☐	☐	
Planning/Expected Outcomes				
1. The catheter will be inserted without trauma to the client. *Comments:*	☐	☐	☐	
2. The client's bladder will be emptied without complication. *Comments:*	☐	☐	☐	
3. The nurse will maintain the sterility of the catheter during insertion. *Comments:*	☐	☐	☐	

continued on the following page

continued from the previous page

Procedure 6-8	Able to Perform	Able to Perform with Assistance	Unable to Perform	Initials and Date
Implementation				
1. Gather the equipment needed. *Comments:*	☐	☐	☐	
2. Provide for privacy and explain procedure to client. *Comments:*	☐	☐	☐	
3. Set the bed to a comfortable height to work, and raise the opposite side rail. *Comments:*	☐	☐	☐	
4. Assist the client to a supine position with legs slightly spread. *Comments:*	☐	☐	☐	
5. Drape the client's abdomen and thighs if needed. *Comments:*	☐	☐	☐	
6. Ensure adequate lighting of the penis and perineal area. *Comments:*	☐	☐	☐	
7. Wash hands, apply disposable gloves, and wash perineal area. *Comments:*	☐	☐	☐	
8. Remove gloves and wash hands. *Comments:*	☐	☐	☐	
9. Open the catheterization kit. Use the wrapper to establish a sterile field. *Comments:*	☐	☐	☐	
10. Add the catheter or any other items needed using sterile technique. *Comments:*	☐	☐	☐	
11. Apply sterile gloves. *Comments:*	☐	☐	☐	

Procedure 6-8	Able to Perform	Able to Perform with Assistance	Unable to Perform	Initials and Date
12. Place the fenestrated drape over the client's perineal area with the penis extending through the opening. *Comments:*	☐	☐	☐	
13. If inserting a retention catheter, attach the syringe filled with sterile water to the Luer-Lok tail of the catheter. Inflate and deflate the retention balloon. Detach the water-filled syringe. *Comments:*	☐	☐	☐	
14. Attach the catheter to the urine drainage bag. *Comments:*	☐	☐	☐	
15. Coat the distal portion of the catheter with water-soluble, sterile lubricant. *Comments:*	☐	☐	☐	
16. With one hand, gently grasp the penis and retract the foreskin (if present). With your other hand, cleanse the glans penis with antimicrobial cleanser. *Comments:*	☐	☐	☐	
17. Hold the penis perpendicular to the body and pull up gently. *Comments:*	☐	☐	☐	
18. Inject 10 ml sterile, water-soluble lubricant into the urethra. *Comments:*	☐	☐	☐	
19. Steadily insert the catheter about 8 inches, until urine is noted. *Comments:*	☐	☐	☐	
20. If the catheter will be removed right away, insert the catheter another inch, place the penis in a comfortable position and hold the catheter in place as the bladder drains. *Comments:*	☐	☐	☐	

continued on the following page

continued from the previous page

Procedure 6-8	Able to Perform	Able to Perform with Assistance	Unable to Perform	Initials and Date
21. If the catheter will be indwelling with a retention balloon, continue inserting until the hub of the catheter is met. *Comments:*	☐	☐	☐	
22. Reattach the water-filled syringe to the inflation port. *Comments:*	☐	☐	☐	
23. Inflate the retention balloon. *Comments:*	☐	☐	☐	
24. If the client experiences pain during balloon inflation, deflate the balloon and insert the catheter farther into the bladder. If the pain continues with balloon inflation, remove the catheter and notify the client's qualified practitioner. *Comments:*	☐	☐	☐	
25. Once the balloon has been inflated, gently pull the catheter until the retention balloon is resting against the bladder neck. *Comments:*	☐	☐	☐	
26. Secure the catheter to either the client's thigh or abdomen. *Comments:*	☐	☐	☐	
27. Place the drainage bag below the level of the bladder. Secure the drainage tubing to prevent pulling. *Comments:*	☐	☐	☐	
28. Remove gloves, dispose of equipment, and wash hands. *Comments:*	☐	☐	☐	
29. Help client adjust position. Lower the bed. *Comments:*	☐	☐	☐	
30. Assess and document properties of the client's urine. *Comments:*	☐	☐	☐	

Checklist for Procedure 6-9 Inserting an Indwelling Catheter: Female

Name _____ Date _____

School _____

Instructor _____

Course _____

Procedure 6-9 Inserting an Indwelling Catheter: Female	Able to Perform	Able to Perform with Assistance	Unable to Perform	Initials and Date
Assessment				
1. Assess the need for catheterization and the type of catheterization ordered. *Comments:*	☐	☐	☐	
2. Assess for the need for peritoneal care prior to catheterization. *Comments:*	☐	☐	☐	
3. Assess the urinary meatus. Ask the client for any history of difficulty with prior catheterizations. *Comments:*	☐	☐	☐	
4. Assess the client's ability to assist with the procedure. *Comments:*	☐	☐	☐	
5. Assess the light. *Comments:*	☐	☐	☐	
6. Assess for an allergy to povidone-iodine. *Comments:*	☐	☐	☐	
7. Watch for indications of distress or embarrassment. *Comments:*	☐	☐	☐	
Planning/Expected Outcomes				
1. The catheter will be inserted without trauma to the client. *Comments:*	☐	☐	☐	
2. The client's bladder will be emptied without complication. *Comments:*	☐	☐	☐	
3. The nurse will maintain the sterility of the catheter during insertion. *Comments:*	☐	☐	☐	

continued on the following page

continued from the previous page

Procedure 6-9	Able to Perform	Able to Perform with Assistance	Unable to Perform	Initials and Date
Implementation				
1. Gather the equipment needed. *Comments:*	☐	☐	☐	
2. Provide for privacy and explain procedure to client. *Comments:*	☐	☐	☐	
3. Set the bed to a comfortable height to work, and raise the opposite side rail. *Comments:*	☐	☐	☐	
4. Assist the client to a supine position with legs spread or to a side-lying position with upper leg flexed. *Comments:*	☐	☐	☐	
5. Drape the client's abdomen and thighs for warmth, if needed. *Comments:*	☐	☐	☐	
6. Ensure adequate lighting of the perineal area. *Comments:*	☐	☐	☐	
7. Wash hands; apply disposable gloves. *Comments:*	☐	☐	☐	
8. Wash perineal area. *Comments:*	☐	☐	☐	
9. Remove gloves and wash hands. *Comments:*	☐	☐	☐	
10. Open the catheterization kit. Use the wrapper to establish a sterile field. *Comments:*	☐	☐	☐	
11. Add the catheter or any other items needed using sterile technique. *Comments:*	☐	☐	☐	
12. Apply sterile gloves. *Comments:*	☐	☐	☐	

Procedure 6-9	Able to Perform	Able to Perform with Assistance	Unable to Perform	Initials and Date
13. If inserting a retention catheter, attach the syringe filled with sterile water to the Luer-Lok tail of the catheter. Inflate and deflate the retention balloon. Detach the water-filled syringe. *Comments:*	☐	☐	☐	
14. Attach the catheter to the urine drainage bag. *Comments:*	☐	☐	☐	
15. Coat the distal portion of the catheter with water-soluble, sterile lubricant. *Comments:*	☐	☐	☐	
16. Place the fenestrated drape over the client's perineal area with the labia visible through the opening. *Comments:*	☐	☐	☐	
17. Gently spread the labia minora with your fingers and visualize the urinary meatus. *Comments:*	☐	☐	☐	
18. Holding the labia apart, use the forceps to pick up a cotton ball soaked in povidone-iodine and cleanse the periurethral mucosa. *Comments:*	☐	☐	☐	
19. Steadily insert the catheter into the meatus until urine is noted. *Comments:*	☐	☐	☐	
20. If the catheter will be removed as soon as the client's bladder is empty, insert the catheter another inch and hold the catheter in place as the bladder drains. *Comments:*	☐	☐	☐	
21. If the catheter will be indwelling with a retention balloon, continue inserting another 1–3 inches. *Comments:*	☐	☐	☐	
22. Reattach the water-filled syringe to the inflation port. *Comments:*	☐	☐	☐	

continued on the following page

continued from the previous page

Procedure 6-9	Able to Perform	Able to Perform with Assistance	Unable to Perform	Initials and Date
23. Inflate the retention balloon. *Comments:*	☐	☐	☐	
24. If the client experiences pain during balloon inflation, deflate the balloon and insert the catheter farther into the bladder. If the pain continues with balloon inflation, remove the catheter and notify the client's qualified practitioner. *Comments:*	☐	☐	☐	
25. Once the balloon has been inflated, gently pull the catheter until the retention balloon is resting against the bladder neck. *Comments:*	☐	☐	☐	
26. Tape the catheter to the abdomen or thigh with enough slack so it will not pull on the bladder. *Comments:*	☐	☐	☐	
27. Place the drainage bag below the level of the bladder. *Comments:*	☐	☐	☐	
28. Remove gloves, dispose of equipment, and wash hands. *Comments:*	☐	☐	☐	
29. Help client adjust position. Lower the bed. *Comments:*	☐	☐	☐	
30. Assess and document the urine's properties. *Comments:*	☐	☐	☐	
31. Wash hands. *Comments:*	☐	☐	☐	

Checklist for Procedure 6-10   Routine Catheter Care

Name _____ Date _____

School _____

Instructor _____

Course _____

Procedure 6-10 Routine Catheter Care	Able to Perform	Able to Perform with Assistance	Unable to Perform	Initials and Date
Assessment				
1. Assess catheter patency and urine color, consistency, and amount while doing the care. *Comments:*	☐	☐	☐	
2. Determine the condition of the urinary meatus and perineal area. *Comments:*	☐	☐	☐	
3. Determine the client's emotional reaction and feelings related to the catheter. *Comments:*	☐	☐	☐	
Planning/Expected Outcomes				
1. The client will be free of symptoms of urinary tract infection. *Comments:*	☐	☐	☐	
2. The client will understand the reason for the catheter and related cares. *Comments:*	☐	☐	☐	
3. The meatus and surrounding area will be clean and intact. *Comments:*	☐	☐	☐	
Implementation				
1. Wash hands. *Comments:*	☐	☐	☐	
2. Check agency protocol or care plan. *Comments:*	☐	☐	☐	

continued on the following page

continued from the previous page

Procedure 6-10	Able to Perform	Able to Perform with Assistance	Unable to Perform	Initials and Date
3. Identify client and explain procedure. *Comments:*	☐	☐	☐	
4. Provide privacy. *Comments:*	☐	☐	☐	
5. Place client in supine position and expose perineal area and catheter. *Comments:*	☐	☐	☐	
6. Put on clean gloves. *Comments:*	☐	☐	☐	
7. Cleanse perineal area with soap and water. *Comments:*	☐	☐	☐	
8. Cleanse meatus in circular motion from the most inner surface to the outside. Use soap and water. *Comments:*	☐	☐	☐	
9. Cleanse catheter from meatus out to end of catheter, taking care not to pull on catheter. *Comments:*	☐	☐	☐	
10. Be sure to repeat catheter care any time it becomes soiled. *Comments:*	☐	☐	☐	
11. Place linen or cotton balls in proper receptacle. *Comments:*	☐	☐	☐	
12. Wash hands. *Comments:*	☐	☐	☐	

Checklist for Procedure 6-11 Obtaining a Residual Urine Specimen from an Indwelling Catheter

Name _____ Date _____

School _____

Instructor _____

Course _____

Procedure 6-11 Obtaining a Residual Urine Specimen from an Indwelling Catheter	Able to Perform	Able to Perform with Assistance	Unable to Perform	Initials and Date
Assessment				
1. Identify the purpose of the urine test. *Comments:*	☐	☐	☐	
2. Assess the client's ability to understand purpose of the test. *Comments:*	☐	☐	☐	
3. Identify the type of collecting tubing attached to the indwelling catheter. *Comments:*	☐	☐	☐	
Planning/Expected Outcomes				
1. Client will understand the reason for the specimen. *Comments:*	☐	☐	☐	
2. Specimen will be obtained in the proper container in a timely manner. *Comments:*	☐	☐	☐	
3. Specimen will remain uncontaminated. *Comments:*	☐	☐	☐	
Implementation				
1. Wash hands. *Comments:*	☐	☐	☐	
2. Check physician's or qualified practitioner's order. *Comments:*	☐	☐	☐	
3. Explain procedure to the client and provide privacy. *Comments:*	☐	☐	☐	

continued on the following page

continued from the previous page

Procedure 6-11	Able to Perform	Able to Perform with Assistance	Unable to Perform	Initials and Date
4. Check for urine in the tubing. *Comments:*	☐	☐	☐	
5. If more urine is needed, clamp the tubing for 10–15 minutes. *Comments:*	☐	☐	☐	
6. Put on clean gloves. *Comments:*	☐	☐	☐	
7. Clean sample port or the catheter with a betadine swab. *Comments:*	☐	☐	☐	
8. Insert sterile needle and syringe into the sample port or catheter at a 45° angle and withdraw 10 ml of urine. *Comments:*	☐	☐	☐	
9. Put urine into sterile container and close tightly. *Comments:*	☐	☐	☐	
10. Remove clamp and rearrange tubing, avoiding dependent loops. *Comments:*	☐	☐	☐	
11. Label specimen container, put it in a plastic bag, and send to the laboratory. *Comments:*	☐	☐	☐	
12. Wash hands *Comments:*	☐	☐	☐	

Checklist for Procedure 6-12   Irrigating a Urinary Catheter

Name _____ Date _____

School _____

Instructor _____

Course _____

Procedure 6-12 Irrigating a Urinary Catheter	Able to Perform	Able to Perform with Assistance	Unable to Perform	Initials and Date
Assessment				
1. Assess the written order for type and purpose of the irrigation. *Comments:*	☐	☐	☐	
2. Assess the condition of the client. *Comments:*	☐	☐	☐	
3. Assess for current pain or bladder spasms. *Comments:*	☐	☐	☐	
4. Assess client's knowledge about the procedure. *Comments:*	☐	☐	☐	
5. If this is a repeat of the procedure, read the charting from previous nurses. *Comments:*	☐	☐	☐	
Planning/Expected Outcomes				
1. Urinary catheter will be patent. *Comments:*	☐	☐	☐	
2. Sediment/blood clots will be passed through the catheter. *Comments:*	☐	☐	☐	
3. Bladder will be free of sources of local irritation. *Comments:*	☐	☐	☐	
4. Urinary pH will be assisted to a more acidic state. *Comments:*	☐	☐	☐	

continued on the following page

continued from the previous page

Procedure 6-12	Able to Perform	Able to Perform with Assistance	Unable to Perform	Initials and Date
Implementation				
1. Verify the need for bladder or catheter irrigation. *Comments:*	☐	☐	☐	
2. For prn irrigation, palpate for full bladder and check current output against previous totals. *Comments:*	☐	☐	☐	
3. Verify written orders for type of irrigation and irrigant, as well as amount. *Comments:*	☐	☐	☐	
4. If repeat procedure, read previous documentation in the record. *Comments:*	☐	☐	☐	
5. Assemble all supplies. *Comments:*	☐	☐	☐	
6. Premedicate client if ordered or needed. *Comments:*	☐	☐	☐	
7. Provide teaching to the client as needed. *Comments:*	☐	☐	☐	
8. Assist the client to a dorsal recumbent position. *Comments:*	☐	☐	☐	
9. Wash your hands. *Comments:*	☐	☐	☐	
10. Provide for client privacy. *Comments:*	☐	☐	☐	
11. Empty the collection bag of urine. *Comments:*	☐	☐	☐	
12. Expose the retention catheter and place the water-resistant drape underneath it. *Comments:*	☐	☐	☐	

Procedure 6-12	Able to Perform	Able to Perform with Assistance	Unable to Perform	Initials and Date
13. Open the sterile syringe and container. Stand sterile container with syringe up and add 100–200 cc sterile diluent. *Comments:*	☐	☐	☐	
14. Open the antiseptic swab package, exposing the swab sticks. *Comments:*	☐	☐	☐	
15. Open the sterile cover for drainage tube. *Comments:*	☐	☐	☐	
16. Apply the sterile gloves. *Comments:*	☐	☐	☐	
17. Disinfect the connection between the catheter and the drainage tubing. *Comments:*	☐	☐	☐	
18. Loosen the ends of the connection. *Comments:*	☐	☐	☐	
19. Grasp the catheter and tubing 1–2 inches from their ends, with the catheter in the nondominant hand. *Comments:*	☐	☐	☐	
20. Pinch the catheter closed; use the thumb and first finger to hold the sterile cap for the drainage tube. *Comments:*	☐	☐	☐	
21. Separate the catheter and tube, covering the tube tightly with the sterile cap. *Comments:*	☐	☐	☐	
22. Fill the syringe with irrigant. Insert the tip of the syringe into the catheter and instill the solution into the catheter. *Comments:*	☐	☐	☐	
23. Clamp catheter if ordered; if not, drain or aspirate irrigant. *Comments:*	☐	☐	☐	

continued on the following page

continued from the previous page

Procedure 6-12	Able to Perform	Able to Perform with Assistance	Unable to Perform	Initials and Date
24. If irrigation is to clear solid material, repeat irrigation until return is clear. *Comments:*	☐	☐	☐	
25. Reconnect system and remove sterile gloves. Wash your hands. *Comments:*	☐	☐	☐	
26. Chart type of returns and total amount of irrigation fluid used. *Comments:*	☐	☐	☐	
27. Monitor client's condition. *Comments:*	☐	☐	☐	
28. Wash hands. *Comments:*	☐	☐	☐	

Checklist for Procedure 6-13   Irrigating the Bladder Using a Closed-System Catheter

Name _____ Date _____

School _____

Instructor _____

Course _____

Procedure 6-13 Irrigating the Bladder Using a Closed-System Catheter	Able to Perform	Able to Perform with Assistance	Unable to Perform	Initials and Date
Assessment				
1. Assess for bladder distention or complaints of fullness. Comments:	☐	☐	☐	
2. Assess the drainage system for equal or larger amounts of drainage versus infused irrigant. Comments:	☐	☐	☐	
3. Assess the bladder drainage noting any clots or debris present. Comments:	☐	☐	☐	
Planning/Expected Outcomes				
1. The client will not exhibit symptoms of infection. Comments:	☐	☐	☐	
2. The client will not experience pain or discomfort. Comments:	☐	☐	☐	
3. The catheter will remain patent, and the bladder will not be distended. Comments:	☐	☐	☐	
Implementation				
Intermittent Bladder Irrigation Using a Standard Retention Catheter and a Y Adapter				
1. Wash hands. Comments:	☐	☐	☐	
2. Close privacy curtain or door. Comments:	☐	☐	☐	
3. Hang the prescribed irrigation solution from an IV pole. Comments:	☐	☐	☐	

continued on the following page

continued from the previous page

Procedure 6-13	Able to Perform	Able to Perform with Assistance	Unable to Perform	Initials and Date
4. Insert the clamped irrigation tubing into the irrigant and prime the tubing with fluid. *Comments:*	☐	☐	☐	
5. Prepare sterile antiseptic swabs and sterile Y connector. *Comments:*	☐	☐	☐	
6. Apply sterile gloves. *Comments:*	☐	☐	☐	
7. Clamp the urinary catheter. *Comments:*	☐	☐	☐	
8. Unhook the drainage bag from the retention catheter. *Comments:*	☐	☐	☐	
9. Cleanse both the drainage tubing and the drainage port with antiseptic swabs. *Comments:*	☐	☐	☐	
10. Connect the Y connector to the drainage port of the retention catheter. *Comments:*	☐	☐	☐	
11. Connect the Y adapter to the drainage tubing and bag. *Comments:*	☐	☐	☐	
12. Attach the third port of the Y adapter to the irrigant tubing. *Comments:*	☐	☐	☐	
13. Unclamp the catheter and reestablish urine drainage. *Comments:*	☐	☐	☐	
14. To irrigate the catheter and bladder, clamp the drainage tubing. *Comments:*	☐	☐	☐	
15. Infuse the prescribed amount of irrigant. *Comments:*	☐	☐	☐	

Procedure 6-13	Able to Perform	Able to Perform with Assistance	Unable to Perform	Initials and Date
16. Clamp the irrigant tubing. *Comments:*	☐	☐	☐	
17. If the irrigant is to remain in the bladder for a measured length of time, wait the prescribed length of time. *Comments:*	☐	☐	☐	
18. Unclamp the drainage tubing and monitor the drainage. *Comments:*	☐	☐	☐	
Closed Bladder Irrigation Using a Three-Way Catheter 19. Wash hands. *Comments:*	☐	☐	☐	
20. Close privacy curtain or door. *Comments:*	☐	☐	☐	
21. Explain the procedure to the client. *Comments:*	☐	☐	☐	
22. Hang the prescribed irrigation solution from an IV pole. *Comments:*	☐	☐	☐	
23. Insert the clamped irrigation tubing into the bottle of irrigant and prime the tubing. *Comments:*	☐	☐	☐	
24. Prepare sterile antiseptic swabs and other sterile equipment. *Comments:*	☐	☐	☐	
25. Apply sterile gloves. *Comments:*	☐	☐	☐	
26. Clamp the urinary catheter. *Comments:*	☐	☐	☐	
27. Remove the cap from the irrigation port of the three-way catheter. *Comments:*	☐	☐	☐	

continued on the following page

continued from the previous page

Procedure 6-13	Able to Perform	Able to Perform with Assistance	Unable to Perform	Initials and Date
28. Cleanse the irrigation port with the sterile antiseptic swabs. *Comments:*	☐	☐	☐	
29. Attach the irrigation tubing to the irrigation port of the three-way catheter. *Comments:*	☐	☐	☐	
30. Remove the clamp from the catheter and observe for urine drainage. *Comments:*	☐	☐	☐	
31. If intermittent irrigation has been ordered: Infuse the prescribed amount of irrigant. *Comments:*	☐	☐	☐	
32. Clamp the irrigant tubing. *Comments:*	☐	☐	☐	
33. If the irrigant is to remain in the bladder for a measured time, clamp the drainage tube prior to infusing the irrigant and wait the prescribed length of time. *Comments:*	☐	☐	☐	
34. Monitor the drainage as it flows into the drainage bag. *Comments:*	☐	☐	☐	
35. If continuous bladder irrigation has been ordered: Adjust the clamp on the irrigation tubing so the prescribed rate of irrigant flows. *Comments:*	☐	☐	☐	
36. Monitor the drainage as it flows back into the drainage bag. *Comments:*	☐	☐	☐	
37. Tape the catheter securely to the thigh. *Comments:*	☐	☐	☐	
38. Wash hands. *Comments:*	☐	☐	☐	

Checklist for Procedure 6-14   Removing an Indwelling Catheter

Name _____ Date _____

School _____

Instructor _____

Course _____

Procedure 6-14 Removing an Indwelling Catheter	Able to Perform	Able to Perform with Assistance	Unable to Perform	Initials and Date
Assessment				
1. Determine previous history and rationale for current treatment. *Comments:*	☐	☐	☐	
2. Assess client for signs of infection and current condition of urinary meatus and perineal area. *Comments:*	☐	☐	☐	
3. Assess client for understanding and ability to cooperate. *Comments:*	☐	☐	☐	
4. Assess room setup for availability of bathroom facilities. *Comments:*	☐	☐	☐	
Planning/Expected Outcomes				
1. Catheter will be removed intact. *Comments:*	☐	☐	☐	
2. Client will void within 8 hours of removal without discomfort. *Comments:*	☐	☐	☐	
3. Client will not develop any complications related to removal. *Comments:*	☐	☐	☐	
4. Client will verbalize understanding of the procedure and will notify staff of voiding or of difficulty with voiding. *Comments:*	☐	☐	☐	

continued on the following page

continued from the previous page

Procedure 6-14	Able to Perform	Able to Perform with Assistance	Unable to Perform	Initials and Date
Implementation				
1. Wash hands. *Comments:*	☐	☐	☐	
2. Check written order and unit protocol. *Comments:*	☐	☐	☐	
3. Identify client and explain procedure. *Comments:*	☐	☐	☐	
4. Provide privacy and position client on back. *Comments:*	☐	☐	☐	
5. Remove covers and drape to expose catheter. *Comments:*	☐	☐	☐	
6. Apply nonsterile gloves. *Comments:*	☐	☐	☐	
7. Place protective pad under client's thighs. *Comments:*	☐	☐	☐	
8. Empty urine in tubing into catheter bag. *Comments:*	☐	☐	☐	
9. Remove any tape holding the catheter to the leg. *Comments:*	☐	☐	☐	
10. Insert syringe end into balloon port and remove all air or fluid from the balloon. *Comments:*	☐	☐	☐	
11. Ask the client to take a deep breath (if able) and remove the catheter on expiration. Stop if you meet resistance. *Comments:*	☐	☐	☐	
12. Note any debris on the catheter. If needed, culture tip of catheter. *Comments:*	☐	☐	☐	

Procedure 6-14	Able to Perform	Able to Perform with Assistance	Unable to Perform	Initials and Date
13. Cleanse the perineal area or allow client to cleanse the area. Remove materials. Assist client to position of comfort. *Comments:*	☐	☐	☐	
14. Instruct the client to drink oral fluids and to call when he or she needs to void. Record time and amount of first voiding. *Comments:*	☐	☐	☐	
15. If unable to void within 8 hours, report to the qualified practitioner. *Comments:*	☐	☐	☐	
16. Wash hands. *Comments:*	☐	☐	☐	

Checklist for Procedure 6-15   Catheterizing a Noncontinent Urinary Diversion

Name _____ Date _____

School _____

Instructor _____

Course _____

Procedure 6-15 **Catheterizing a Noncontinent Urinary Diversion**	Able to Perform	Able to Perform with Assistance	Unable to Perform	Initials and Date
Assessment				
1. Inspect the stoma for color and texture. *Comments:*	☐	☐	☐	
2. Observe the color and odor of the urine. *Comments:*	☐	☐	☐	
Planning/Expected Outcomes				
1. Client will express positive feelings about self. *Comments:*	☐	☐	☐	
2. Client will voice understanding of the procedure. *Comments:*	☐	☐	☐	
3. The stoma and peristomal skin will not be traumatized. *Comments:*	☐	☐	☐	
4. The client will not suffer infection secondary to this procedure. *Comments:*	☐	☐	☐	
Implementation				
1. Wash hands. *Comments:*	☐	☐	☐	
2. Assemble equipment. *Comments:*	☐	☐	☐	
3. Apply clean gloves. *Comments:*	☐	☐	☐	
4. Remove current ostomy appliance. *Comments:*	☐	☐	☐	

continued on the following page

continued from the previous page

Procedure 6-15	Able to Perform	Able to Perform with Assistance	Unable to Perform	Initials and Date
5. Dispose of appliance appropriately. *Comments:*	☐	☐	☐	
6. Wash hands. *Comments:*	☐	☐	☐	
7. Open all sterile equipment. *Comments:*	☐	☐	☐	
8. Squeeze water-soluble jelly onto sterile field of an opened package. *Comments:*	☐	☐	☐	
9. Apply sterile gloves. *Comments:*	☐	☐	☐	
10. Lubricate one gloved finger and insert into orifice of stoma. *Comments:*	☐	☐	☐	
11. Cleanse stoma with povidone-iodine. Pat dry. *Comments:*	☐	☐	☐	
12. Wipe excess povidone-iodine off of stoma. *Comments:*	☐	☐	☐	
13. Holding catheter, lubricate tip with water-soluble jelly. *Comments:*	☐	☐	☐	
14. Gently insert catheter into orifice of stoma. *Comments:*	☐	☐	☐	
15. Place other end of catheter into sterile container to collect urine. *Comments:*	☐	☐	☐	
16. If urine does not readily drain, apply slight suction using a sterile syringe. *Comments:*	☐	☐	☐	

continued from the previous page

Procedure 6-15	Able to Perform	Able to Perform with Assistance	Unable to Perform	Initials and Date
17. After collecting a sample, remove and dispose of catheter appropriately. *Comments:*	☐	☐	☐	
18. Label container and send to laboratory. *Comments:*	☐	☐	☐	
19. Cleanse stoma and skin with warm tap water. Pat dry. *Comments:*	☐	☐	☐	
20. If replacing the entire appliance, measure stoma at base. *Comments:*	☐	☐	☐	
21. Place gauze or slender tampon into orifice of stoma to wick urine. *Comments:*	☐	☐	☐	
22. Trace pattern onto paper backing of wafer. *Comments:*	☐	☐	☐	
23. Cut wafer as traced. *Comments:*	☐	☐	☐	
24. Attach clean pouch to wafer. Make sure port is closed. *Comments:*	☐	☐	☐	
25. Remove wick from orifice of stoma. *Comments:*	☐	☐	☐	
26. Remove paper backing from wafer and place on skin with stoma centered in cutout of wafer. *Comments:*	☐	☐	☐	
27. Remove gloves; wash hands. *Comments:*	☐	☐	☐	

Checklist for Procedure 6-16   Maintaining a Continent Urinary Diversion

Name _____ Date _____

School _____

Instructor _____

Course _____

Procedure 6-16 **Maintaining a Continent Urinary Diversion**	Able to Perform	Able to Perform with Assistance	Unable to Perform	Initials and Date
Assessment				
1. Inspect the stoma for color and texture, if present. *Comments:*	☐	☐	☐	
2. Inspect the condition of the skin surrounding the stoma. *Comments:*	☐	☐	☐	
3. Inspect all tubes and drains. *Comments:*	☐	☐	☐	
Planning/Expected Outcomes				
1. Peristomal skin integrity will remain intact. *Comments:*	☐	☐	☐	
2. Irritated or denuded peristomal skin integrity will heal. *Comments:*	☐	☐	☐	
3. Client will acknowledge the change in body image and express positive feelings about self. *Comments:*	☐	☐	☐	
4. Client will maintain fluid balance. *Comments:*	☐	☐	☐	
5. Client will express understanding regarding the urinary diversion. *Comments:*	☐	☐	☐	
6. Instruct client to report changes in urine flow or difficulty catheterizing and/or flushing nonbladder to wound/ostomy care nurse. *Comments:*	☐	☐	☐	

continued on the following page

continued from the previous page

Procedure 6-16	Able to Perform	Able to Perform with Assistance	Unable to Perform	Initials and Date
Implementation				
Flushing Tubes and Drains				
1. Wash hands. *Comments:*	☐	☐	☐	
2. Assemble equipment. *Comments:*	☐	☐	☐	
3. Pour normal saline into a basin. *Comments:*	☐	☐	☐	
4. Open remaining sterile packages. *Comments:*	☐	☐	☐	
5. Apply sterile gloves. *Comments:*	☐	☐	☐	
6. Draw up 30 ml of normal saline into piston syringe. *Comments:*	☐	☐	☐	
7. Disconnect the tube into the stoma from the drainage system. *Comments:*	☐	☐	☐	
8. Attach syringe to catheter marked for the stoma. *Comments:*	☐	☐	☐	
9. Flush catheter until irrigant is free of mucus strands. *Comments:*	☐	☐	☐	
10. Reconnect Foley/tube to drainage system. *Comments:*	☐	☐	☐	
11. Repeat for additional catheters or stents using a new sterile syringe for each catheter. *Comments:*	☐	☐	☐	
12. Wash hands. *Comments:*	☐	☐	☐	

Procedure 6-16	Able to Perform	Able to Perform with Assistance	Unable to Perform	Initials and Date
Catheterizing Continent Urinary Diversion 13. Wash hands. Comments:	☐	☐	☐	
14. Assemble equipment. Comments:	☐	☐	☐	
15. Open packages. Comments:	☐	☐	☐	
16. Apply sterile gloves. Comments:	☐	☐	☐	
17. Draw up 30 ml of normal saline into piston syringe. Comments:	☐	☐	☐	
18. Gently insert catheter into new bladder. Comments:	☐	☐	☐	
19. Place other end of catheter into container. Comments:	☐	☐	☐	
20. Irrigate new bladder with normal saline until irrigant is free of mucus strands. Comments:	☐	☐	☐	
21. Remove catheter. Comments:	☐	☐	☐	
22. Apply Band-Aid over stoma. Comments:	☐	☐	☐	
23. In hospital, dispose of catheter. At home, client can reuse catheters. Comments:	☐	☐	☐	
24. Wash hands. Comments:	☐	☐	☐	

Checklist for Procedure 6-17   Pouching a Noncontinent Urinary Diversion

Name _____ Date _____

School _____

Instructor _____

Course _____

Procedure 6-17 **Pouching a Noncontinent Urinary Diversion**	Able to Perform	Able to Perform with Assistance	Unable to Perform	Initials and Date
Assessment				
1. Inspect the stoma for color and texture. *Comments:*	☐	☐	☐	
2. Inspect the condition of the skin surrounding the stoma. *Comments:*	☐	☐	☐	
3. Measure the dimensions of the stoma. *Comments:*	☐	☐	☐	
4. Inspect stents for appropriate placement and drainage. *Comments:*	☐	☐	☐	
Planning/Expected Outcomes				
1. Peristomal skin integrity will remain intact. *Comments:*	☐	☐	☐	
2. Irritated or denuded peristomal skin integrity will heal. *Comments:*	☐	☐	☐	
3. Client will acknowledge the change in body image. *Comments:*	☐	☐	☐	
4. Client will express positive feelings about self. *Comments:*	☐	☐	☐	
5. Client will maintain fluid balance. *Comments:*	☐	☐	☐	
Implementation				
1. Wash hands. *Comments:*	☐	☐	☐	

continued on the following page

continued from the previous page

Procedure 6-17	Able to Perform	Able to Perform with Assistance	Unable to Perform	Initials and Date
2. Assemble clean urinary pouch and wafer. *Comments:*	☐	☐	☐	
3. Apply clean gloves. *Comments:*	☐	☐	☐	
4. Empty urine and remove current ostomy appliance. *Comments:*	☐	☐	☐	
5. Dispose of old appliance and contaminated gloves appropriately. *Comments:*	☐	☐	☐	
6. Wash hands. *Comments:*	☐	☐	☐	
7. Apply clean gloves. *Comments:*	☐	☐	☐	
8. Cleanse stoma and skin with warm tap water. Pat dry. *Comments:*	☐	☐	☐	
9. Measure stoma at base. *Comments:*	☐	☐	☐	
10. Place gauze or slender tampon into orifice of stoma to wick urine. *Comments:*	☐	☐	☐	
11. Trace pattern onto paper backing of wafer. *Comments:*	☐	☐	☐	
12. Cut wafer as traced. *Comments:*	☐	☐	☐	
13. Remove paper backing from wafer and place on skin with stoma centered in opening of wafer. *Comments:*	☐	☐	☐	

Procedure 6-17	Able to Perform	Able to Perform with Assistance	Unable to Perform	Initials and Date
14. Remove wick from orifice of stoma. *Comments:*	☐	☐	☐	
15. Attach clean pouch to wafer. Make sure drainage port is closed. *Comments:*	☐	☐	☐	
16. Remove gloves and wash hands. *Comments:*	☐	☐	☐	

Checklist for Procedure 6-18   Administering Peritoneal Dialysis

Name _____ Date _____

School _____

Instructor _____

Course _____

Procedure 6-18 **Administering Peritoneal Dialysis**	Able to Perform	Able to Perform with Assistance	Unable to Perform	Initials and Date
Assessment				
1. Assess the client's cardiovascular and respiratory status. *Comments:*	☐	☐	☐	
2. Measure the client's abdominal girth. *Comments:*	☐	☐	☐	
3. Assess the client's abdomen. *Comments:*	☐	☐	☐	
Planning/Expected Outcomes				
1. Client will experience relief of respiratory symptoms. *Comments:*	☐	☐	☐	
2. Client will experience relief of symptoms from nitrogenous waste products. *Comments:*	☐	☐	☐	
3. Client will not suffer from fluid volume overload or deficit. *Comments:*	☐	☐	☐	
4. Client will not exhibit any signs or symptoms of infection. *Comments:*	☐	☐	☐	
5. The skin at the catheter entry site will remain intact. *Comments:*	☐	☐	☐	
6. Client will not experience pain or discomfort. *Comments:*	☐	☐	☐	

continued on the following page

continued from the previous page

Procedure 6-18	Able to Perform	Able to Perform with Assistance	Unable to Perform	Initials and Date
Implementation				
1. Warm the dialysate to body temperature. Gather needed equipment and bring it to the bedside. *Comments:*	☐	☐	☐	
2. Wash hands; apply clean gloves. *Comments:*	☐	☐	☐	
3. Position the client in a comfortable position. *Comments:*	☐	☐	☐	
4. Weigh the dialysate. *Comments:*	☐	☐	☐	
5. Spike the dialysate bag with the tubing, hang the bag from an IV pole, and prime the tubing. *Comments:*	☐	☐	☐	
6. Establish a sterile field under the peritoneal catheter, using the sterile drape. *Comments:*	☐	☐	☐	
7. Open the povidone-iodine swabs aseptically and drop them onto the sterile field. If using sterile 4 × 4s, pour povidone-iodine into the sterile basin. Aseptically drop the 4 × 4s into the povidone-iodine in the basin. *Comments:*	☐	☐	☐	
8. Apply sterile gloves. *Comments:*	☐	☐	☐	
9. Using the povidone-iodine swabs, cleanse the proximal end of the catheter. Allow the povidone-iodine to dry. *Comments:*	☐	☐	☐	
10. Attach the infusion tubing and dialysate to the dialysis catheter. Hang the dialysate on a pole. *Comments:*	☐	☐	☐	
11. Unclamp the tubing and allow dialysate to enter the abdomen. *Comments:*	☐	☐	☐	

Procedure 6-18	Able to Perform	Able to Perform with Assistance	Unable to Perform	Initials and Date
12. Assess the client for pain or discomfort. *Comments:*	☐	☐	☐	
13. When the ordered amount of dialysate has been infused, clamp the dialysis tubing for the ordered amount of dwell time. *Comments:*	☐	☐	☐	
14. Wash hands after infusing the dialysate and prior to draining the effluent. *Comments:*	☐	☐	☐	
15. After the specified dwell time, place the empty bag below the level of the peritoneum. Unclamp the tubing and allow the effluent to drain into the empty bag. *Comments:*	☐	☐	☐	
16. Periodically weigh the effluent as the abdomen drains. When the effluent weight has been stable for 10–15 minutes, clamp the drainage tubing. *Comments:*	☐	☐	☐	
17. Hold the full bag up to the light and inspect the fluid. *Comments:*	☐	☐	☐	
18. Compare the weight of the returned fluid with the preinfusion weight. *Comments:*	☐	☐	☐	
19. Ensure that any laboratory tests ordered are performed. *Comments:*	☐	☐	☐	
20. Wash hands after disconnecting the effluent and prior to connecting a new bag of dialysate. *Comments:*	☐	☐	☐	
21. Warm and connect the next bag of dialysate and repeat the process. Use new tubing for each bag. *Comments:*	☐	☐	☐	

Checklist for Procedure 6-19   Administering an Enema

Name _____ Date _____

School _____

Instructor _____

Course _____

Procedure 6-19 Administering an Enema	Able to Perform	Able to Perform with Assistance	Unable to Perform	Initials and Date
Assessment				
1. Identify the type of enema and rationale of the ordered enema. *Comments:*	☐	☐	☐	
2. Assess the physical condition of the client. *Comments:*	☐	☐	☐	
3. Assess the client's mental state. *Comments:*	☐	☐	☐	
Planning/Expected Outcomes				
1. The client's rectum will be free of feces and flatus. *Comments:*	☐	☐	☐	
2. The client will experience a minimum of trauma and embarrassment. *Comments:*	☐	☐	☐	
Implementation				
Large Volume, Cleansing Enema 1. Wash hands. *Comments:*	☐	☐	☐	
2. Assess client's understanding of procedure. Provide privacy. *Comments:*	☐	☐	☐	
3. Apply gloves. *Comments:*	☐	☐	☐	
4. Prepare equipment. *Comments:*	☐	☐	☐	

continued on the following page

continued from the previous page

Procedure 6-19	Able to Perform	Able to Perform with Assistance	Unable to Perform	Initials and Date
5. Place absorbent pad on bed under client. Assist client into left lateral position. *Comments:*	☐	☐	☐	
6. Heat solution to desired temperature. *Comments:*	☐	☐	☐	
7. Pour solution into the bag or bucket. Open clamp and prime tubing. *Comments:*	☐	☐	☐	
8. Lubricate 5 cm of the rectal tube unless the tube is prelubricated. *Comments:*	☐	☐	☐	
9. Hold the enema container level with the rectum. Have the client take a deep breath. Simultaneously insert rectal tube into rectum. *Comments:*	☐	☐	☐	
10. Squeeze the solution container or raise it to the appropriate height and open clamp. *Comments:*	☐	☐	☐	
11. Slowly administer the fluid. *Comments:*	☐	☐	☐	
12. When solution has been administered or the client cannot hold more fluid, clamp and remove the rectal tube, disposing of it properly. *Comments:*	☐	☐	☐	
13. Clean lubricant, solution, and any feces from the anus with toilet tissue. *Comments:*	☐	☐	☐	
14. Have the client continue to lie on the left side for the prescribed length of time. *Comments:*	☐	☐	☐	

Procedure 6-19	Able to Perform	Able to Perform with Assistance	Unable to Perform	Initials and Date
15. When the enema has been retained the prescribed amount of time, assist client to the bedside commode, toilet, or bedpan. *Comments:*	☐	☐	☐	
16. When the client is finished, assist to clean the perineal area. *Comments:*	☐	☐	☐	
17. Return the client to a comfortable position with a protective pad in place. *Comments:*	☐	☐	☐	
18. Observe feces and document data. *Comments:*	☐	☐	☐	
19. Remove gloves and wash hands. *Comments:*	☐	☐	☐	
Small Volume, Prepackaged Enema 20. Wash hands. *Comments:*	☐	☐	☐	
21. Remove prepackaged enema from packaging. Warm the fluid prior to use. *Comments:*	☐	☐	☐	
22. Apply gloves. *Comments:*	☐	☐	☐	
23. Place absorbent pad under client. Assist client into left lateral position. *Comments:*	☐	☐	☐	
24. Remove the protective cap from the nozzle. Lubricate as needed. *Comments:*	☐	☐	☐	
25. Squeeze the container to remove any air and prime the nozzle. *Comments:*	☐	☐	☐	

continued on the following page

continued from the previous page

Procedure 6-19	Able to Perform	Able to Perform with Assistance	Unable to Perform	Initials and Date
26. Have the client take a deep breath and insert the enema nozzle into the anus. Comments:	☐	☐	☐	
27. Squeeze the container until all the solution is instilled. Comments:	☐	☐	☐	
28. Remove the nozzle from the anus and dispose of the container appropriately. Comments:	☐	☐	☐	
29. Clean lubricant, solution, and any feces from the anus with toilet tissue. Comments:	☐	☐	☐	
30. Have the client continue to lie on the left side for the prescribed length of time. Comments:	☐	☐	☐	
31. After the prescribed amount of time, assist client to the commode, toilet, or bedpan. Comments:	☐	☐	☐	
32. When the client is finished, assist to clean the perineal area. Comments:	☐	☐	☐	
33. Return the client to a comfortable position on a protective pad. Comments:	☐	☐	☐	
34. Observe feces and document data. Comments:	☐	☐	☐	
35. Remove gloves and wash hands. Comments:	☐	☐	☐	
Return-Flow Enema 36. Wash hands. Comments:	☐	☐	☐	

Procedure 6-19	Able to Perform	Able to Perform with Assistance	Unable to Perform	Initials and Date
37. Assess if client understands procedure. *Comments:*	☐	☐	☐	
38. Apply gloves. *Comments:*	☐	☐	☐	
39. Place absorbent pad on bed under client and assist into left lateral position. *Comments:*	☐	☐	☐	
40. Heat solution to desired temperature. *Comments:*	☐	☐	☐	
41. Pour solution into the bag or bucket, open clamp, and prime tubing. Clamp tubing when primed. *Comments:*	☐	☐	☐	
42. Lubricate 5 cm of the rectal tube unless the tube is prelubricated. *Comments:*	☐	☐	☐	
43. Hold the enema container level with the rectum. Have the client take a deep breath. Simultaneously insert rectal tube into rectum. *Comments:*	☐	☐	☐	
44. Raise the solution container to the appropriate height and open clamp. *Comments:*	☐	☐	☐	
45. Slowly administer approximately 200 cc of solution. *Comments:*	☐	☐	☐	
46. Clamp the tubing and lower the enema container 12–18 inches below the client's rectum. Open the clamp. *Comments:*	☐	☐	☐	
47. Observe the solution container for air bubbles and fecal particles as the solution returns. *Comments:*	☐	☐	☐	

continued on the following page

continued from the previous page

Procedure 6-19	Able to Perform	Able to Perform with Assistance	Unable to Perform	Initials and Date
48. When no further solution is returned, clamp the tubing and raise the enema container as before. Open the clamp and instill approximately 200 cc of fluid. *Comments:*	☐	☐	☐	
49. Repeat until no further flatus is seen or the institutional guidelines have been met. *Comments:*	☐	☐	☐	
50. After the final return, clamp and remove the tubing. Clean the anus with tissue. *Comments:*	☐	☐	☐	
51. If the client needs to empty the rectum, assist him or her to the bedpan, bathroom, or commode. *Comments:*	☐	☐	☐	
52. When the client is finished, assist in cleaning the perineal area. *Comments:*	☐	☐	☐	
53. Return the client to a comfortable position on a protective pad. *Comments:*	☐	☐	☐	
54. Observe any expelled solution and document the results of the enema. *Comments:*	☐	☐	☐	
55. Remove gloves and wash hands. *Comments:*	☐	☐	☐	

Checklist for Procedure 6-20   Digital Removal of Fecal Impaction

Name _____ Date _____

School _____

Instructor _____

Course _____

Procedure 6-20 **Digital Removal of Fecal Impaction**	Able to Perform	Able to Perform with Assistance	Unable to Perform	Initials and Date
Assessment				
1. Assess the date and quality of client's last bowel movement. *Comments:*	☐	☐	☐	
2. Assess the client for signs of fecal impaction. *Comments:*	☐	☐	☐	
3. Assess the condition of the client's perianal area. *Comments:*	☐	☐	☐	
4. Auscultate bowel sounds. *Comments:*	☐	☐	☐	
Planning/Expected Outcomes				
1. The client's rectum will be free of feces. *Comments:*	☐	☐	☐	
2. The client will experience a minimum of discomfort and embarrassment. *Comments:*	☐	☐	☐	
3. The client will not experience any adverse side effects. *Comments:*	☐	☐	☐	
Implementation				
1. Wash hands. *Comments:*	☐	☐	☐	
2. Assemble equipment. *Comments:*	☐	☐	☐	
3. Explain procedure to client. *Comments:*	☐	☐	☐	

continued on the following page

continued from the previous page

Procedure 6-20	Able to Perform	Able to Perform with Assistance	Unable to Perform	Initials and Date
4. Position client in the left lateral position with upper leg bent over lower leg. *Comments:*	☐	☐	☐	
5. Place disposable pads underneath client. Position a bedpan nearby. *Comments:*	☐	☐	☐	
6. Use odor eliminator per manufacturer. *Comments:*	☐	☐	☐	
7. Apply gloves. *Comments:*	☐	☐	☐	
8. Apply lubricant to a gloved finger. *Comments:*	☐	☐	☐	
9. Insert lubricated finger into rectum to check for impaction. *Comments:*	☐	☐	☐	
10. Gently probe for and dislodge stool. *Comments:*	☐	☐	☐	
11. Once anus relaxes, several lubricated fingers can be inserted to assist in removal of stool. *Comments:*	☐	☐	☐	
12. Manipulate the stool mass, breaking it up into small pieces. *Comments:*	☐	☐	☐	
13. Remove the stool pieces and place them into an appropriate receptacle. *Comments:*	☐	☐	☐	
14. Monitor the client for complications. *Comments:*	☐	☐	☐	
15. With clean gloves, provide pericare. *Comments:*	☐	☐	☐	

Procedure 6-20	Able to Perform	Able to Perform with Assistance	Unable to Perform	Initials and Date
16. Dispose of stool in appropriate receptacle. *Comments:*	☐	☐	☐	
17. Assist client with use of the bedpan or commode if he or she needs to defecate. *Comments:*	☐	☐	☐	
18. Remove gloves; wash hands. *Comments:*	☐	☐	☐	

Checklist for Procedure 6-21   Inserting a Rectal Tube

Name _____ Date _____

School _____

Instructor _____

Course _____

Procedure 6-21 Inserting a Rectal Tube	Able to Perform	Able to Perform with Assistance	Unable to Perform	Initials and Date
Assessment				
1. Auscultate bowel sounds. *Comments:*	☐	☐	☐	
2. Assess fluid intake and output status. *Comments:*	☐	☐	☐	
3. Assess nutritional intake. *Comments:*	☐	☐	☐	
4. Inspect the perianal skin. *Comments:*	☐	☐	☐	
5. Assess for abdominal distress. *Comments:*	☐	☐	☐	
Planning/Expected Outcomes				
1. Elimination pattern will return to normal. *Comments:*	☐	☐	☐	
2. Client's abdominal girth will return to normal limits. *Comments:*	☐	☐	☐	
3. Client's skin will not be damaged by the procedure. *Comments:*	☐	☐	☐	
Implementation				
1. Wash hands. *Comments:*	☐	☐	☐	
2. Assemble equipment. *Comments:*	☐	☐	☐	
3. Explain procedure to client. *Comments:*	☐	☐	☐	

continued on the following page

continued from the previous page

Procedure 6-21	Able to Perform	Able to Perform with Assistance	Unable to Perform	Initials and Date
4. Position client in left lateral position with upper leg bent over lower leg. *Comments:*	☐	☐	☐	
5. Place disposable pads. *Comments:*	☐	☐	☐	
6. Use odor eliminator per manufacturer's directions. *Comments:*	☐	☐	☐	
7. Apply gloves. *Comments:*	☐	☐	☐	
8. Apply lubricant to a gloved finger. *Comments:*	☐	☐	☐	
9. Insert lubricated finger into rectum to check for possible obstructions. *Comments:*	☐	☐	☐	
10. Change gloves if soiled from rectal exam. *Comments:*	☐	☐	☐	
11. Lubricate end of catheter. *Comments:*	☐	☐	☐	
12. Gently insert catheter into anal canal approximately 10–15 cm. *Comments:*	☐	☐	☐	
13. Attach plastic bag or drainage bag to end of catheter if needed. *Comments:*	☐	☐	☐	
14. Inflate balloon or tape tube to the lower buttock if rectal tube is to be retained. *Comments:*	☐	☐	☐	
15. Dispose of pad and soiled gloves appropriately. *Comments:*	☐	☐	☐	
16. Wash hands. *Comments:*	☐	☐	☐	

continued from the previous page

Checklist for Procedure 6-22 Irrigating and Cleaning a Stoma

Name _____ Date _____

School _____

Instructor _____

Course _____

Procedure 6-22 Irrigating and Cleaning a Stoma	Able to Perform	Able to Perform with Assistance	Unable to Perform	Initials and Date
Assessment				
1. Inspect the stoma for color and texture. *Comments:*	☐	☐	☐	
2. Inspect the condition of the skin surrounding the stoma. *Comments:*	☐	☐	☐	
3. Determine the direction of the intestine. *Comments:*	☐	☐	☐	
4. Measure the dimensions of the stoma. *Comments:*	☐	☐	☐	
Planning/Expected Outcomes				
1. Client will experience bowel movement after irrigation. *Comments:*	☐	☐	☐	
2. Client and/or caregiver will demonstrate skill in performing irrigation of colon. *Comments:*	☐	☐	☐	
3. Peristomal skin integrity will remain intact. *Comments:*	☐	☐	☐	
4. Irritated or denuded peristomal skin integrity will heal. *Comments:*	☐	☐	☐	
5. Client will acknowledge the change in body image. *Comments:*	☐	☐	☐	
6. Client will express positive feelings about self. *Comments:*	☐	☐	☐	
7. Client will maintain fluid balance. *Comments:*	☐	☐	☐	

continued on the following page

continued from the previous page

Procedure 6-22	Able to Perform	Able to Perform with Assistance	Unable to Perform	Initials and Date
Implementation				
1. Wash hands. *Comments:*	☐	☐	☐	
2. Apply clean gloves. *Comments:*	☐	☐	☐	
3. Assemble irrigation kit: Attach cone or catheter to irrigation bag tubing. *Comments:*	☐	☐	☐	
4. Fill irrigation bag with 1000 cc tepid tap water. *Comments:*	☐	☐	☐	
5. Open clamp and prime the irrigation bag tubing. *Comments:*	☐	☐	☐	
6. Hang bottom of irrigation bag 18 inches above the stoma. *Comments:*	☐	☐	☐	
7. Check direction of intestine by inserting a gloved finger into orifice of stoma. *Comments:*	☐	☐	☐	
8. Place irrigation sleeve over stoma and hold in place with belt. *Comments:*	☐	☐	☐	
9. Spray inside of irrigation sleeve and bathroom with odor eliminator. *Comments:*	☐	☐	☐	
10. Cuff end of irrigation sleeve and place into toilet bowl or bedpan. *Comments:*	☐	☐	☐	
11. Lubricate the irrigation cone and insert into stoma through the top opening of irrigation sleeve. *Comments:*	☐	☐	☐	

Procedure 6-22	Able to Perform	Able to Perform with Assistance	Unable to Perform	Initials and Date
12. Close top of irrigation sleeve over the tubing. *Comments:*	☐	☐	☐	
13. Slowly run water through tubing into colon. *Comments:*	☐	☐	☐	
14. Remove cone after all water has emptied out of irrigation bag. *Comments:*	☐	☐	☐	
15. Close end of irrigation sleeve. *Comments:*	☐	☐	☐	
16. Encourage client to ambulate to facilitate emptying of colon. *Comments:*	☐	☐	☐	
17. Remove irrigation sleeve after 20–30 minutes. *Comments:*	☐	☐	☐	
18. Cleanse stoma and skin with warm tap water. Pat dry. *Comments:*	☐	☐	☐	
19. Place gauze pad over stoma to absorb mucus from stoma. *Comments:*	☐	☐	☐	
20. Secure gauze with hypoallergenic tape. *Comments:*	☐	☐	☐	
21. Wash hands. *Comments:*	☐	☐	☐	

Checklist for Procedure 6-23   Changing a Bowel Diversion Ostomy Appliance: Pouching a Stoma

Name _____ Date _____

School _____

Instructor _____

Course _____

Procedure 6-23 Changing a Bowel Diversion Ostomy Appliance: Pouching a Stoma	Able to Perform	Able to Perform with Assistance	Unable to Perform	Initials and Date
Assessment				
1. Inspect the stoma for color and texture. *Comments:*	☐	☐	☐	
2. Inspect the condition of the skin surrounding the stoma. *Comments:*	☐	☐	☐	
3. Measure the dimensions of the stoma. *Comments:*	☐	☐	☐	
Planning/Expected Outcomes				
1. Peristomal skin integrity will remain intact. *Comments:*	☐	☐	☐	
2. Irritated or denuded peristomal skin integrity will heal. *Comments:*	☐	☐	☐	
3. Client will acknowledge the change in body image. *Comments:*	☐	☐	☐	
4. Client will express positive feelings about self. *Comments:*	☐	☐	☐	
5. Client will maintain fluid balance. *Comments:*	☐	☐	☐	
Implementation				
1. Wash hands. *Comments:*	☐	☐	☐	
2. Assemble drainable pouch and wafer. *Comments:*	☐	☐	☐	

continued on the following page

continued from the previous page

Procedure 6-23	Able to Perform	Able to Perform with Assistance	Unable to Perform	Initials and Date
3. Apply gloves. *Comments:*	☐	☐	☐	
4. Remove current ostomy appliance after emptying pouch. *Comments:*	☐	☐	☐	
5. Dispose of appliance appropriately. *Comments:*	☐	☐	☐	
6. Wash hands. *Comments:*	☐	☐	☐	
7. Apply clean gloves. *Comments:*	☐	☐	☐	
8. Cleanse stoma and skin with warm tap water. Pat dry. *Comments:*	☐	☐	☐	
9. Measure stoma at base. *Comments:*	☐	☐	☐	
10. Place gauze pad over stoma while you are preparing the new wafer and pouch. *Comments:*	☐	☐	☐	
11. Trace pattern onto paper backing of wafer. *Comments:*	☐	☐	☐	
12. Cut wafer as traced. *Comments:*	☐	☐	☐	
13. Attach clean pouch to wafer. Make sure port is closed. *Comments:*	☐	☐	☐	
14. Remove gauze pad from orifice of stoma. *Comments:*	☐	☐	☐	
15. Remove paper backing from wafer and place on skin with stoma centered in cutout opening of wafer. *Comments:*	☐	☐	☐	

Procedure 6-23	Able to Perform	Able to Perform with Assistance	Unable to Perform	Initials and Date
16. Tape the wafer edges down with hypoallergenic tape. *Comments:*	☐	☐	☐	
17. Wash hands. *Comments:*	☐	☐	☐	

Checklist for Procedure 7-1   Administering Oxygen Therapy

Name _____ Date _____

School _____

Instructor _____

Course _____

Procedure 7-1 Administering Oxygen Therapy	Able to Perform	Able to Perform with Assistance	Unable to Perform	Initials and Date
Assessment				
1. Determine client history and acute and chronic health problems. *Comments:*	☐	☐	☐	
2. Assess the client's baseline respiratory signs. *Comments:*	☐	☐	☐	
3. Check the extremities and mucous membranes for color. *Comments:*	☐	☐	☐	
4. Review arterial blood gas (ABG) and pulse oximetry results. *Comments:*	☐	☐	☐	
5. Note lung sounds for rales and rhonchi. *Comments:*	☐	☐	☐	
6. Assess the skin in places where tubing or equipment touches the skin. *Comments:*	☐	☐	☐	
Planning/Expected Outcomes				
1. Oxygen levels will return to normal in blood and tissues. *Comments:*	☐	☐	☐	
2. Respiratory rate, pattern, and depth will be within the normal range. *Comments:*	☐	☐	☐	
3. The client will not develop any skin breakdown. *Comments:*	☐	☐	☐	
4. The client will demonstrate methods to clear secretions and maintain optimal oxygenation. *Comments:*	☐	☐	☐	

continued on the following page

continued from the previous page

Procedure 7-1	Able to Perform	Able to Perform with Assistance	Unable to Perform	Initials and Date
5. Breathing efficiency and activity tolerance will be increased. *Comments:*	☐	☐	☐	
6. The client will understand the rationale for the therapy. *Comments:*	☐	☐	☐	
Implementation				
Nasal Cannula 1. Wash hands. *Comments:*	☐	☐	☐	
2. Verify the written order. *Comments:*	☐	☐	☐	
3. Explain procedure and hazards to the client. *Comments:*	☐	☐	☐	
4. Fill humidifier to fill line with distilled water and close container. *Comments:*	☐	☐	☐	
5. Attach humidifier to oxygen flow meter. *Comments:*	☐	☐	☐	
6. Insert humidifier and flow meter into oxygen source. *Comments:*	☐	☐	☐	
7. Attach the oxygen tubing and nasal cannula to the flow meter and turn it on to the prescribed flow rate. *Comments:*	☐	☐	☐	
8. Check for bubbling in the humidifier. *Comments:*	☐	☐	☐	
9. Place the nasal prongs in the client's nostrils and secure the cannula over the client's ears. *Comments:*	☐	☐	☐	
10. Check for proper flow rate every 4 hours. *Comments:*	☐	☐	☐	

Procedure 7-1	Able to Perform	Able to Perform with Assistance	Unable to Perform	Initials and Date
11. Assess client nostrils every 8 hours. *Comments:*	☐	☐	☐	
12. Monitor vital signs, oxygen saturation, and client condition every 4–8 hours. *Comments:*	☐	☐	☐	
13. Wean clients from oxygen as soon as possible using standard protocols. *Comments:*	☐	☐	☐	
Mask 14. Wash hands. *Comments:*	☐	☐	☐	
15. Repeat Actions 2–6. *Comments:*	☐	☐	☐	
16. Attach appropriately sized mask or face tent to oxygen tubing and turn on flow meter to prescribed flow rate. *Comments:*	☐	☐	☐	
17. Check for bubbling in the humidifier. *Comments:*	☐	☐	☐	
18. Place the mask or tent on the client's face and fasten snugly with elastic band. *Comments:*	☐	☐	☐	
19. Check for proper flow rate every 4 hours. *Comments:*	☐	☐	☐	
20. Ensure that the ports of the Venturi mask are not blocked. *Comments:*	☐	☐	☐	
21. Assess client's skin for pressure areas and pad as needed. *Comments:*	☐	☐	☐	
22. Wean client to nasal cannula and then off oxygen per protocol. *Comments:*	☐	☐	☐	

continued on the following page

continued from the previous page

Procedure 7-1	Able to Perform	Able to Perform with Assistance	Unable to Perform	Initials and Date
Oxygen via an Artificial Airway				
23. Wash hands. *Comments:*	☐	☐	☐	
24. Verify the written order. *Comments:*	☐	☐	☐	
25. Fill the humidifier with water and close the container. *Comments:*	☐	☐	☐	
26. Attach humidifier and warmer to the oxygen flow meter. *Comments:*	☐	☐	☐	
27. Attach wide-bore oxygen tubing and T-tube adapter or tracheostomy mask to the flow meter. Initiate oxygen at the prescribed rate. *Comments:*	☐	☐	☐	
28. Check for bubbling in the humidifier and a fine mist from the adapter. *Comments:*	☐	☐	☐	
29. Attach the T-piece to the client's artificial airway or place the mask over the client's airway. *Comments:*	☐	☐	☐	
30. Position tubing so that it is not pulling client's airway. *Comments:*	☐	☐	☐	
31. Check for proper flow rate and patency of the system every 1–2 hours. Suction as needed to maintain a patent airway. *Comments:*	☐	☐	☐	
32. Monitor for signs and symptoms of hypoxia every 2 hours. Monitor breath sounds and tube position every 4 hours. *Comments:*	☐	☐	☐	
33. Wean client from therapy as ordered by qualified practitioner. *Comments:*	☐	☐	☐	

Checklist for Procedure 7-2 Assisting a Client with Controlled Coughing and Deep Breathing

Name _____ Date _____

School _____

Instructor _____

Course _____

Procedure 7-2 Assisting a Client with Controlled Coughing and Deep Breathing	Able to Perform	Able to Perform with Assistance	Unable to Perform	Initials and Date
Assessment				
1. Identify need for controlled coughing. *Comments:*	☐	☐	☐	
2. Assess breath sounds by auscultation. *Comments:*	☐	☐	☐	
3. Assess breath sounds by percussion (if necessary). *Comments:*	☐	☐	☐	
4. Assess by tactile means for fremitus. *Comments:*	☐	☐	☐	
5. Assess the client for understanding, ability, and cooperation. *Comments:*	☐	☐	☐	
Planning/Expected Outcomes				
1. The client will be able to breathe deeply and clearly. *Comments:*	☐	☐	☐	
2. The client will be able to use effective breathing techniques. *Comments:*	☐	☐	☐	
3. The client will be able to cough productively if secretions are present. *Comments:*	☐	☐	☐	
4. The lung fields will be clear to auscultation. *Comments:*	☐	☐	☐	

continued on the following page

continued from the previous page

Procedure 7-2	Able to Perform	Able to Perform with Assistance	Unable to Perform	Initials and Date
5. The client's respiratory rate will be normal. *Comments:*	☐	☐	☐	
6. The client will have good skin color and mentation. *Comments:*	☐	☐	☐	
Implementation				
1. Wash hands. *Comments:*	☐	☐	☐	
2. Assess the client's pain status. *Comments:*	☐	☐	☐	
3. Explain the purpose and importance of the procedure to the client. *Comments:*	☐	☐	☐	
4. Help the client sit in a high-Fowler's position if able. *Comments:*	☐	☐	☐	
5. Auscultate lungs before procedure. *Comments:*	☐	☐	☐	
6. Place the palms of your hands on the client's rib cage. *Comments:*	☐	☐	☐	
7. Use pillow or folded towels to splint the abdomen or chest. *Comments:*	☐	☐	☐	
8. Practice deep breathing with client: • Instruct the client to cover the mouth with tissue. • Take a deep breath in and exhale slowly 2–3 times. • Repeat 10 times every 1–2 hours as needed. *Comments:*	☐	☐	☐	
9. Reassess lung fields after procedure. *Comments:*	☐	☐	☐	

Procedure 7-2	Able to Perform	Able to Perform with Assistance	Unable to Perform	Initials and Date
10. Assist the client to cough: • Follow the deep breathing procedure and have the client hold breath for 1–2 seconds. • Have client contract abdominal muscles, cough forcefully, and expectorate secretions. • Splint the client's abdomen and chest as he or she coughs. *Comments:*	☐	☐	☐	
11. Repeat as necessary to clear lung fields. *Comments:*	☐	☐	☐	
12. Observe for dizziness, shortness of breath, or other respiratory problems. *Comments:*	☐	☐	☐	
13. Dispose of all tissues and wash hands. *Comments:*	☐	☐	☐	

Checklist for Procedure 7-3   Assisting a Client with an Incentive Spirometer

Name _____ Date _____

School _____

Instructor _____

Course _____

Procedure 7-3 **Assisting a Client with an Incentive Spirometer**	Able to Perform	Able to Perform with Assistance	Unable to Perform	Initials and Date
Assessment				
1. Assess need for incentive spirometry. *Comments:*	☐	☐	☐	
2. Assess the client's respiratory status. *Comments:*	☐	☐	☐	
3. Review medical record for recent arterial blood gases. *Comments:*	☐	☐	☐	
Planning/Expected Outcomes				
1. The client has clear breath sounds throughout lung fields. *Comments:*	☐	☐	☐	
2. The client has normal depth and rate of respiration. *Comments:*	☐	☐	☐	
3. Inspiratory lung expansion returned to pre-event status. *Comments:*	☐	☐	☐	
4. The client's arterial blood gases are normal. *Comments:*	☐	☐	☐	
5. There is an absence of consolidation or atelectasis. *Comments:*	☐	☐	☐	
6. Respirations are not labored. *Comments:*	☐	☐	☐	
Implementation				
1. Wash hands. *Comments:*	☐	☐	☐	

continued on the following page

continued from the previous page

Procedure 7-3	Able to Perform	Able to Perform with Assistance	Unable to Perform	Initials and Date
2. Check chart for previous respiratory assessment. *Comments:*	☐	☐	☐	
3. Gather equipment. *Comments:*	☐	☐	☐	
4. Explain procedure to client. *Comments:*	☐	☐	☐	
5. Demonstrate deep, sustained inspiration. *Comments:*	☐	☐	☐	
6. Have client assume semi-Fowler's or high-Fowler's position. *Comments:*	☐	☐	☐	
7. Set pointer on incentive spirometer (IS) or point to level where disk or ball should reach. *Comments:*	☐	☐	☐	
8. Use incentive spirometer: • Have client breathe in and exhale completely. • Hold unit upright. • Have client seal lips around mouthpiece and inhale slowly and deeply until desired volume is attained. • Sustain inspiration for at least 3 seconds. • Exhale slowly. *Comments:*	☐	☐	☐	
9. Repeat 10–20 times every hour while awake for 72 hours. *Comments:*	☐	☐	☐	
10. Teach client to perform IS every hour and verify compliance. *Comments:*	☐	☐	☐	
11. Dispose of soiled equipment or tissues and wash hands. *Comments:*	☐	☐	☐	

Checklist for Procedure 7-4   Administering Pulmonary Therapy and Postural Drainage

Name _____ Date _____

School _____

Instructor _____

Course _____

Procedure 7-4 Administering Pulmonary Therapy and Postural Drainage	Able to Perform	Able to Perform with Assistance	Unable to Perform	Initials and Date
Assessment				
1. Assess the client's breath sounds and ability to clear secretions. *Comments:*	☐	☐	☐	
2. Determine the client's rhythm, depth, and rate of breathing. *Comments:*	☐	☐	☐	
3. Observe the quality of the secretions. *Comments:*	☐	☐	☐	
4. Take note of any complicating conditions. *Comments:*	☐	☐	☐	
Planning/Expected Outcomes				
1. Clearance of pulmonary secretions will be improved. *Comments:*	☐	☐	☐	
2. Ventilation will be improved. *Comments:*	☐	☐	☐	
3. Potential complications will be minimized. *Comments:*	☐	☐	☐	
4. Client will experience an improved sense of well-being. *Comments:*	☐	☐	☐	
Implementation				
1. Wash hands. *Comments:*	☐	☐	☐	

continued on the following page

continued from the previous page

Procedure 7-4	Able to Perform	Able to Perform with Assistance	Unable to Perform	Initials and Date
2. Auscultate client's lungs. *Comments:*	☐	☐	☐	
3. Confirm presence of appropriate equipment. *Comments:*	☐	☐	☐	
4. Turn off tube feeding. *Comments:*	☐	☐	☐	
5. Position client properly. *Comments:*	☐	☐	☐	
6. Initiate chest pulmonary therapy (CPT). *Comments:*	☐	☐	☐	
7. Move the percussor around the chest area where CPT has been ordered. *Comments:*	☐	☐	☐	
8. Monitor the client during the therapy for signs of distress. *Comments:*	☐	☐	☐	
9. Auscultate after the therapy is completed. *Comments:*	☐	☐	☐	
10. Suction secretions as necessary. *Comments:*	☐	☐	☐	
11. Wash hands. *Comments:*	☐	☐	☐	

Checklist for Procedure 7-5 Administering Pulse Oximetry

Name _____ Date _____

School _____

Instructor _____

Course _____

Procedure 7-5 Administering Pulse Oximetry	Able to Perform	Able to Perform with Assistance	Unable to Perform	Initials and Date
Assessment				
1. Assess the client's hemoglobin level. *Comments:*	☐	☐	☐	
2. Assess the client's color. *Comments:*	☐	☐	☐	
3. Assess the client's mental status. *Comments:*	☐	☐	☐	
4. Assess the client's pulse rate. *Comments:*	☐	☐	☐	
5. Assess the area where the sensors will be placed. *Comments:*	☐	☐	☐	
6. Remove nail polish and/or acrylic nails. *Comments:*	☐	☐	☐	
Planning/Expected Outcomes				
1. The SaO_2 will be in a normal range for the client. *Comments:*	☐	☐	☐	
2. The client will be alert and oriented. *Comments:*	☐	☐	☐	
3. The client's color will remain normal. *Comments:*	☐	☐	☐	
4. The client will tolerate the placement of sensors. *Comments:*	☐	☐	☐	
5. There will not be any skin irritation at area of sensors. *Comments:*	☐	☐	☐	

continued on the following page

continued from the previous page

Procedure 7-5	Able to Perform	Able to Perform with Assistance	Unable to Perform	Initials and Date
Implementation				
1. Wash hands. *Comments:*	☐	☐	☐	
2. Select an appropriate sensor. *Comments:*	☐	☐	☐	
3. Select an appropriate site for the sensor. *Comments:*	☐	☐	☐	
4. Clean the site with an alcohol wipe or soap and water. *Comments:*	☐	☐	☐	
5. Apply the sensor. *Comments:*	☐	☐	☐	
6. Connect the sensor to the oximeter with a sensor cable. Turn on the machine. *Comments:*	☐	☐	☐	
7. Adjust the alarm limits. Adjust volume. *Comments:*	☐	☐	☐	
8. If taking a single reading, note the results. For constant monitoring, move spring sensors every 2 hours and adhesive sensors every 4 hours. *Comments:*	☐	☐	☐	
9. Cover the sensor with a sheet or towel. *Comments:*	☐	☐	☐	
10. Notify the qualified practitioner of abnormal results. *Comments:*	☐	☐	☐	
11. Record the results of O_2 saturation measurements. *Comments:*	☐	☐	☐	

Checklist for Procedure 7-6   Measuring Peak Expiratory Flow Rates

Name _____ Date _____

School _____

Instructor _____

Course _____

Procedure 7-6 Measuring Peak Expiratory Flow Rates	Able to Perform	Able to Perform with Assistance	Unable to Perform	Initials and Date
Assessment				
1. Take a history regarding the frequency and signs and symptoms of the attacks. *Comments:*	☐	☐	☐	
2. Ask about all medications the client is taking. *Comments:*	☐	☐	☐	
3. Assess the client's ability to cooperate with testing. *Comments:*	☐	☐	☐	
Planning/Expected Outcomes				
1. The client will use the peak flow monitor to assess the course and treatment of the attack. *Comments:*	☐	☐	☐	
2. The client will detect early stages of airway obstruction. *Comments:*	☐	☐	☐	
3. The client will have an accurate perception of the severity of the obstruction. *Comments:*	☐	☐	☐	
4. The client will accurately determine when emergency medical care is needed. *Comments:*	☐	☐	☐	
5. The client will be able to distinguish between asthma and other causes of breathlessness. *Comments:*	☐	☐	☐	
6. The effectiveness of client communication will be improved. *Comments:*	☐	☐	☐	

continued on the following page

continued from the previous page

Procedure 7-6	Able to Perform	Able to Perform with Assistance	Unable to Perform	Initials and Date
Implementation				
1. Set up all the equipment needed before going to the client's room. *Comments:*	☐	☐	☐	
2. Identify the client and check client's height, age, and sex. *Comments:*	☐	☐	☐	
3. Explain and demonstrate the procedure. *Comments:*	☐	☐	☐	
4. Have the client stand up with the chin slightly raised. *Comments:*	☐	☐	☐	
5. Show the client how and where to place the indicator/pointer. *Comments:*	☐	☐	☐	
6. Have the client take a deep breath through the mouth. *Comments:*	☐	☐	☐	
7. Have the client hold the peak flow meter without touching the pointer. *Comments:*	☐	☐	☐	
8. Have the client place the peak flow meter in the mouth, sealing the lips and teeth around the mouthpiece. *Comments:*	☐	☐	☐	
9. Have the client blow out as hard and as fast as possible over about a second. *Comments:*	☐	☐	☐	
10. Teach the client how to read the meter and where to record the reading. *Comments:*	☐	☐	☐	
11. Have the client slide the pointer down to 0 and repeat Actions 5–10 two more times. *Comments:*	☐	☐	☐	

Procedure 7-6	Able to Perform	Able to Perform with Assistance	Unable to Perform	Initials and Date
12. Allow the client to rest between attempts, if necessary. *Comments:*	☐	☐	☐	
13. Record the highest of the three numbers achieved. *Comments:*	☐	☐	☐	
14. Use the zone determination to evaluate what course of treatment should be followed. *Comments:*	☐	☐	☐	

Checklist for Procedure 7-7   Administering Intermittent Positive-Pressure Breathing (IPPB)

Name _____ Date _____

School _____

Instructor _____

Course _____

Procedure 7-7 Administering Intermittent Positive-Pressure Breathing (IPPB)	Able to Perform	Able to Perform with Assistance	Unable to Perform	Initials and Date
Assessment				
1. Assess the client's ability to understand and cooperate with the procedure. *Comments:*	☐	☐	☐	
2. Assess the orders for IPPB. *Comments:*	☐	☐	☐	
3. Assess the equipment being used. *Comments:*	☐	☐	☐	
Planning/Expected Outcomes				
1. The client will have improved tidal breathing. *Comments:*	☐	☐	☐	
2. The client will have a more effective cough. *Comments:*	☐	☐	☐	
3. The client will have increased sputum production. *Comments:*	☐	☐	☐	
4. The client will have improved breath sounds and an improved chest X-ray. *Comments:*	☐	☐	☐	
Implementation				
1. Review and verify written order. *Comments:*	☐	☐	☐	
2. Wash hands. Apply protective clothing as needed. *Comments:*	☐	☐	☐	
3. Explain treatment and technique to client. *Comments:*	☐	☐	☐	

continued on the following page

continued from the previous page

Procedure 7-7	Able to Perform	Able to Perform with Assistance	Unable to Perform	Initials and Date
4. Set up equipment and connect to gas source. *Comments:*	☐	☐	☐	
5. Set parameters on IPPB device. *Comments:*	☐	☐	☐	
6. Fill nebulizer with sterile normal saline or medication. *Comments:*	☐	☐	☐	
7. Assist the client to an upright sitting position. *Comments:*	☐	☐	☐	
8. Assess client's breath sounds, respiratory rate, and pulse, and obtain inspiratory capacity. *Comments:*	☐	☐	☐	
9. Initiate therapy and monitor effectiveness of treatment. *Comments:*	☐	☐	☐	
10. Discontinue treatment when medication is administered or time limit is reached. *Comments:*	☐	☐	☐	
11. Assess breath sounds, respiratory rate, pulse, and inspiratory capacity. *Comments:*	☐	☐	☐	
12. Disconnect IPPB from gas source. *Comments:*	☐	☐	☐	
13. Rinse nebulizer with sterile water or sterile saline and air dry. *Comments:*	☐	☐	☐	
14. Document treatment. *Comments:*	☐	☐	☐	
15. Wash hands. *Comments:*	☐	☐	☐	

Checklist for Procedure 7-8   Assisting with Continuous Positive Airway Pressure (CPAP)

Name _____ Date _____

School _____

Instructor _____

Course _____

Procedure 7-8 **Assisting with Continuous Positive Airway Pressure (CPAP)**	Able to Perform	Able to Perform with Assistance	Unable to Perform	Initials and Date
Assessment				
1. Assess for breath sounds. *Comments:*	☐	☐	☐	
2. Assess client's response to therapy before, during, and after. *Comments:*	☐	☐	☐	
3. Assess changes in vital signs. *Comments:*	☐	☐	☐	
4. Assess changes in arterial blood gas values or oxygen saturation. *Comments:*	☐	☐	☐	
5. Assess changes in chest x-rays as per orders. *Comments:*	☐	☐	☐	
Planning/Expected Outcomes				
1. The client will have a reduction in the work of breathing. *Comments:*	☐	☐	☐	
2. The client will have a decrease in the severity of retractions, grunting, and nasal flaring. *Comments:*	☐	☐	☐	
3. The client will have improvement in lung volumes and appearance. *Comments:*	☐	☐	☐	
4. The client will have increased comfort in breathing. *Comments:*	☐	☐	☐	
5. The client will have an improvement in oxygen saturation. *Comments:*	☐	☐	☐	

continued on the following page

continued from the previous page

Procedure 7-8	Able to Perform	Able to Perform with Assistance	Unable to Perform	Initials and Date
Implementation				
1. Wash hands. *Comments:*	☐	☐	☐	
2. Check orders regarding CPAP administration. *Comments:*	☐	☐	☐	
3. Assess breath sounds, vital signs, and oxygen saturation. *Comments:*	☐	☐	☐	
4. Assist client into position of comfort. *Comments:*	☐	☐	☐	
5. Secure mask over the nose and/or mouth of the client. Check connections. *Comments:*	☐	☐	☐	
6. Turn CPAP machine on and check settings. *Comments:*	☐	☐	☐	
7. Maintain CPAP for prescribed length of time. *Comments:*	☐	☐	☐	
8. Assess breath sounds, vital signs, and oxygen saturation. *Comments:*	☐	☐	☐	
9. Observe the client for side effects. *Comments:*	☐	☐	☐	
10. Wash hands. *Comments:*	☐	☐	☐	

Checklist for Procedure 7-9   Preparing the Chest Drainage System

Name _____ Date _____

School _____

Instructor _____

Course _____

Procedure 7-9 Preparing the Chest Drainage System	Able to Perform	Able to Perform with Assistance	Unable to Perform	Initials and Date
Assessment				
1. Assess the written orders. *Comments:*	☐	☐	☐	
2. Assess the available equipment. *Comments:*	☐	☐	☐	
3. Assess the client's environment. *Comments:*	☐	☐	☐	
Planning/Expected Outcomes				
1. The drainage system will be appropriate for the client and consistent with the written orders. *Comments:*	☐	☐	☐	
2. The drainage system setup will be in accord with institutional policy. *Comments:*	☐	☐	☐	
3. The chest drainage system will not pose a hazard to the client. *Comments:*	☐	☐	☐	
Implementation				
Disposable Chest Tube Drainage System				
1. Gather equipment. *Comments:*	☐	☐	☐	
2. Wash hands. *Comments:*	☐	☐	☐	
3. Open the disposable chest tube system using aseptic technique. *Comments:*	☐	☐	☐	
4. Set the unit upright. *Comments:*	☐	☐	☐	

continued on the following page

continued from the previous page

Procedure 7-9	Able to Perform	Able to Perform with Assistance	Unable to Perform	Initials and Date
5. For water seal only, pour the measured amount of sterile water or saline into the funnel provided. *Comments:*	☐	☐	☐	
6. For suction, fill the suction control chamber to the ordered level of fluid. *Comments:*	☐	☐	☐	
7. For suction, attach suction tubing to the marked port and to the suction source. *Comments:*	☐	☐	☐	
8. Turn the suction up until there is gentle bubbling in the suction control chamber. *Comments:*	☐	☐	☐	
9. Set the system up at the client's bedside below the level of the client. *Comments:*	☐	☐	☐	
10. Wash hands. *Comments:*	☐	☐	☐	
Reusable Bottle Chest Drainage System 11. Repeat Actions 1–3. *Comments:*	☐	☐	☐	
12. Apply sterile gloves. *Comments:*	☐	☐	☐	
13. One-bottle water seal: • Insert a long glass tube and a short glass tube into a two-hole rubber stopper. • Pour sterile saline or water into the water seal bottle to a depth of at least 4 cm. • Put the rubber stopper onto the bottle. • Submerge the long glass tube 2 cm into the water. • Attach the client's chest tube to the long glass tube. • Place a measuring guide on the side of the drainage bottle. *Comments:*	☐	☐	☐	

Procedure 7-9	Able to Perform	Able to Perform with Assistance	Unable to Perform	Initials and Date
14. Two-bottle drainage and water seal: • Insert a long glass tube and a short glass tube into a two-hole rubber stopper. • Insert two short glass tubes into a two-hole rubber stopper. • Pour sterile water or saline into the water seal bottle to a depth of about 4 cm. • Put the rubber stopper with two short glass tubes on the drainage bottle. • Put the second rubber stopper onto the water seal bottle. • Submerge the long glass tube 2 cm into the water. • Place rubber tubing between one of the two short glass tubes on the drainage bottle and the long glass tube in the water seal bottle. • Attach the client's chest tube to the second glass tube in the drainage bottle. • Place a measuring guide on the side of the drainage bottle. *Comments:*	☐	☐	☐	
15. Two-bottle drainage and suction control: • Insert a long glass tube and a short glass tube into a two-hole rubber stopper. • In the three-hole stopper, insert a long glass tube in the middle hole and short glass tubes in the other two holes. • Pour sterile water or saline into the water seal/drainage bottle to a depth of about 4 cm. • Pour sterile saline or water into the suction control bottle to the ordered depth. • Put the two-hole rubber stopper onto the water seal/drainage bottle. • Submerge the long glass tube 2 cm into the water. • Place the three-hole stopper onto the suction control bottle. • The long glass tube must extend into the water but cannot touch the bottom of the bottle. • Attach rubber tubing to the outer end of the short glass tube in the water seal/drainage bottle and connect it to the outer end of one of the short glass tubes in the suction control bottle. • Attach suction tubing between the second short glass tube in the suction control bottle and the suction source. • Do not attach anything to the long glass tube in the suction control bottle. • Attach the client's chest tube to the long glass tube in the water seal/drainage bottle. • Turn the suction up until a gentle bubbling is noted in the suction control bottle. • Place a measuring guide on the side of the drainage bottle. *Comments:*	☐	☐	☐	

continued on the following page

continued from the previous page

Procedure 7-9	Able to Perform	Able to Perform with Assistance	Unable to Perform	Initials and Date
16. Three-bottle drainage, water seal, and suction control: • Insert a long glass tube and a short glass tube into a two-hole rubber stopper. • Insert short glass tubes into a two-hole rubber stopper. • In the three-hole stopper, insert a long glass tube in the middle hole and short glass tubes in the other two holes. • Pour sterile water or saline into the water seal bottle to a depth of about 4 cm. • Pour sterile saline or water into the suction control bottle to the ordered depth. • Put the rubber stopper with two short glass tubes on the drainage bottle. • Put the second rubber stopper onto the water seal bottle. • Submerge the long glass tube 2 cm into the water. • Place the three-hole rubber stopper onto the suction control bottle. • The long glass tube must extend into the water but cannot touch the bottom of the bottle. • Place rubber tubing between one of the short glass tubes in the drainage bottle and the long glass tube in the water seal bottle. • Attach rubber tubing between the short glass tube in the water seal/drainage bottle and one of the short glass tubes in the suction control bottle. • Attach suction tubing between the second short glass tube in the suction control bottle and the suction source. • Do not attach anything to the long glass tube in the suction control bottle. • Attach the client's chest tube to one of the short glass tubes extending from the drainage bottle. • Turn the suction up until a gentle bubbling is noted in the suction control bottle. • Place a measuring guide on the side of the drainage bottle. *Comments:*	☐	☐	☐	
17. Tape all connections. *Comments:*	☐	☐	☐	
18. Dispose of gloves in the proper container. *Comments:*	☐	☐	☐	
19. Arrange the drainage system at the client's bedside below the level of the client. *Comments:*	☐	☐	☐	
20. Wash hands. *Comments:*	☐	☐	☐	

Checklist for Procedure 7-10   Maintaining the Chest Tube and Chest Drainage System

Name _____ Date _____

School _____

Instructor _____

Course _____

Procedure 7-10 **Maintaining the Chest Tube and Chest Drainage System**	Able to Perform	Able to Perform with Assistance	Unable to Perform	Initials and Date
Assessment				
1. Assess that the chest tube is set to the ordered amount of suction. *Comments:*	☐	☐	☐	
2. Assess that the water seal is maintained at the marked line. *Comments:*	☐	☐	☐	
3. Assess for an air leak in the water seal chamber. *Comments:*	☐	☐	☐	
4. Assess that all connections are taped. *Comments:*	☐	☐	☐	
5. Assess the chest tube dressing and change every 24–48 hours. *Comments:*	☐	☐	☐	
6. Assess the drainage system and drainage. *Comments:*	☐	☐	☐	
7. Assess the chest drain tubing. *Comments:*	☐	☐	☐	
8. Ensure that the drainage system has not been compromised. *Comments:*	☐	☐	☐	
9. Identify risk factors for a tension pneumothorax. *Comments:*	☐	☐	☐	

continued on the following page

continued from the previous page

Procedure 7-10	Able to Perform	Able to Perform with Assistance	Unable to Perform	Initials and Date
Planning/Expected Outcomes				
1. The chest tube and drainage system will be maintained without pneumothorax. *Comments:*	☐	☐	☐	
2. Client will be free of infection related to the chest tube. *Comments:*	☐	☐	☐	
3. Chest tube and drainage system will be maintained safely. *Comments:*	☐	☐	☐	
Implementation				
1. Assess that the drainage system is set to the ordered amount of suction. *Comments:*	☐	☐	☐	
2. Assess that the water seal chamber is filled to the marked level. *Comments:*	☐	☐	☐	
3. Assess for an air leak. *Comments:*	☐	☐	☐	
4. If there is a new air leak, you may have to assess where the air leak is. *Comments:*	☐	☐	☐	
5. Assess that all connections are spiral-wrapped with silk tape. *Comments:*	☐	☐	☐	
6. Assess the chest tube dressing every shift and change the dressing every 24–48 hours. *Comments:*	☐	☐	☐	
7. Assess drainage every 1–8 hours. *Comments:*	☐	☐	☐	
8. Assess that the drainage system is anchored safely, lower than the client. *Comments:*	☐	☐	☐	

Procedure 7-10	Able to Perform	Able to Perform with Assistance	Unable to Perform	Initials and Date
9. Assess the tubing for kinks and dependent loops. *Comments:*	☐	☐	☐	
10. Have a bottle of sterile water or saline at the client's bedside. *Comments:*	☐	☐	☐	
11. Ensure that an occlusive dressing is applied at the site. *Comments:*	☐	☐	☐	
12. Ensure that the chest tube is never milked or stripped. *Comments:*	☐	☐	☐	

Checklist for Procedure 7-11   Measuring the Output from a Chest Drainage System

Name _____ Date _____

School _____

Instructor _____

Course _____

Procedure 7-11 **Measuring the Output from a** **Chest Drainage System**	Able to Perform	Able to Perform with Assistance	Unable to Perform	Initials and Date
Assessment				
1. Assess the chest drainage system. *Comments:*	☐	☐	☐	
2. Assess the drainage. *Comments:*	☐	☐	☐	
Planning/Expected Outcomes				
1. The amount of drainage will be accurately determined and recorded. *Comments:*	☐	☐	☐	
Implementation				
1. Wash hands. *Comments:*	☐	☐	☐	
2. Determine which bottle or chamber contains the drainage. *Comments:*	☐	☐	☐	
3. With the meniscus at eye level, note the level of the drainage. *Comments:*	☐	☐	☐	
4. Use the pen or marker to mark the current fluid level. *Comments:*	☐	☐	☐	
5. Note the level of drainage marked just prior to this measurement. *Comments:*	☐	☐	☐	
6. Note the amount of drainage since the last measurement. *Comments:*	☐	☐	☐	
7. Wash hands. *Comments:*	☐	☐	☐	

Checklist for Procedure 7-12 Obtaining a Specimen from a Chest Drainage System

Name _____ Date _____

School _____

Instructor _____

Course _____

Procedure 7-12 Obtaining a Specimen from a Chest Drainage System	Able to Perform	Able to Perform with Assistance	Unable to Perform	Initials and Date
Assessment				
1. Assess the written order. *Comments:*	☐	☐	☐	
2. Assess the available equipment. *Comments:*	☐	☐	☐	
Planning/Expected Outcomes				
1. The chest drainage specimen will be obtained without compromising client safety. *Comments:*	☐	☐	☐	
Implementation				
1. Wash hands. *Comments:*	☐	☐	☐	
2. Determine if there is drainage in the tubing. *Comments:*	☐	☐	☐	
3. Apply clean gloves. *Comments:*	☐	☐	☐	
4. Cleanse access port or rubber tubing with Betadine or alcohol. *Comments:*	☐	☐	☐	
5. Using the syringe and needle, puncture the port or tubing at a 45° angle. *Comments:*	☐	☐	☐	
6. Gently withdraw the needed amount of drainage from the tubing. *Comments:*	☐	☐	☐	

continued on the following page

continued from the previous page

Procedure 7-12	Able to Perform	Able to Perform with Assistance	Unable to Perform	Initials and Date
7. Place the drainage into a laboratory specimen container. *Comments:*	☐	☐	☐	
8. Dispose of the syringe and needle appropriately. *Comments:*	☐	☐	☐	
9. Label the specimen container. *Comments:*	☐	☐	☐	
10. Remove gloves and dispose of in the proper container. *Comments:*	☐	☐	☐	
11. Wash hands. *Comments:*	☐	☐	☐	

Checklist for Procedure 7-13   Removing a Chest Tube

Name _____ Date _____

School _____

Instructor _____

Course _____

Procedure 7-13 **Removing a Chest Tube**	Able to Perform	Able to Perform with Assistance	Unable to Perform	Initials and Date
Assessment				
1. Assess whether the client has a new or larger air leak present. *Comments:*	☐	☐	☐	
2. Ensure that the client has had a chest x-ray. *Comments:*	☐	☐	☐	
3. Check that your client has received pain medication. *Comments:*	☐	☐	☐	
4. Assess the client's anxiety level. *Comments:*	☐	☐	☐	
5. Assess client's tolerance of the absence of chest tube suction for 1–2 days. *Comments:*	☐	☐	☐	
6. Check when the qualified practitioner is planning to remove the tube. *Comments:*	☐	☐	☐	
7. Assess the client's ability to perform Valsalva's maneuver. *Comments:*	☐	☐	☐	
Planning/Expected Outcomes				
1. The chest tube will be removed without complication. *Comments:*	☐	☐	☐	
2. The nurse will assist with the procedure and avoid exposure to bodily fluids. *Comments:*	☐	☐	☐	
3. Client will not experience undue pain or anxiety during the procedure. *Comments:*	☐	☐	☐	

continued on the following page

continued from the previous page

Procedure 7-13	Able to Perform	Able to Perform with Assistance	Unable to Perform	Initials and Date
Implementation				
1. Gather all equipment in the client's room. *Comments:*	☐	☐	☐	
2. Wash hands. *Comments:*	☐	☐	☐	
3. Premedicate the client. *Comments:*	☐	☐	☐	
4. Assist the client into an accessible and comfortable position. *Comments:*	☐	☐	☐	
5. Explain what you are doing as you proceed. *Comments:*	☐	☐	☐	
6. Assess for effects of premedication on respiratory status. *Comments:*	☐	☐	☐	
7. Apply gloves. *Comments:*	☐	☐	☐	
8. Assist physician or qualified practitioner as directed. *Comments:*	☐	☐	☐	
9. After removal, check that the dressing is secure and airtight. Do not remove dressing for 24 hours. *Comments:*	☐	☐	☐	
10. Order post-chest tube removal x-ray. *Comments:*	☐	☐	☐	
11. Ensure that waste has been properly disposed of. *Comments:*	☐	☐	☐	
12. Dispose of gloves and wash hands. *Comments:*	☐	☐	☐	
13. Assess client in 30 minutes for signs of a pneumothorax. Assess the dressing. *Comments:*	☐	☐	☐	

Checklist for Procedure 7-14 Ventilating the Client with an Ambu Bag®

Name _____ Date _____

School _____

Instructor _____

Course _____

Procedure 7-14 Ventilating the Client with an Ambu Bag®	Able to Perform	Able to Perform with Assistance	Unable to Perform	Initials and Date
Assessment				
1. Determine the need to use manual ventilation. *Comments:*	☐	☐	☐	
2. Identify symptoms that may indicate the need for manual ventilation. *Comments:*	☐	☐	☐	
3. Review the client's medical history. *Comments:*	☐	☐	☐	
4. If the client is alert, assess the client's ability to cooperate with the procedure. *Comments:*	☐	☐	☐	
Planning/Expected Outcomes				
1. The client will have adequate respirations spontaneously or mechanically. *Comments:*	☐	☐	☐	
2. Laboratory tests and monitors will indicate appropriate CO_2 and O_2 levels. *Comments:*	☐	☐	☐	
3. Intracranial pressure will be within normal limits. *Comments:*	☐	☐	☐	
4. The client will maintain effective ventilation during transportation. *Comments:*	☐	☐	☐	
5. The client will have improved airway clearance. *Comments:*	☐	☐	☐	
6. The client will report minimal anxiety related to the procedure. *Comments:*	☐	☐	☐	

continued on the following page

continued from the previous page

Procedure 7-14	Able to Perform	Able to Perform with Assistance	Unable to Perform	Initials and Date
Implementation				
1. Obtain baseline assessment of client including vital signs. *Comments:*	☐	☐	☐	
2. Prepare, connect, and check functioning of equipment. *Comments:*	☐	☐	☐	
3. Adjust bed or cart to a comfortable working height. *Comments:*	☐	☐	☐	
4. Wash hands, apply gloves and face shield. *Comments:*	☐	☐	☐	
5. For the client who is mechanically ventilated: • Remove the mechanical ventilation system. • For transfer, attach Ambu bag® to airway and compress bag to administer one breath every 3–5 seconds. • Adjust the flow meter to adequate inspiratory volume. • The Ambu bag® may be compressed with two hands if the airway is stable. • For suction, instill normal saline. • Suction the client, reattach the Ambu bag®, and repeat the three preceding steps. • End suctioning by administering several breaths and reconnecting client to mechanical ventilation. • Assess the chest to verify equal air flow. *Comments:*	☐	☐	☐	
6. For the client who is unconscious and not intubated: • Assess need for Ambu bag® or immediate intubation. • Clear oral cavity of vomit, mucus, or other debris. • Insert an oropharyngeal airway. • Position client to open the airway. • Position Ambu bag® over the client's nose and mouth. • The dominant hand is used to compress the Ambu bag and deliver breaths to the client. • The chest is assessed to verify adequate, equal inspiratory flow. • Assess for the need to insert a nasogastric tube. • Suction as necessary. *Comments:*	☐	☐	☐	

Procedure 7-14	Able to Perform	Able to Perform with Assistance	Unable to Perform	Initials and Date
7. Assess to determine need to discontinue procedure by: • Secretions minimal and artificial airway patent. • Client no longer coughing or "bucking" ventilation. • Stable vital signs. • Client no longer dusky or cyanotic. • Return of spontaneous respirations. • Decreased intracranial pressure. *Comments:*	☐	☐	☐	
8. Remove Ambu bag and reattach client to mechanical ventilation system. *Comments:*	☐	☐	☐	
9. Discontinue oxygen flow to the Ambu bag. *Comments:*	☐	☐	☐	
10. Reposition client, return bed and guard rails to safe position. *Comments:*	☐	☐	☐	
11. Clean supplies per institution protocol. *Comments:*	☐	☐	☐	
12. Dispose of used supplies appropriately. *Comments:*	☐	☐	☐	
13. Document tolerance of procedure. *Comments:*	☐	☐	☐	

Checklist for Procedure 7-15   Inserting the Pharyngeal Airway

Name _____ Date _____

School _____

Instructor _____

Course _____

Procedure 7-15 Inserting the Pharyngeal Airway	Able to Perform	Able to Perform with Assistance	Unable to Perform	Initials and Date
Assessment				
1. Assess need for pharyngeal intubation. *Comments:*	☐	☐	☐	
2. Assess the age and size of the client. *Comments:*	☐	☐	☐	
3. Assess response to pharyngeal tube placement. *Comments:*	☐	☐	☐	
Planning/Expected Outcomes				
1. Airway patency will be established and maintained. *Comments:*	☐	☐	☐	
2. Suctioning equipment can be passed into the airway as needed. *Comments:*	☐	☐	☐	
3. The client will not bite the equipment. *Comments:*	☐	☐	☐	
Implementation				
1. Wash hands. *Comments:*	☐	☐	☐	
2. Apply clean gloves. Put on mask, eyewear, and gown if appropriate. *Comments:*	☐	☐	☐	
3. Clear the mouth and pharynx using a suction catheter. *Comments:*	☐	☐	☐	

continued on the following page

continued from the previous page

Procedure 7-15	Able to Perform	Able to Perform with Assistance	Unable to Perform	Initials and Date
4. Nasopharyngeal airway insertion: • Lubricate the nasopharyngeal airway. • Gently insert nasopharyngeal airway. *Comments:*	☐	☐	☐	
5. Oropharyngeal airway insertion: • Gently insert oropharyngeal airway by turning it upside down and sliding it into the mouth. • Rotate the airway after it transverses the oral cavity. *Comments:*	☐	☐	☐	
6. Maintain head slightly tilted back with chin elevated. *Comments:*	☐	☐	☐	
7. Ensure airway position by visually inspecting the mouth and auscultating the lungs. *Comments:*	☐	☐	☐	
8. Dispose of all soiled material and wash hands. *Comments:*	☐	☐	☐	

Checklist for Procedure 7-16   Maintaining Mechanical Ventilation

Name _____ Date _____

School _____

Instructor _____

Course _____

Procedure 7-16 Maintaining Mechanical Ventilation	Able to Perform	Able to Perform with Assistance	Unable to Perform	Initials and Date
Assessment				
1. Assess the need for mechanical support, as well as the ordered ventilator settings. *Comments:*	☐	☐	☐	
2. Assess the client's vital signs, ABG results, and airway. *Comments:*	☐	☐	☐	
3. Assess the client's level of comfort. *Comments:*	☐	☐	☐	
Planning/Expected Outcomes				
1. Client's pain and anxiety will be controlled. *Comments:*	☐	☐	☐	
2. Client's ABGs and O_2 saturation levels will be within normal limits. *Comments:*	☐	☐	☐	
3. Client will understand the need for mechanical oxygenation. *Comments:*	☐	☐	☐	
Implementation				
1. Wash hands; apply gloves. *Comments:*	☐	☐	☐	
2. Attach the mechanical ventilator to the secure airway. *Comments:*	☐	☐	☐	
3. Compare ventilator settings with ordered settings, and observe ventilator function. *Comments:*	☐	☐	☐	

continued on the following page

continued from the previous page

Procedure 7-16	Able to Perform	Able to Perform with Assistance	Unable to Perform	Initials and Date
4. Monitor vital signs; observe for distress and discomfort. *Comments:*	☐	☐	☐	
5. Set up suction equipment. *Comments:*	☐	☐	☐	
6. Draw ABGs or assist in drawing up the ABGs. *Comments:*	☐	☐	☐	
7. Remove gloves and wash hands. *Comments:*	☐	☐	☐	
8. Periodically empty accumulated water from tubing. *Comments:*	☐	☐	☐	
9. Periodically verify that the Ambu bag is at hand. *Comments:*	☐	☐	☐	
10. Provide oral care to client as needed. *Comments:*	☐	☐	☐	
11. Provide skin care to client as needed. *Comments:*	☐	☐	☐	
12. Document interventions. *Comments:*	☐	☐	☐	

Checklist for Procedure 7-17   Suctioning Endotracheal and Tracheal Tubes

Name _____ Date _____

School _____

Instructor _____

Course _____

Procedure 7-17 Suctioning Endotracheal and Tracheal Tubes	Able to Perform	Able to Perform with Assistance	Unable to Perform	Initials and Date
Assessment				
1. Assess respirations for rate, rhythm, and depth. *Comments:*	☐	☐	☐	
2. Auscultate lung fields. *Comments:*	☐	☐	☐	
3. Monitor arterial blood gas and/or pulse oximetry values. *Comments:*	☐	☐	☐	
4. Assess passage of air through the endotracheal/tracheal tube. *Comments:*	☐	☐	☐	
5. Monitor secretions for amount, color, consistency, and odor. *Comments:*	☐	☐	☐	
6. Assess for anxiety and restlessness. *Comments:*	☐	☐	☐	
7. Assess the client's understanding of the suctioning procedure. *Comments:*	☐	☐	☐	
Planning/Expected Outcomes				
1. The client will have no crackles or wheezes in large airways and no cyanosis. *Comments:*	☐	☐	☐	
2. The client will appear to breathe comfortably. *Comments:*	☐	☐	☐	
3. The client will have minimal amount of thin secretions. *Comments:*	☐	☐	☐	

continued on the following page

continued from the previous page

Procedure 7-17	Able to Perform	Able to Perform with Assistance	Unable to Perform	Initials and Date
4. The client will maintain a patent airway. *Comments:*	☐	☐	☐	

Implementation

Suctioning Tracheal Tube

1. Assess respirations and breath sounds. *Comments:*	☐	☐	☐	
2. Assemble supplies on bedside table. *Comments:*	☐	☐	☐	
3. Wash hands. *Comments:*	☐	☐	☐	
4. Connect suction tube to source of negative pressure. *Comments:*	☐	☐	☐	
5. Administer oxygen or use Ambu bag. *Comments:*	☐	☐	☐	
6. Remove inner cannula and clean, if reusable, or set aside if disposable. *Comments:*	☐	☐	☐	
7. Apply sterile glove to your dominant hand. *Comments:*	☐	☐	☐	
8. Open sterile suction catheter, remove it from package with your sterile hand, and wrap the catheter around your sterile hand from the tip down to the port end. Or use the reusable closed system catheter. Attach catheter to suction. *Comments:*	☐	☐	☐	
9. Insert the catheter into the trachea without suction. *Comments:*	☐	☐	☐	
10. Apply suction while gently rotating the catheter and removing it. • Disposable catheter: Apply suction by placing your thumb over the open port of the catheter. • Closed system catheter: Apply suction by depressing the white button at the catheter connector. *Comments:*	☐	☐	☐	

Procedure 7-17	Able to Perform	Able to Perform with Assistance	Unable to Perform	Initials and Date
11. Wrap the disposable suction catheter around your sterile hand while withdrawing it from the tube. *Comments:*	☐	☐	☐	
12. Suction for no more than 10 seconds. *Comments:*	☐	☐	☐	
13. Administer oxygen using the ventilator or using an Ambu bag. *Comments:*	☐	☐	☐	
14. Assess airway and repeat suctioning as necessary. *Comments:*	☐	☐	☐	
15. Clean inner cannula or replace disposable inner cannula. *Comments:*	☐	☐	☐	
16. Reinsert inner cannula and lock into place. *Comments:*	☐	☐	☐	
17. Apply humidified oxygen or compressed air. *Comments:*	☐	☐	☐	
18. Remove gloves and discard. *Comments:*	☐	☐	☐	
19. Wash hands. *Comments:*	☐	☐	☐	
20. Record the procedure. *Comments:*	☐	☐	☐	
Suctioning an Endotracheal Tube 21. Repeat Actions 1–14. *Comments:*	☐	☐	☐	
22. Remove gloves and discard. *Comments:*	☐	☐	☐	

continued on the following page

continued from the previous page

Procedure 7-17	Able to Perform	Able to Perform with Assistance	Unable to Perform	Initials and Date
23. Wash hands. *Comments:*	☐	☐	☐	
24. Record the procedure. *Comments:*	☐	☐	☐	

Checklist for Procedure 7-18   Maintaining and Cleaning Endotracheal Tubes

Name _____ Date _____

School _____

Instructor _____

Course _____

Procedure 7-18 **Maintaining and Cleaning Endotracheal Tubes**	Able to Perform	Able to Perform with Assistance	Unable to Perform	Initials and Date
Assessment				
1. Assess the need for endotracheal intubation. *Comments:*	☐	☐	☐	
2. Assess placement of the endotracheal tube. *Comments:*	☐	☐	☐	
3. Assess response to endotracheal tube placement. *Comments:*	☐	☐	☐	
4. Assess cuff pressure. *Comments:*	☐	☐	☐	
Planning/Expected Outcomes				
1. Client will have adequate oxygenation of tissues. *Comments:*	☐	☐	☐	
2. Cuff will be inflated and deflated at designated intervals. Endotracheal tube will be rotated at regular intervals. *Comments:*	☐	☐	☐	
3. Client will be sedated as needed and will be comfortable. *Comments:*	☐	☐	☐	
Implementation				
1. Wash hands. *Comments:*	☐	☐	☐	
2. Prepare tape to be used when endotracheal tube is rotated. *Comments:*	☐	☐	☐	
3. Apply gloves. *Comments:*	☐	☐	☐	

continued on the following page

continued from the previous page

Procedure 7-18	Able to Perform	Able to Perform with Assistance	Unable to Perform	Initials and Date
4. Clean any secretions and old tape from the endotracheal tube. *Comments:*	☐	☐	☐	
5. Gently move the endotracheal tube to the other side of the client's mouth and secure. Assess inside and outside of mouth. *Comments:*	☐	☐	☐	
6. Suction oral cavity as needed. Deflate the cuff. *Comments:*	☐	☐	☐	
7. Reinflate the cuff to a maximum pressure of 15–20 mm Hg. *Comments:*	☐	☐	☐	
8. Remove gloves. *Comments:*	☐	☐	☐	
9. Monitor client for adverse effects; place the call light within reach. *Comments:*	☐	☐	☐	
10. Wash hands. *Comments:*	☐	☐	☐	
11. Document the procedure. *Comments:*	☐	☐	☐	

Checklist for Procedure 7-19   Maintaining and Cleaning the Tracheostomy Tube

Name _____ Date _____

School _____

Instructor _____

Course _____

Procedure 7-19 **Maintaining and Cleaning the Tracheostomy Tube**	Able to Perform	Able to Perform with Assistance	Unable to Perform	Initials and Date
Assessment				
1. Assess respirations for rate, rhythm, and depth. *Comments:*	☐	☐	☐	
2. Auscultate lung fields. *Comments:*	☐	☐	☐	
3. Monitor arterial blood gas and/or pulse oximetry values. *Comments:*	☐	☐	☐	
4. Assess passage of air through tracheostomy tube. *Comments:*	☐	☐	☐	
5. Evaluate amount and color of tracheal secretions. *Comments:*	☐	☐	☐	
6. Assess anxiety, restlessness, and fear. *Comments:*	☐	☐	☐	
7. Assess the client's understanding of the procedure. *Comments:*	☐	☐	☐	
Planning/Expected Outcomes				
1. The tracheostomy site will heal with minimal drainage and erythema. *Comments:*	☐	☐	☐	
2. There will be no evidence of infection. *Comments:*	☐	☐	☐	
3. The client will maintain a patent airway. *Comments:*	☐	☐	☐	

continued on the following page

continued from the previous page

Procedure 7-19	Able to Perform	Able to Perform with Assistance	Unable to Perform	Initials and Date
4. The inner and outer cannulas will be free of secretions. The ties will be clean and secure. *Comments:*	☐	☐	☐	
Implementation				
Cleaning Trach Tube Site 1. Wash hands and apply gloves. *Comments:*	☐	☐	☐	
2. Remove soiled dressing and discard. *Comments:*	☐	☐	☐	
3. Cleanse neck plate with cotton applicators and hydrogen peroxide. *Comments:*	☐	☐	☐	
4. Rinse neck plate with applicators and sterile water or saline. *Comments:*	☐	☐	☐	
5. Cleanse skin under neck plate with cotton applicators and hydrogen peroxide. *Comments:*	☐	☐	☐	
6. Rinse skin under neck plate with applicators and sterile water or saline. *Comments:*	☐	☐	☐	
7. Dry skin under neck plate with dry cotton applicators. *Comments:*	☐	☐	☐	
One-Person Technique of Changing Tracheostomy Ties 8. Prepare clean tracheostomy ties. • Cut twill tape to fit around the client's neck plus 6 inches. Cut the ends of the tape on the diagonal. • Open Velcro ties on continuous neck band. *Comments:*	☐	☐	☐	
9. Leave the old ties in place. Insert one end of the new tie through the neck plate from back to front. Pull the tie ends even, and bring both ends around the back of the neck to the other side. *Comments:*	☐	☐	☐	

Procedure 7-19	Able to Perform	Able to Perform with Assistance	Unable to Perform	Initials and Date
10. Insert the end of the tape through the second opening of the neck plate from back to front. *Comments:*	☐	☐	☐	
11. Securely tie the two ends of the new tape at side of neck. *Comments:*	☐	☐	☐	
12. Cut and remove old tracheostomy tapes and discard. *Comments:*	☐	☐	☐	
13. Place one finger under tracheostomy ties to test security. *Comments:*	☐	☐	☐	
Two-Person Technique of Changing Tracheostomy Ties 14. Cut two pieces of twill tape about 12–14 inches in length. *Comments:*	☐	☐	☐	
15. Fold about 1 inch at the end of twill tape and cut a half-inch slit lengthwise in the center of the fold. Repeat for other tape. *Comments:*	☐	☐	☐	
16. The second person holds the tracheostomy tube in place with fingers on both sides of the neck plate. *Comments:*	☐	☐	☐	
17. Cut old tracheostomy ties and discard. *Comments:*	☐	☐	☐	
18. Insert the split end of the twill tape through the opening on one side of the neck plate. Pull the distal end of the tie through the cut and pull tightly. *Comments:*	☐	☐	☐	
19. Repeat procedure with second piece of twill tape. *Comments:*	☐	☐	☐	
20. Tie tracheostomy tapes securely at the side of the neck. *Comments:*	☐	☐	☐	

continued on the following page

continued from the previous page

Procedure 7-19	Able to Perform	Able to Perform with Assistance	Unable to Perform	Initials and Date
21. Insert one finger under tracheostomy tapes. *Comments:*	☐	☐	☐	
22. Insert lint-free tracheostomy gauze under neck plate of tube. *Comments:*	☐	☐	☐	
23. Discard all used materials and wash hands. *Comments:*	☐	☐	☐	

Checklist for Procedure 7-20   Maintaining a Double Cannula Tracheostomy Tube

Name _____ Date _____

School _____

Instructor _____

Course _____

Procedure 7-20 Maintaining a Double Cannula Tracheostomy Tube	Able to Perform	Able to Perform with Assistance	Unable to Perform	Initials and Date
Assessment				
1. Assess respirations for rate, rhythm, and depth. *Comments:*	☐	☐	☐	
2. Assess the client's lung sounds. *Comments:*	☐	☐	☐	
3. Assess the client's ABGs and/or pulse oximetry values. *Comments:*	☐	☐	☐	
4. Assess the movement of air through the tracheostomy tube. *Comments:*	☐	☐	☐	
5. Assess the amount and color of tracheal secretions. *Comments:*	☐	☐	☐	
6. Assess the client's level of consciousness. *Comments:*	☐	☐	☐	
7. Assess the client's understanding of the procedure. *Comments:*	☐	☐	☐	
Planning/Expected Outcomes				
1. The client's airway will be free of obstruction. *Comments:*	☐	☐	☐	
2. The procedure will be performed with minimum client anxiety. *Comments:*	☐	☐	☐	
3. The client's skin will remain intact. *Comments:*	☐	☐	☐	

continued on the following page

continued from the previous page

Procedure 7-20	Able to Perform	Able to Perform with Assistance	Unable to Perform	Initials and Date
4. The client will remain free of symptoms of infection. *Comments:*	☐	☐	☐	
Implementation				
1. Wash hands. *Comments:*	☐	☐	☐	
Conventional/Reusable Inner Cannula 2. Open tracheostomy care set. *Comments:*	☐	☐	☐	
3. Place hydrogen peroxide solution and sterile water or saline in separate basins. *Comments:*	☐	☐	☐	
4. Apply sterile gloves. *Comments:*	☐	☐	☐	
5. Remove inner cannula. *Comments:*	☐	☐	☐	
6. Place inner cannula in basin of hydrogen peroxide. *Comments:*	☐	☐	☐	
7. Clean the area under the neck plate using a cotton applicator and hydrogen peroxide. *Comments:*	☐	☐	☐	
8. Rinse area under neck plate with a cotton applicator and sterile water or saline. *Comments:*	☐	☐	☐	
9. Dry skin under neck plate with a cotton-tip applicator. *Comments:*	☐	☐	☐	
10. Apply lint free tracheostomy gauze under neck plate. *Comments:*	☐	☐	☐	
11. Use a tracheostomy brush or sterile cotton-tip applicator to clean inner cannula. *Comments:*	☐	☐	☐	

Procedure 7-20	Able to Perform	Able to Perform with Assistance	Unable to Perform	Initials and Date
12. Rinse inner cannula with sterile water or sterile saline. *Comments:*	☐	☐	☐	
13. Dry inner cannula. *Comments:*	☐	☐	☐	
14. Reinsert inner cannula and lock it into place. *Comments:*	☐	☐	☐	
15. Remove gloves and discard. *Comments:*	☐	☐	☐	
16. Wash hands. *Comments:*	☐	☐	☐	
17. Record the procedure. *Comments:*	☐	☐	☐	
Disposable Inner Cannula 18. Wash hands. Open disposable cannula without touching cannula. *Comments:*	☐	☐	☐	
19. Apply sterile gloves. *Comments:*	☐	☐	☐	
20. Remove used inner cannula and discard. *Comments:*	☐	☐	☐	
21. Replace inner cannula with new disposable cannula. *Comments:*	☐	☐	☐	
22. Remove gloves and discard. *Comments:*	☐	☐	☐	
23. Wash hands. *Comments:*	☐	☐	☐	
24. Record the procedure *Comments:*	☐	☐	☐	

Checklist for Procedure 7-21   Plugging the Tracheostomy Tube

Name _____   Date _____

School _____

Instructor _____

Course _____

Procedure 7-21 Plugging the Tracheostomy Tube	Able to Perform	Able to Perform with Assistance	Unable to Perform	Initials and Date
Assessment				
1. Assess respirations for rate, rhythm, and depth. *Comments:*	☐	☐	☐	
2. Assess client's ability to speak. *Comments:*	☐	☐	☐	
Planning/Expected Outcomes				
1. The client will tolerate plugging of the tracheostomy tube while maintaining an adequate airway. *Comments:*	☐	☐	☐	
Implementation				
1. Deflate the cuff on a cuffed tracheostomy tube. *Comments:*	☐	☐	☐	
2. Change the tracheostomy tube to a smaller uncuffed tube. *Comments:*	☐	☐	☐	
3. Replace the inner cannula with a capped inner cannula. *Comments:*	☐	☐	☐	

Checklist for Procedure 8-1   Performing Venipuncture (Blood Drawing)

Name _____ Date _____

School _____

Instructor _____

Course _____

Procedure 8-1 Performing Venipuncture (Blood Drawing)	Able to Perform	Able to Perform with Assistance	Unable to Perform	Initials and Date
Assessment				
1. Determine which test(s) is (are) ordered and any special conditions for the collection or handling of the specimen. *Comments:*	☐	☐	☐	
2. Assess the integrity of the veins to be used in the procedure. *Comments:*	☐	☐	☐	
3. Review the client's medical history. *Comments:*	☐	☐	☐	
4. Determine the client's ability to cooperate with the procedure. *Comments:*	☐	☐	☐	
5. Review the physician's or qualified practitioner's order. *Comments:*	☐	☐	☐	
Planning/Expected Outcomes				
1. Puncture site will not continue to bleed or bruise. *Comments:*	☐	☐	☐	
2. Puncture site will show no evidence of infection. *Comments:*	☐	☐	☐	
3. The specimen will be properly acquired and appropriately handled. *Comments:*	☐	☐	☐	
4. The client will understand the test's purpose and the procedure. *Comments:*	☐	☐	☐	
5. The client will report minimal anxiety from the procedure. *Comments:*	☐	☐	☐	

continued on the following page

continued from the previous page

Procedure 8-1	Able to Perform	Able to Perform with Assistance	Unable to Perform	Initials and Date
Implementation				
1. Greet client by name and validate client's identification. *Comments:*	☐	☐	☐	
2. Explain the procedure to the client. *Comments:*	☐	☐	☐	
3. Wash hands. *Comments:*	☐	☐	☐	
4. Bring equipment to bedside, or client exam room. *Comments:*	☐	☐	☐	
5. Close curtain or door. *Comments:*	☐	☐	☐	
6. Raise or lower bed/table to a comfortable working height. *Comments:*	☐	☐	☐	
7. Position client's arm. *Comments:*	☐	☐	☐	
8. Apply disposable gloves. *Comments:*	☐	☐	☐	
9. Apply the tourniquet 3–4 inches above the venipuncture site. *Comments:*	☐	☐	☐	
10. Check for the distal pulse. *Comments:*	☐	☐	☐	
11. Have client open and close fist several times, leaving fist clenched prior to venipuncture. *Comments:*	☐	☐	☐	
12. Maintain tourniquet only for 1–2 minutes. *Comments:*	☐	☐	☐	
13. Identify the best venipuncture site through palpation. *Comments:*	☐	☐	☐	

Procedure 8-1	Able to Perform	Able to Perform with Assistance	Unable to Perform	Initials and Date
14. Select the vein for venipuncture. *Comments:*	☐	☐	☐	
15. Prepare to obtain the blood sample: • Syringe method: Have appropriate sized syringe and needle. • Vacutainer method: Attach double-ended needle to Vacutainer holder with the blood specimen tube resting inside the holder, without puncturing the stopper. *Comments:*	☐	☐	☐	
16. Cleanse the site with alcohol swab using a circular motion. *Comments:*	☐	☐	☐	
17. Remove the needle cover and warn the client about the needle stick. *Comments:*	☐	☐	☐	
18. Pull the skin taut below the site. *Comments:*	☐	☐	☐	
19. Hold the needle at 15–30° angle to the skin with the bevel up. *Comments:*	☐	☐	☐	
20. Slowly insert needle. *Comments:*	☐	☐	☐	
21. Technique varies depending on equipment used: • Syringe method: Gently pull back on syringe plunger and look for blood return. Obtain desired amount of blood. • Vacutainer method: Advance specimen tube onto double-ended needle. After the tube is full of blood, grasp the holder firmly, remove the tube, and insert additional tubes as indicated. *Comments:*	☐	☐	☐	
22. After the specimen is collected, release the tourniquet. *Comments:*	☐	☐	☐	
23. Place gauze over the puncture site, without pressure, and withdraw the needle from the vein. *Comments:*	☐	☐	☐	

continued on the following page

continued from the previous page

Procedure 8-1	Able to Perform	Able to Perform with Assistance	Unable to Perform	Initials and Date
24. Apply pressure over the venipuncture site until the bleeding has stopped. Tape the gauze or a Band-Aid over the site. *Comments:*	☐	☐	☐	
25. Syringe method: • Insert the syringe needle into the appropriate collection tubes and allow to fill. *Comments:*	☐	☐	☐	
26. Gently rotate tubes with additives 8–10 times. *Comments:*	☐	☐	☐	
27. Inspect the puncture site for bleeding. Reapply gauze and tape as needed. *Comments:*	☐	☐	☐	
28. Assist client for comfort. Return bed to safe, comfortable position. *Comments:*	☐	☐	☐	
29. Check tubes for external blood and decontaminate as appropriate. *Comments:*	☐	☐	☐	
30. Check for proper labeling and packaging for transport to laboratory. *Comments:*	☐	☐	☐	
31. Dispose of soiled equipment appropriately. *Comments:*	☐	☐	☐	
32. Remove and dispose of gloves. *Comments:*	☐	☐	☐	
33. Wash hands after the procedure. *Comments:*	☐	☐	☐	
34. Send specimens to the laboratory. *Comments:*	☐	☐	☐	

Checklist for Procedure 8-2 Starting an IV

Name _____ Date _____

School _____

Instructor _____

Course _____

Procedure 8-2 Starting an IV	Able to Perform	Able to Perform with Assistance	Unable to Perform	Initials and Date
Assessment				
1. Check the written order for the type of IV therapy planned. *Comments:*	☐	☐	☐	
2. Review information regarding the insertion of the IV. *Comments:*	☐	☐	☐	
3. Know the agency's policy regarding who may start an IV. *Comments:*	☐	☐	☐	
4. Assess the client's veins. *Comments:*	☐	☐	☐	
5. Check the client's fluid, electrolyte, and nutritional status. *Comments:*	☐	☐	☐	
6. Assess the client's understanding of the procedure. *Comments:*	☐	☐	☐	
Planning/Expected Outcomes				
1. The IV will be inserted without complications and will remain patent. *Comments:*	☐	☐	☐	
2. Fluid and electrolyte balance will be restored to the client. *Comments:*	☐	☐	☐	
3. Nutrition will be restored or maintained. *Comments:*	☐	☐	☐	
4. The IV site will remain free of swelling and inflammation. *Comments:*	☐	☐	☐	

continued on the following page

continued from the previous page

Procedure 8-2	Able to Perform	Able to Perform with Assistance	Unable to Perform	Initials and Date
Implementation				
1. Check physician's or qualified practitioner's order for an IV. *Comments:*	☐	☐	☐	
2. Wash hands, and put on mask and gown if needed. *Comments:*	☐	☐	☐	
3. Organize all equipment at bedside. *Comments:*	☐	☐	☐	
4. Explain procedure and reason the catheter is being inserted. *Comments:*	☐	☐	☐	
5. Inspect potential sites: • Place a tourniquet around the upper arm. • Examine the veins as they dilate. • Palpate the vein to test for firmness. • Release the tourniquet. *Comments:*	☐	☐	☐	
6. Select vein for venipuncture. *Comments:*	☐	☐	☐	
7. Select appropriate IV needle or catheter. *Comments:*	☐	☐	☐	
8. Prepare supplies: • Place towel or drape on table and place supplies on field. • Open needle adapter end of IV tubing set. *Comments:*	☐	☐	☐	
9. Clip hair on skin at site if necessary. *Comments:*	☐	☐	☐	
10. Ask client to rest arm in a dependent position. *Comments:*	☐	☐	☐	
11. Put on disposable gloves. *Comments:*	☐	☐	☐	

Procedure 8-2	Able to Perform	Able to Perform with Assistance	Unable to Perform	Initials and Date
12. Prepare insertion site: • Place absorbent drape under the arm. • Scrub the insertion site with alcohol and povidone-iodine. • Allow the povidone-iodine to dry. *Comments:*	☐	☐	☐	
13. Apply tourniquet 5–6 inches above the insertion site: • Secure tightly enough to occlude venous flow. • Check presence of distal pulse. *Comments:*	☐	☐	☐	
14. Perform the venipuncture: • Anchor the vein by stretching the skin distal to the site. • Insert the stylet needle at a 20–30° angle, bevel up. • Watch for blood return in the flashback chamber. • Advance stylet into the vein while it is parallel to the skin. • Loosen stylet and advance catheter into vein until the hub rests at the site. • Release the tourniquet. *Comments:*	☐	☐	☐	
15. Attach IV tubing to the IV catheter. • Stabilize the catheter with one hand. • Remove the stylet from catheter. • Connect IV set to hub of catheter. • Begin infusion. *Comments:*	☐	☐	☐	
16. Secure catheter in place: • Tape over the hub of the catheter. • Place gauze pads and tape or transparent dressing over insertion site. *Comments:*	☐	☐	☐	
17. Remove gloves and dispose with all used materials. *Comments:*	☐	☐	☐	
18. Label dressing with date, time, size, and gauge of catheter. *Comments:*	☐	☐	☐	
19. Wash hands. *Comments:*	☐	☐	☐	

Checklist for Procedure 8-3   Inserting a Butterfly Needle

Name _____ Date _____

School _____

Instructor _____

Course _____

Procedure 8-3 Inserting a Butterfly Needle	Able to Perform	Able to Perform with Assistance	Unable to Perform	Initials and Date
Assessment				
1. Assess the purpose of the IV. *Comments:*	☐	☐	☐	
2. Assess the client's veins. *Comments:*	☐	☐	☐	
3. Check the client's fluid, electrolyte, and nutritional status. *Comments:*	☐	☐	☐	
4. Assess the client's understanding of the procedure. *Comments:*	☐	☐	☐	
Planning/Expected Outcomes				
1. The IV will be inserted without complications and will remain patent. *Comments:*	☐	☐	☐	
2. The IV site will be without signs or symptoms of infiltration. *Comments:*	☐	☐	☐	
3. The IV will start and infuse with a minimum of trauma to the client. *Comments:*	☐	☐	☐	
Implementation				
1. Check physician's or qualified practitioner's order for an IV. *Comments:*	☐	☐	☐	
2. Wash hands; put on mask and gown, if needed. *Comments:*	☐	☐	☐	

continued on the following page

continued from the previous page

Procedure 8-3	Able to Perform	Able to Perform with Assistance	Unable to Perform	Initials and Date
3. Organize all equipment at bedside. *Comments:*	☐	☐	☐	
4. Explain procedure and reason the IV needle is being inserted. *Comments:*	☐	☐	☐	
5. Inspect potential sites: • Place a tourniquet around the right upper arm. • Examine the veins as they dilate. • Palpate the vein to test for firmness. • Release the tourniquet. *Comments:*	☐	☐	☐	
6. Select vein for venipuncture. *Comments:*	☐	☐	☐	
7. Select appropriate gauge butterfly needle. *Comments:*	☐	☐	☐	
8. Prepare supplies and sterile field: • Place towel with supplies on table. • Open needle adapter end of IV tubing set. *Comments:*	☐	☐	☐	
9. Clip hair on skin at site if necessary. *Comments:*	☐	☐	☐	
10. Ask client to rest arm in a dependent position. *Comments:*	☐	☐	☐	
11. Apply disposable gloves. *Comments:*	☐	☐	☐	
12. Prepare insertion site: • Place towel or absorbent drape under the arm. • Scrub the insertion site with alcohol and povidone-iodine. • Allow the povidone-iodine to dry. *Comments:*	☐	☐	☐	

Procedure 8-3	Able to Perform	Able to Perform with Assistance	Unable to Perform	Initials and Date
13. Apply tourniquet 5–6 inches above the insertion site: • Check presence of distal pulse. *Comments:*	☐	☐	☐	
14. Perform the venipuncture: • Anchor the vein by stretching the skin distal to the site. • Grasping the needle wings, insert needle, bevel up, at a 20–30° angle slightly distal to the site. • Watch for a blood return through the attached tubing. • Advance needle into the vein until the hub rests at the site. • Release the tourniquet. *Comments:*	☐	☐	☐	
15. Attach IV tubing to butterfly needle: • Stabilize the needle with one hand. • Connect IV set to hub of butterfly needle tubing. • Begin infusion. *Comments:*	☐	☐	☐	
16. Secure needle in place: • Place tape over the wings of the butterfly needle. • Place gauze over site and secure with tape or transparent dressing. *Comments:*	☐	☐	☐	
17. Remove gloves and dispose of all used materials. *Comments:*	☐	☐	☐	
18. Label dressing with date, time, size, and gauge of needle. *Comments:*	☐	☐	☐	
19. Wash hands. *Comments:*	☐	☐	☐	

① pt.
② med.
③ dose
④ time
⑤
⑥ documentation

Checklist for Procedure 8-4 Preparing the IV Bag and Tubing

Name _____ Date _____

School _____

Instructor _____

Course _____

Procedure 8-4 Preparing the IV Bag and Tubing	Able to Perform	Able to Perform with Assistance	Unable to Perform	Initials and Date
Assessment				
1. Check the written order for the IV to be infused and the flow rate. *Comments:*	☐	☐	☐	
2. Review information regarding the solution and nursing implications. *Comments:*	☐	☐	☐	
3. Check all additives in the solution and other medications. *Comments:*	☐	☐	☐	
4. Assess the patency of the IV. *Comments:* (site)	☐	☐	☐	
5. Assess the skin at the IV site. *Comments:*	☐	☐	☐	
6. Assess the client's understanding of the procedure. *Comments:*	☐	☐	☐	
Planning/Expected Outcomes				
1. The IV tubing will be replaced without compromising sterility. *Comments:*	☐	☐	☐	
2. The tubing will infuse the solution without leaks or air bubbles. *Comments:*	☐	☐	☐	
3. The IV solution will infuse at the prescribed rate. *Comments:*	☐	☐	☐	
4. The client will understand the purpose of the IV therapy. *Comments:*	☐	☐	☐	

continued on the following page

continued from the previous page

Procedure 8-4	Able to Perform	Able to Perform with Assistance	Unable to Perform	Initials and Date
Implementation				
1. Check the written order for the IV solution. *Comments:*	☐	☐	☐	
2. Wash hands. *Comments:*	☐	☐	☐	
3. Check client's identification bracelet. *Comments:*	☐	☐	☐	
4. Remove cover from bag or bottle. Check the expiration date and assess for cloudiness or leakage. *Comments:*	☐	☐	☐	
5. Open new infusion set. Unroll tubing and close roller clamp. *Comments:*	☐	☐	☐	
6. Spike bag with new tubing and fill drip chamber halfway. *Comments:*	☐	☐	☐	
7. Open roller clamp and flush the tubing with solution. *Comments:*	☐	☐	☐	
8. Close roller clamp and replace cap protector. *Comments:*	☐	☐	☐	
9. Apply clean gloves. *Comments:*	☐	☐	☐	
10. Remove old tubing and replace with new tubing: • Place sterile gauze under IV catheter. • Stabilize hub of IV and gently pull out old tubing. • Insert new tubing into hub of catheter or needle. • Open roller clamp to establish flow of IV solution. • Reestablish drip rate. • Apply new dressing to IV site. *Comments:*	☐	☐	☐	
11. Discard old tubing and IV bag. *Comments:*	☐	☐	☐	

Procedure 8-4	Able to Perform	Able to Perform with Assistance	Unable to Perform	Initials and Date
12. Remove gloves and dispose with all used materials. *Comments:*	☐	☐	☐	
13. Apply a label with date and time of tubing change. *Comments:*	☐	☐	☐	
14. Wash hands. *Comments:*	☐	☐	☐	

Checklist for Procedure 8-5   Setting the IV Flow Rate

Name _____ Date _____

School _____

Instructor _____

Course _____

Procedure 8-5 Setting the IV Flow Rate	Able to Perform	Able to Perform with Assistance	Unable to Perform	Initials and Date
Assessment				
1. Check the written order for the IV to be infused and flow rate. *Comments:*	☐	☐	☐	
2. Review information regarding the solution and nursing implications. *Comments:*	☐	☐	☐	
3. Assess the patency of the IV. *Comments:*	☐	☐	☐	
4. Assess the skin at the IV site. *Comments:*	☐	☐	☐	
5. Assess the client's understanding of the IV infusion. *Comments:*	☐	☐	☐	
Planning/Expected Outcomes				
1. The fluid will be infused into the vein without complications. *Comments:*	☐	☐	☐	
2. The IV catheter will remain patent. *Comments:*	☐	☐	☐	
3. The fluid and electrolyte balance will return to normal. *Comments:*	☐	☐	☐	
4. The client will be able to discuss the purpose of the IV therapy. *Comments:*	☐	☐	☐	

continued on the following page

continued from the previous page

Procedure 8-5	Able to Perform	Able to Perform with Assistance	Unable to Perform	Initials and Date
Implementation				
1. Check written order for the IV solution and rate of infusion. *Comments:*	☐	☐	☐	
2. Wash hands. *Comments:*	☐	☐	☐	
3. Check client's identification bracelet. *Comments:*	☐	☐	☐	
4. Prepare to set flow rate: • Have paper and pencil ready to calculate flow rate. • Review calibration (gtt/ml) of each infusion set. *Comments:*	☐	☐	☐	
5. Determine hourly rate by dividing total volume by total hours. *Comments:*	☐	☐	☐	
6. Label the IV bag or bottle with the hourly time periods. *Comments:*	☐	☐	☐	
7. Calculate the minute rate based on the drop factor of the infusion set. *Comments:*	☐	☐	☐	
8. Set flow rate: • Regular tubing; no device: Count drops in drip chamber for 1 minute and adjust the roller clamp. • Infusion pump: Insert the tubing into the pump, select the rate, open the roller clamp, and push start button. • Controller: Place bag 36 inches above the IV site, select the drops per minute, open the roller clamp, and count drops for 1 minute to verify the rate. • Volume control device: Place device between IV bag and IV tubing, fill with 1–2 hours of IV fluid, and count drops for 1 minute. *Comments:*	☐	☐	☐	
9. Monitor infusion rate and IV site for infiltration. *Comments:*	☐	☐	☐	
10. Assess infusion when alarm sounds. *Comments:*	☐	☐	☐	
11. Wash hands. *Comments:*	☐	☐	☐	

Checklist for Procedure 8-6   Assessing and Maintaining an IV Insertion Site

Name _____ Date _____

School _____

Instructor _____

Course _____

Procedure 8-6 **Assessing and Maintaining an IV Insertion Site**	Able to Perform	Able to Perform with Assistance	Unable to Perform	Initials and Date
Assessment				
1. Review the order for IV therapy. *Comments:*	☐	☐	☐	
2. Identify potential risk factors for fluid and electrolyte imbalances. *Comments:*	☐	☐	☐	
3. Assess for dehydration. *Comments:*	☐	☐	☐	
4. Assess for fluid overload. *Comments:*	☐	☐	☐	
5. Determine the client's risk for complications from IV therapy. *Comments:*	☐	☐	☐	
6. Observe IV site for complications. *Comments:*	☐	☐	☐	
7. Observe IV site for patency. *Comments:*	☐	☐	☐	
8. Assess the client's knowledge regarding the IV therapy. *Comments:*	☐	☐	☐	
Planning/Expected Outcomes				
1. The IV will be patent, without infection or inflammation. *Comments:*	☐	☐	☐	
2. The fluid and electrolyte balance will return to and remain normal. *Comments:*	☐	☐	☐	

continued on the following page

continued from the previous page

Procedure 8-6	Able to Perform	Able to Perform with Assistance	Unable to Perform	Initials and Date
3. The client will be able to report signs of inflammation or infiltration. *Comments:*	☐	☐	☐	
4. The client's IV will be administered per order. *Comments:*	☐	☐	☐	
5. The client's IV dressing will remain intact, clean, and dry. *Comments:*	☐	☐	☐	
Implementation				
1. Review the written order for IV therapy. *Comments:*	☐	☐	☐	
2. Review client's history for medical conditions or allergies. *Comments:*	☐	☐	☐	
3. Review client's IV site record and intake and output record. *Comments:*	☐	☐	☐	
4. Wash hands. *Comments:*	☐	☐	☐	
5. Obtain client's vital signs. *Comments:*	☐	☐	☐	
6. Check IV for correct fluid, additives, rate, and volume at the beginning of your shift. *Comments:*	☐	☐	☐	
7. Check IV tubing for tight connections every 4 hours. *Comments:*	☐	☐	☐	
8. Check gauze IV dressing hourly to be sure it is dry and intact. *Comments:*	☐	☐	☐	
9. If gauze is not dry and intact, observe site for redness, swelling, or drainage every hour. *Comments:*	☐	☐	☐	

Procedure 8-6	Able to Perform	Able to Perform with Assistance	Unable to Perform	Initials and Date
10. If an occlusive dressing is used, do not remove dressing when assessing the site. *Comments:*	☐	☐	☐	
11. Observe vein track hourly. *Comments:*	☐	☐	☐	
12. Document findings in the nursing record or IV flow sheet. *Comments:*	☐	☐	☐	
13. Wash hands. *Comments:*	☐	☐	☐	

Checklist for Procedure 8-7   Changing the IV Solution

Name _____ Date _____

School _____

Instructor _____

Course _____

Procedure 8-7 Changing the IV Solution	Able to Perform	Able to Perform with Assistance	Unable to Perform	Initials and Date
Assessment				
1. Check the written order for the solution, rate, and medications to be given. *Comments:*	☐	☐	☐	
2. Review information regarding nursing implications. *Comments:*	☐	☐	☐	
3. Check all additives in the solution and other medications. *Comments:*	☐	☐	☐	
4. Assess the patency of the IV. *Comments:*	☐	☐	☐	
5. Assess the skin at the IV site. *Comments:*	☐	☐	☐	
6. Assess the client's understanding of the IV infusion. *Comments:*	☐	☐	☐	
Planning/Expected Outcomes				
1. The ordered solution will be infused correctly without complications. *Comments:*	☐	☐	☐	
2. The IV catheter will remain patent. *Comments:*	☐	☐	☐	
3. The client will understand the purpose of the IV therapy. *Comments:*	☐	☐	☐	
4. The solution infused will not harm the client. *Comments:*	☐	☐	☐	

continued on the following page

continued from the previous page

Procedure 8-7	Able to Perform	Able to Perform with Assistance	Unable to Perform	Initials and Date
Implementation				
1. Check the written order for the IV solution. *Comments:*	☐	☐	☐	
2. Wash hands and put on clean gloves. *Comments:*	☐	☐	☐	
3. Check client's identification bracelet. *Comments:*	☐	☐	☐	
4. Prepare new bag with additives, as ordered, one hour before needed. *Comments:*	☐	☐	☐	
5. Be sure drip chamber is at least half full. *Comments:*	☐	☐	☐	
6. Change IV solution: • Close roller clamp to stop flow of fluid. • Remove old IV from pole, and hang new bag. • Spike new bag or bottle with tubing. • Reestablish prescribed flow rate. *Comments:*	☐	☐	☐	
7. Check for air in tubing. Remove air bubbles if found. *Comments:*	☐	☐	☐	
8. Empty remaining fluid from old IV if needed. *Comments:*	☐	☐	☐	
9. Remove gloves and dispose of all used materials. *Comments:*	☐	☐	☐	
10. Label IV with date, time, and type of solution. *Comments:*	☐	☐	☐	
11. Wash hands. *Comments:*	☐	☐	☐	

Checklist for Procedure 8-8   Discontinuing the IV and Changing to a Saline or Heparin Lock

Name _____ Date _____

School _____

Instructor _____

Course _____

Procedure 8-8 Discontinuing the IV and Changing to a Saline or Heparin Lock	Able to Perform	Able to Perform with Assistance	Unable to Perform	Initials and Date
Assessment				
1. Check the written order for the insertion of the saline or heparin lock. *Comments:*	☐	☐	☐	
2. For existing IVs, assess the patency of the IV. *Comments:*	☐	☐	☐	
3. For existing IVs, assess the skin at the IV site. *Comments:*	☐	☐	☐	
4. Check the client's drug allergy history. *Comments:*	☐	☐	☐	
5. Assess the client's understanding of the heparin lock. *Comments:*	☐	☐	☐	
Planning/Expected Outcomes				
1. The IV is discontinued and heparin lock placed without complications. *Comments:*	☐	☐	☐	
2. The IV site remains patent and free of complications. *Comments:*	☐	☐	☐	
3. The IV will be converted with a minimum of trauma. *Comments:*	☐	☐	☐	
4. For new sites, the heparin lock is placed with a minimum of trauma. *Comments:*	☐	☐	☐	

continued on the following page

continued from the previous page

Procedure 8-8	Able to Perform	Able to Perform with Assistance	Unable to Perform	Initials and Date
Implementation				
1. Check the written order to discontinue IV and to insert a heparin lock. *Comments:*	☐	☐	☐	
2. Wash hands and put on clean gloves. *Comments:*	☐	☐	☐	
3. Check client's identification bracelet. *Comments:*	☐	☐	☐	
4. Explain procedure and reason for discontinuing IV to client. *Comments:*	☐	☐	☐	
5. Prepare supplies at bedside. *Comments:*	☐	☐	☐	
6. For a new saline lock: • Prime the extension tubing with a saline lock cap on it. • Follow the procedure for starting an IV. • Attach the catheter to the extension tubing. • Dress the site. *Comments:*	☐	☐	☐	
7. If discontinuing an IV and converting to a heparin lock: • Stop IV infusion. • Close roller clamp on IV tubing. • Turn off infusion pump. *Comments:*	☐	☐	☐	
8. Place saline lock: • Open sterile package with heparin lock. • For existing IV, loosen and remove IV tubing. • Screw heparin lock into hub of catheter. *Comments:*	☐	☐	☐	
9. Check for patency of IV: • Clean heparin lock with antiseptic solution. • Insert saline syringe into center of diaphragm. • Pull back on syringe and watch for blood return. • Inject saline slowly into lock. *Comments:*	☐	☐	☐	

Procedure 8-8	Able to Perform	Able to Perform with Assistance	Unable to Perform	Initials and Date
10. Every 8 hours or at every use: • Clean the rubber diaphragm with an antiseptic swab. • Insert the syringe with saline into the diaphragm. • Inject saline slowly into lock. *Comments:*	☐	☐	☐	
11. Remove the syringe and swab the diaphragm with antiseptic. *Comments:*	☐	☐	☐	
12. Assess the site for leakage, irritation, or infiltration. *Comments:*	☐	☐	☐	
13. Remove gloves and dispose with all used materials. *Comments:*	☐	☐	☐	
14. Wash hands. *Comments:*	☐	☐	☐	

Checklist for Procedure 8-9   Administering a Blood Transfusion

Name _____ Date _____

School _____

Instructor _____

Course _____

Procedure 8-9 Administering a Blood Transfusion	Able to Perform	Able to Perform with Assistance	Unable to Perform	Initials and Date
Assessment				
1. Assess the client for indications requiring the blood product to be given. *Comments:*	☐	☐	☐	
2. Verify the written order for the blood product to be given. *Comments:*	☐	☐	☐	
3. Review the client's transfusion history. *Comments:*	☐	☐	☐	
4. Review the client's baseline vital signs. *Comments:*	☐	☐	☐	
5. Assess the type, integrity, and patency of venous access. *Comments:*	☐	☐	☐	
6. Verify that a large-bore IV catheter is to be used. *Comments:*	☐	☐	☐	
7. Review hospital policy and procedure for the administration of blood products. *Comments:*	☐	☐	☐	
8. Ensure that the client has signed an informed consent release that includes potential risks and benefits. *Comments:*	☐	☐	☐	
Planning/Expected Outcomes				
1. The client receives the transfusion without adverse reactions or with successfully managed reactions. *Comments:*	☐	☐	☐	
2. The client demonstrates desired benefit from transfusion. *Comments:*	☐	☐	☐	

continued on the following page

continued from the previous page

Procedure 8-9	Able to Perform	Able to Perform with Assistance	Unable to Perform	Initials and Date
3. The client understands the purpose and procedure of the transfusion. *Comments:*	☐	☐	☐	
4. The client describes the possible complications of a transfusion. *Comments:*	☐	☐	☐	

Implementation

Procedure 8-9	Able to Perform	Able to Perform with Assistance	Unable to Perform	Initials and Date
1. Verify the written order for the transfusion. *Comments:*	☐	☐	☐	
2. If a venipuncture is necessary, refer to Skill 8-1. *Comments:*	☐	☐	☐	
3. Explain procedure to the client. *Comments:*	☐	☐	☐	
4. Review side effects with client and instruct the client to report any to the nurse. *Comments:*	☐	☐	☐	
5. Have the client sign consent forms. *Comments:*	☐	☐	☐	
6. Obtain baseline vital signs. *Comments:*	☐	☐	☐	
7. Obtain the blood product from the blood bank within 30 minutes of initiation. *Comments:*	☐	☐	☐	
8. Verify the blood product and the client with another nurse. • Client's name, blood group, Rh type • Cross-match compatibility • Donor blood group and Rh type • Unit and hospital number • Expiration date and time on blood bag • Type of blood product compared with written order • Presence of clots in blood *Comments:*	☐	☐	☐	

Procedure 8-9	Able to Perform	Able to Perform with Assistance	Unable to Perform	Initials and Date
9. Instruct client to empty the bladder. *Comments:*	☐	☐	☐	
10. Wash hands and put on gloves. *Comments:*	☐	☐	☐	
11. Open blood administration kit and close roller clamps. *Comments:*	☐	☐	☐	
12. For Y-tubing set: • Spike the normal saline bag and prime the tubing between the saline bag and the filter. • Squeeze sides of drip chamber and allow filter to partially fill. • Open lower roller clamp and prime tubing to the hub. • Close lower clamp. • Invert blood bag once or twice. Spike blood bag, open clamps, and fill tubing completely, covering the filter with blood. • Close lower clamp. *Comments:*	☐	☐	☐	
13. For single-tubing set: • Spike blood unit using filter tubing. • Squeeze drip chamber and allow the filter to fill with blood. • Open roller clamp and allow tubing to fill with blood. • Piggyback a saline line into the blood administration tubing. • Secure all connections with tape. *Comments:*	☐	☐	☐	
14. Attach tubing to venous catheter aseptically and open clamps on blood tubing. *Comments:*	☐	☐	☐	
15. Infuse the blood product at the ordered rate. *Comments:*	☐	☐	☐	
16. Remain with client for first 15–30 minutes, monitoring vital signs frequently according to institutional policy. *Comments:*	☐	☐	☐	

continued on the following page

continued from the previous page

Procedure 8-9	Able to Perform	Able to Perform with Assistance	Unable to Perform	Initials and Date
17. After blood has infused, flush the tubing with normal saline. *Comments:*	☐	☐	☐	
18. Dispose of bag, tubing, and gloves appropriately. Wash hands. *Comments:*	☐	☐	☐	
19. Document the procedure. *Comments:*	☐	☐	☐	

Checklist for Procedure 8-10 Assessing and Responding to Transfusion Reactions

Name _____ Date _____

School _____

Instructor _____

Course _____

Procedure 8-10 Assessing and Responding to Transfusion Reactions	Able to Perform	Able to Perform with Assistance	Unable to Perform	Initials and Date
Assessment				
1. Assess for symptoms of an acute hemolytic reaction. *Comments:*	☐	☐	☐	
2. Assess for a nonhemolytic reaction. *Comments:*	☐	☐	☐	
3. Assess for an allergic reaction. *Comments:*	☐	☐	☐	
4. Assess for a citrate reaction. *Comments:*	☐	☐	☐	
5. Assess for sepsis. *Comments:*	☐	☐	☐	
6. Assess for circulatory overload. Assess for hypothermia and cardiac dysrhythmias. *Comments:*	☐	☐	☐	
7. Assess for graft-versus-host disease (GVHD) in the immunocompromised client. *Comments:*	☐	☐	☐	
8. Assess for a delayed hemolytic reaction. *Comments:*	☐	☐	☐	
Planning/Expected Outcomes				
1. The client will have a normal temperature and no chills. *Comments:*	☐	☐	☐	

continued on the following page

continued from the previous page

Procedure 8-10	Able to Perform	Able to Perform with Assistance	Unable to Perform	Initials and Date
2. The client will have normal tissue perfusion and cardiac output. *Comments:*	☐	☐	☐	
3. The client will be calm and comfortable. *Comments:*	☐	☐	☐	
4. The client will show no signs of infection. *Comments:*	☐	☐	☐	
Implementation				
1. Stop the transfusion. *Comments:*	☐	☐	☐	
2. Using gloved hangs, remove tubing with blood and replace with new tubing. *Comments:*	☐	☐	☐	
3. Maintain a patent IV with normal saline. *Comments:*	☐	☐	☐	
4. Obtain vital signs, including oxygen saturation. *Comments:*	☐	☐	☐	
5. Remove gloves and wash hands. *Comments:*	☐	☐	☐	
6. Notify physician of client's transfusion reaction. *Comments:*	☐	☐	☐	
7. Monitor client's vital signs at least every 15 minutes. *Comments:*	☐	☐	☐	
8. Read the blood component bag to ensure that the correct unit was given to the correct client. *Comments:*	☐	☐	☐	
9. Administer medications as prescribed. *Comments:*	☐	☐	☐	
10. Start cardiopulmonary resuscitation if indicated. *Comments:*	☐	☐	☐	

Procedure 8-10	Able to Perform	Able to Perform with Assistance	Unable to Perform	Initials and Date
11. Obtain two blood samples from arm opposite transfusion. *Comments:*	☐	☐	☐	
12. Return the remaining blood and tubing to blood bank. *Comments:*	☐	☐	☐	
13. Obtain first voided urine. *Comments:*	☐	☐	☐	

Checklist for Procedure 8-11 Assisting with the Insertion of a Central Venous Catheter

Name _____ Date _____

School _____

Instructor _____

Course _____

Procedure 8-11 **Assisting with the Insertion of a Central Venous Catheter**	Able to Perform	Able to Perform with Assistance	Unable to Perform	Initials and Date
Assessment				
1. Verify policy regarding central venous catheter insertion. *Comments:*	☐	☐	☐	
2. Review client's past medical history. *Comments:*	☐	☐	☐	
3. Assess client's knowledge regarding central venous catheter insertion and care. *Comments:*	☐	☐	☐	
4. Assess the client's ability to cooperate with the procedure. *Comments:*	☐	☐	☐	
5. Assess whether or not consent is needed and signed. *Comments:*	☐	☐	☐	
Planning/Expected Outcomes				
1. Central venous catheter will be placed in an optimal position for the client. *Comments:*	☐	☐	☐	
2. The client will not experience any adverse effects from the catheter insertion. *Comments:*	☐	☐	☐	
3. The client will experience a minimum of anxiety and pain. *Comments:*	☐	☐	☐	
Implementation				
1. Wash hands. *Comments:*	☐	☐	☐	

continued on the following page

continued from the previous page

Procedure 8-11	Able to Perform	Able to Perform with Assistance	Unable to Perform	Initials and Date
2. Check the written order for type of catheter to be placed. *Comments:*	☐	☐	☐	
3. Check for drug or iodine allergies. *Comments:*	☐	☐	☐	
4. Clean chest area with Betadine and drape appropriately. *Comments:*	☐	☐	☐	
5. Assist with administration of subcutaneous lidocaine. *Comments:*	☐	☐	☐	
6. Prior to insertion, prime the central venous catheter lumens. *Comments:*	☐	☐	☐	
7. The qualified practitioner will thread the catheter into the superior vena cava through a small incision. *Comments:*	☐	☐	☐	
8. Following insertion, the practitioner will secure and dress the catheter. *Comments:*	☐	☐	☐	
9. The practitioner will flush each lumen of the catheter. *Comments:*	☐	☐	☐	
10. Chest x-ray is performed. *Comments:*	☐	☐	☐	
11. Wash hands. *Comments:*	☐	☐	☐	

Checklist for Procedure 8-12   Changing the Central Venous Dressing

Name _____   Date _____

School _____

Instructor _____

Course _____

Procedure 8-12 Changing the Central Venous Dressing	Able to Perform	Able to Perform with Assistance	Unable to Perform	Initials and Date
Assessment				
1. Assess the need for dressing change. *Comments:*	☐	☐	☐	
2. Assess the timing of the dressing change. *Comments:*	☐	☐	☐	
3. Assess the type of central venous access in place. *Comments:*	☐	☐	☐	
4. Assess the integrity of the skin at the site. *Comments:*	☐	☐	☐	
5. Assess the client's and caregiver's knowledge of the purpose and care of the catheter. *Comments:*	☐	☐	☐	
Planning/Expected Outcomes				
1. Skin is intact and not edematous at the catheter site. *Comments:*	☐	☐	☐	
2. Client has no signs of systemic infection. *Comments:*	☐	☐	☐	
3. Catheter and tubing are intact. *Comments:*	☐	☐	☐	
4. Client and caregiver are able to perform skin care and dressing change. *Comments:*	☐	☐	☐	

continued on the following page

continued from the previous page

Procedure 8-12	Able to Perform	Able to Perform with Assistance	Unable to Perform	Initials and Date
Implementation				
1. Wash hands and put on clean gloves. *Comments:*	☐	☐	☐	
2. Remove old dressing carefully. Do not dislodge the catheter. *Comments:*	☐	☐	☐	
3. Note drainage on dressing. *Comments:*	☐	☐	☐	
4. Inspect skin at insertion site. *Comments:*	☐	☐	☐	
5. Palpate tunneled catheter for presence of Dacron cuff. *Comments:*	☐	☐	☐	
6. Inspect catheter from hub to skin. *Comments:*	☐	☐	☐	
7. Remove gloves and put on sterile gloves. *Comments:*	☐	☐	☐	
8. Clean exit site with povidone-iodine swab. *Comments:*	☐	☐	☐	
9. Apply povidone-iodine ointment to exit site. *Comments:*	☐	☐	☐	
10. Apply transparent dressing. *Comments:*	☐	☐	☐	
11. Label with date and time of dressing change. *Comments:*	☐	☐	☐	
12. Secure tubing to client's clothing. *Comments:*	☐	☐	☐	

Procedure 8-12	Able to Perform	Able to Perform with Assistance	Unable to Perform	Initials and Date
13. Remove gloves and dispose of all used materials. *Comments:*	☐	☐	☐	
14. Wash hands. *Comments:*	☐	☐	☐	

Checklist for Procedure 8-13   Changing the Central Venous Tubing

Name _____ Date _____

School _____

Instructor _____

Course _____

Procedure 8-13 Changing the Central Venous Tubing	Able to Perform	Able to Perform with Assistance	Unable to Perform	Initials and Date
Assessment				
1. Verify policy regarding frequency of central venous catheter tubing changes. *Comments:*	☐	☐	☐	
2. Check original orders regarding rate of infusion and duration. *Comments:*	☐	☐	☐	
3. Assess client's knowledge regarding fluid or medications. *Comments:*	☐	☐	☐	
4. Assess client's catheter site. *Comments:*	☐	☐	☐	
Planning/Expected Outcomes				
1. Central venous catheter tubing will be changed according to policy. *Comments:*	☐	☐	☐	
2. The client will remain free of infection secondary to the central venous catheter tubing. *Comments:*	☐	☐	☐	
3. The client will remain free of infection secondary to the central venous catheter tubing change. *Comments:*	☐	☐	☐	
Implementation				
1. Wash hands. *Comments:*	☐	☐	☐	
2. Check MAR against the written orders. *Comments:*	☐	☐	☐	

continued on the following page

continued from the previous page

Procedure 8-13	Able to Perform	Able to Perform with Assistance	Unable to Perform	Initials and Date
3. Check for drug allergies. *Comments:*	☐	☐	☐	
4. Assemble the equipment needed. *Comments:*	☐	☐	☐	
5. Check the client's armband. *Comments:*	☐	☐	☐	
6. Identify the fluids for the client and their therapeutic purpose. *Comments:*	☐	☐	☐	
7. Clamp off new tubing. Spike bag with new tubing. Fill drip chamber about half full. Prime new tubing. *Comments:*	☐	☐	☐	
8. Clamp off the central venous catheter and old tubing. Disconnect old tubing and connect new tubing aseptically. Secure the connection. *Comments:*	☐	☐	☐	
9. Insert tubing into pump and unclamp new tubing. Set pump or adjust drip rate to infuse at ordered rate. *Comments:*	☐	☐	☐	
10. Label tubing with next date to be changed. Document tubing change. *Comments:*	☐	☐	☐	
11. Wash hands. *Comments:*	☐	☐	☐	

Checklist for Procedure 8-14   Flushing a Central Venous Catheter

Name _____ Date _____

School _____

Instructor _____

Course _____

Procedure 8-14 Flushing a Central Venous Catheter	Able to Perform	Able to Perform with Assistance	Unable to Perform	Initials and Date
Assessment				
1. Assess the type of central venous line in place. *Comments:*	☐	☐	☐	
2. Assess the function and patency of the catheter. *Comments:*	☐	☐	☐	
3. Assess client's knowledge of the purpose of the central venous line. *Comments:*	☐	☐	☐	
Planning/Expected Outcomes				
1. The nurse will be able to aspirate blood through the catheter. *Comments:*	☐	☐	☐	
2. The nurse will be able to infuse fluid through the catheter. *Comments:*	☐	☐	☐	
3. The client will not exhibit any symptoms of systemic infection. *Comments:*	☐	☐	☐	
4. The visible portion of the catheter will be intact. *Comments:*	☐	☐	☐	
Implementation				
1. Wash hands. Apply gloves and protective equipment as needed. *Comments:*	☐	☐	☐	
2. Prepare two syringes: one with saline and one with heparin solution. *Comments:*	☐	☐	☐	

continued on the following page

continued from the previous page

Procedure 8-14	Able to Perform	Able to Perform with Assistance	Unable to Perform	Initials and Date
3. Swab injection cap or hub with povidone-iodine and alcohol. *Comments:*	☐	☐	☐	
4. Clamp catheter and remove cap. *Comments:*	☐	☐	☐	
5. Check catheter for patency: • Attach syringe with normal saline. • Release clamp. • Aspirate heparin solution from catheter. • Observe blood return. • Flush with normal saline. • Reclamp. • Remove empty syringe. • Attach syringe filled with heparin solution to catheter. • Release clamp. • Flush quickly. • Reclamp. *Comments:*	☐	☐	☐	
6. Place new cap on catheter, tape all connections, and attach tubing to client's clothing. *Comments:*	☐	☐	☐	
7. Dispose of soiled equipment and used supplies. *Comments:*	☐	☐	☐	
8. Wash hands. *Comments:*	☐	☐	☐	

Checklist for Procedure 8-15   Measuring Central Venous Pressure (CVP)

Name _____ Date _____

School _____

Instructor _____

Course _____

Procedure 8-15 Measuring Central Venous Pressure (CVP)	Able to Perform	Able to Perform with Assistance	Unable to Perform	Initials and Date
Assessment				
1. Assess the client's ability to lie in a supine position without a pillow. Comments:	☐	☐	☐	
2. Assess the client's vital signs and intake and output. Comments:	☐	☐	☐	
Planning/Expected Outcomes				
1. The client's CVP will be measured accurately. Comments:	☐	☐	☐	
2. Aseptic technique will be maintained. Comments:	☐	☐	☐	
3. The client will not suffer any complications. Comments:	☐	☐	☐	
Implementation				
Taking a CVP with a Manometer 1. Wash hands and apply nonsterile gloves. Comments:	☐	☐	☐	
2. Explain procedure to client. Comments:	☐	☐	☐	
3. Gather equipment needed at bedside. Comments:	☐	☐	☐	
4. Mark the right atrium with an "X" using indelible ink pen. Comments:	☐	☐	☐	
5. Connect the IV fluid to a three-way stopcock and flush the ports. Comments:	☐	☐	☐	

continued on the following page

continued from the previous page

Procedure 8-15	Able to Perform	Able to Perform with Assistance	Unable to Perform	Initials and Date
6. Apply sterile gloves and mask. *Comments:*	☐	☐	☐	
7. Connect the CVP manometer to the upper port of the stopcock. *Comments:*	☐	☐	☐	
8. Connect the tubing from the client to the remaining stopcock port. *Comments:*	☐	☐	☐	
9. Allow normal saline to flow rapidly for a few seconds, with stopcock closed to manometer. *Comments:*	☐	☐	☐	
10. Turn stopcock off to client and fill manometer with normal saline above the anticipated reading. *Comments:*	☐	☐	☐	
11. Hold manometer at the phlebostatic axis and turn the stopcock off to the saline. *Comments:*	☐	☐	☐	
12. As the fluid falls in the manometer, take the pressure reading when the fluid stabilizes. *Comments:*	☐	☐	☐	
13. Turn the stopcock off to the manometer. *Comments:*	☐	☐	☐	
14. Store the manometer in an upright position. *Comments:*	☐	☐	☐	
15. Wash hands. *Comments:*	☐	☐	☐	
16. Document reading. *Comments:*	☐	☐	☐	

Procedure 8-15	Able to Perform	Able to Perform with Assistance	Unable to Perform	Initials and Date
Taking a CVP Using a Transducer				
17. Wash hands. *Comments:*	☐	☐	☐	
18. Prime the transducer and the attached IV lines. *Comments:*	☐	☐	☐	
19. Place the IV bag into a pressure bag and pressurize the IV solution. *Comments:*	☐	☐	☐	
20. Attach the IV pressure tubing from the transducer to the central line. *Comments:*	☐	☐	☐	
21. Attach the transducer to the pressure monitoring equipment. *Comments:*	☐	☐	☐	
22. Place the client in the supine position with the bed flat. *Comments:*	☐	☐	☐	
23. Level the pressure transducer to the phlebostatic axis. *Comments:*	☐	☐	☐	
24. Zero the monitor according to the manufacturer's instructions. *Comments:*	☐	☐	☐	
25. The CVP will appear on the monitor. *Comments:*	☐	☐	☐	
26. Return the client to a position of comfort. *Comments:*	☐	☐	☐	
27. Wash hands. *Comments:*	☐	☐	☐	
28. Document CVP reading. *Comments:*	☐	☐	☐	

Checklist for Procedure 8-16   Drawing Blood from a Central Venous Catheter

Name _____ Date _____

School _____

Instructor _____

Course _____

Procedure 8-16 **Drawing Blood from a Central Venous Catheter**	Able to Perform	Able to Perform with Assistance	Unable to Perform	Initials and Date
Assessment				
1. Assess the type of central venous line in place. *Comments:*	☐	☐	☐	
2. Assess the need to use the central line for blood samples. *Comments:*	☐	☐	☐	
3. Assess the function and patency of the catheter. *Comments:*	☐	☐	☐	
4. Assess client's knowledge of the central line in relation to obtaining blood samples. *Comments:*	☐	☐	☐	
5. Check the written order for blood sampling. *Comments:*	☐	☐	☐	
Planning/Expected Outcomes				
1. The blood sample obtained will be representative of the client's circulating blood. *Comments:*	☐	☐	☐	
2. The blood sample will not be contaminated. *Comments:*	☐	☐	☐	
3. The blood will be collected in the appropriate containers. *Comments:*	☐	☐	☐	
4. The client will not suffer any infection or complications. *Comments:*	☐	☐	☐	
5. The client's central venous catheter will remain intact and patent. *Comments:*	☐	☐	☐	

continued on the following page

continued from the previous page

Procedure 8-16	Able to Perform	Able to Perform with Assistance	Unable to Perform	Initials and Date
Implementation				
1. Wash hands. Apply gown and gloves. *Comments:*	☐	☐	☐	
2. Prepare two syringes: one with saline and one with heparin solution. *Comments:*	☐	☐	☐	
3. Swab injection site with povidone-iodine and alcohol. *Comments:*	☐	☐	☐	
4. Shut off IV solutions infusing through the other ports of the central line. *Comments:*	☐	☐	☐	
5. Clamp catheter and remove cap, if appropriate. *Comments:*	☐	☐	☐	
6. Aspirate heparin solution in catheter: • Attach empty syringe or vacutainer adapter and tube to catheter. • Release clamp. • Aspirate 5 ml of blood. • Clamp catheter. • Remove syringe or vacutainer tube and discard. *Comments:*	☐	☐	☐	
7. Obtain blood samples: • Attach empty syringe or place appropriate vacutainer tube into the adapter. • Release clamp. • Collect blood. • Clamp catheter. • Remove syringe or adapter and attach new capped needle. *Comments:*	☐	☐	☐	
8. Flush catheter: • Attach syringe filled with saline to catheter. • Release clamp. • Flush quickly. • Reclamp. • Attach syringe filled with heparin solution to catheter. • Release clamp. • Flush quickly. • Reclamp. *Comments:*	☐	☐	☐	

Procedure 8-16	Able to Perform	Able to Perform with Assistance	Unable to Perform	Initials and Date
9. Place new cap on catheter, tape all connections, and attach tubing to client's clothing. *Comments:*	☐	☐	☐	
10. Prepare blood samples: • Insert blood-filled syringe into blood tube and allow to fill. Repeat for all tubes ordered. • Label blood tubes with client's identification. • Fill out requisition forms. • Send to laboratory. *Comments:*	☐	☐	☐	
11. Dispose of soiled equipment and used supplies. Wash hands. *Comments:*	☐	☐	☐	

Checklist for Procedure 8-17   Infusing Total Parenteral Nutrition (TPN) and Fat Emulsion through a Central Venous Catheter

Name _____ Date _____

School _____

Instructor _____

Course _____

Procedure 8-17 Infusing Total Parenteral Nutrition (TPN) and Fat Emulsion through a Central Venous Catheter	Able to Perform	Able to Perform with Assistance	Unable to Perform	Initials and Date
Assessment				
1. Determine the presence of an ongoing nutritional plan. *Comments:*	☐	☐	☐	
2. Determine the type of venous access to be utilized for TPN. *Comments:*	☐	☐	☐	
3. Review the written orders. Compare the ordered solution with the venous access to be utilized. *Comments:*	☐	☐	☐	
4. Review the client's medical history and rationale for central parenteral nutrition (CPN). *Comments:*	☐	☐	☐	
5. Review the client's baseline vital signs and laboratory values. *Comments:*	☐	☐	☐	
6. If lipid emulsion is ordered, review the client's history of food allergies. *Comments:*	☐	☐	☐	
Planning/Expected Outcomes				
1. Client maintains ideal body weight. *Comments:*	☐	☐	☐	
2. Client gains weight to reach ideal body weight as appropriate. *Comments:*	☐	☐	☐	
3. Serum glucose levels are less than 200 mg/dl. *Comments:*	☐	☐	☐	

continued on the following page

continued from the previous page

Procedure 8-17	Able to Perform	Able to Perform with Assistance	Unable to Perform	Initials and Date
4. Venous access site remains patent and free of infection. Comments:	☐	☐	☐	
5. Client masters self-administration of CPN as needed. Comments:	☐	☐	☐	

Implementation

1. Remove TPN from refrigerator an hour before hanging. Comments:	☐	☐	☐	
2. Inspect fluid for precipitate, discoloration, or cream separation. Comments:	☐	☐	☐	
3. Wash hands. Comments:	☐	☐	☐	
4. Using aseptic technique, attach and prime filter tubing. Comments:	☐	☐	☐	
5. Insert tubing into the infusion pump and connect it to the catheter. Comments:	☐	☐	☐	
6. Regulate flow rate based on client's needs and written orders. Comments:	☐	☐	☐	
7. Check to see that all IV connections are secured. Comments:	☐	☐	☐	
8. Recheck flow rate and function of infusion pump. Comments:	☐	☐	☐	
9. Wash hands. Comments:	☐	☐	☐	

Checklist for Procedure 8-18   Removing the Central Venous Catheter

Name _____ Date _____

School _____

Instructor _____

Course _____

Procedure 8-18 Removing the Central Venous Catheter	Able to Perform	Able to Perform with Assistance	Unable to Perform	Initials and Date
Assessment				
1. Verify policy regarding removal of central venous catheter. *Comments:*	☐	☐	☐	
2. Check original order regarding removal of catheter. *Comments:*	☐	☐	☐	
3. Assess client's knowledge regarding catheter removal. *Comments:*	☐	☐	☐	
Planning/Expected Outcomes				
1. Central venous catheter will be removed in accordance with institutional policy. *Comments:*	☐	☐	☐	
Implementation				
1. Wash hands and apply gloves. *Comments:*	☐	☐	☐	
2. Check written orders regarding removal of catheter. *Comments:*	☐	☐	☐	
3. Check the client's armband before removing catheter. *Comments:*	☐	☐	☐	
4. Set up equipment and supplies aseptically. *Comments:*	☐	☐	☐	
5. Remove tape and dressings from around catheter. *Comments:*	☐	☐	☐	
6. Free the cuff from the tissue and pull the catheter smoothly. *Comments:*	☐	☐	☐	

continued on the following page

continued from the previous page

Procedure 8-18	Able to Perform	Able to Perform with Assistance	Unable to Perform	Initials and Date
7. Apply pressure to the site. Assess for bleeding. *Comments:*	☐	☐	☐	
8. For culture, cut off tip of catheter into a sterile container. *Comments:*	☐	☐	☐	
9. Place gauze over exit site and hold pressure until bleeding stops. Apply a gauze dressing. *Comments:*	☐	☐	☐	
10. Wash hands. *Comments:*	☐	☐	☐	

Checklist for Procedure 8-19   Inserting a Peripherally Inserted Central Catheter (PICC)

Name _____ Date _____

School _____

Instructor _____

Course _____

Procedure 8-19 **Inserting a Peripherally Inserted Central Catheter (PICC)**	Able to Perform	Able to Perform with Assistance	Unable to Perform	Initials and Date
Assessment				
1. Check the written order for the type of catheter. *Comments:*	☐	☐	☐	
2. Review information regarding the insertion of the catheter. *Comments:*	☐	☐	☐	
3. Know the agency's policy regarding who may insert a PICC. *Comments:*	☐	☐	☐	
4. Assess the pulse in the antecubital fossa. *Comments:*	☐	☐	☐	
5. Check the client's fluid, electrolyte, and nutritional status. *Comments:*	☐	☐	☐	
6. Assess the client's understanding of the procedure. *Comments:*	☐	☐	☐	
Planning/Expected Outcomes				
1. The PICC will be inserted without complications and will remain patent. *Comments:*	☐	☐	☐	
2. The client will remain free of complications secondary to the insertion of a PICC. *Comments:*	☐	☐	☐	
3. The client will not suffer neurovascular damage secondary to the PICC insertion. *Comments:*	☐	☐	☐	
4. The client will be able to discuss the purpose of the PICC. *Comments:*	☐	☐	☐	

continued on the following page

continued from the previous page

Procedure 8-19	Able to Perform	Able to Perform with Assistance	Unable to Perform	Initials and Date
Implementation				
1. Check physician's or qualified practitioner's order for PICC. *Comments:*	☐	☐	☐	
2. Wash hands; put on mask and gown. *Comments:*	☐	☐	☐	
3. Organize all equipment at bedside. *Comments:*	☐	☐	☐	
4. Explain procedure and reason the catheter is being inserted. *Comments:*	☐	☐	☐	
5. Identify vein to be used: • Place a tourniquet around the right upper arm. • Examine the veins in the antecubital fossa. • Release the tourniquet. *Comments:*	☐	☐	☐	
6. Have client lie flat with arm extended at a 90° angle. Have client apply mask. *Comments:*	☐	☐	☐	
7. Determine the length of catheter. The measurement method varies depending on the vein used. *Comments:*	☐	☐	☐	
8. Prepare supplies and sterile field: • Open sterile towel and place on table for the sterile field. • Open sterile supplies and drop onto sterile field. • Place heparin and saline vials next to sterile field. *Comments:*	☐	☐	☐	

Procedure 8-19	Able to Perform	Able to Perform with Assistance	Unable to Perform	Initials and Date
9. Clip hair on skin at site if necessary. *Comments:*	☐	☐	☐	
10. Put on sterile gloves. *Comments:*	☐	☐	☐	
11. Prepare catheter and tubing: • Measure the determined length of catheter plus 1 inch. • Cut the catheter with sterile scissors at the appropriate length. • Attach the injection cap to the extension tubing. • Draw up saline into a syringe. • Flush each cap and tubing with sterile saline and leave the syringe in place. • Inspect the catheter for cracks or kinks. • Verify patency of introducer. *Comments:*	☐	☐	☐	
12. Prepare insertion site: • Place sterile drapes under the arm. • Scrub the insertion site with alcohol and povidone-iodine. • Allow the povidone-iodine to dry. *Comments:*	☐	☐	☐	
13. Remove gloves and reapply tourniquet. • Place sterile 4 × 4 gauze over tourniquet. *Comments:*	☐	☐	☐	
14. Put on new pair of sterile gloves without powder. *Comments:*	☐	☐	☐	
15. Place sterile drapes over the insertion site. *Comments:*	☐	☐	☐	
16. Inject local anesthetic at the insertion site. *Comments:*	☐	☐	☐	

continued on the following page

continued from the previous page

Procedure 8-19	Able to Perform	Able to Perform with Assistance	Unable to Perform	Initials and Date
17. Insert the PICC: • Insert the introducer needle with the bevel up. • Watch for a blood return through the introducer. • Verify its placement in a vein, not an artery. • Advance the introducer one-quarter to one-half inch further into the vein. • Insert the catheter through the introducer needle. • Advance the catheter slowly 2–3 inches using the nontoothed forceps. • Be sure the guidewire remains within the lumen of the PICC during insertion. • Release the tourniquet using the sterile 4 × 4 gauze. • Advance the catheter until the tip is at the client's shoulder. • Instruct the client to turn his or her head toward the venous access site and drop chin to chest. • Continue to advance the catheter the predetermined length. • Withdraw the introducer needle using the forceps. • Tell the client to expect to hear a snapping sound. • Press the wings together until they snap; then remove the needle. • Remove the guidewire with a gentle twisting motion. *Comments:*	☐	☐	☐	
18. Check catheter placement: • Attach a syringe filled with normal saline to the lumen. • Aspirate blood. • Flush the catheter with normal saline. • Repeat if there is more than one lumen. *Comments:*	☐	☐	☐	
19. Secure catheter in place: • Attach the extension tubing and cap to the lumen. • Place Steri-strips over the catheter or suture in place. • Place gauze pads and a transparent dressing over insertion site. • Coil the extension tubing and tape to client's arm. *Comments:*	☐	☐	☐	
20. Fill syringe with 3 ml heparin and flush each lumen. *Comments:*	☐	☐	☐	
21. Remove gloves and dispose with all used materials. *Comments:*	☐	☐	☐	

Procedure 8-19	Able to Perform	Able to Perform with Assistance	Unable to Perform	Initials and Date
22. Label dressing with date, time, size, and gauge of catheter. *Comments:*	☐	☐	☐	
23. Wash hands. *Comments:*	☐	☐	☐	
24. Order chest x-ray to document correct placement of PICC. *Comments:*	☐	☐	☐	
25. Postinsertion care of the PICC: • Replace gauze with transparent occlusive dressing 24 hours after insertion. • Change dressing every 3–7 days. • Check length of external tubing with each dressing change. • Flush the catheter with saline and heparin after any infusion. *Comments:*	☐	☐	☐	

Checklist for Procedure 8-20   Administering Peripheral Vein Total Parenteral Nutrition

Name _____ Date _____

School _____

Instructor _____

Course _____

Procedure 8-20 **Administering Peripheral Vein Total Parenteral Nutrition**	Able to Perform	Able to Perform with Assistance	Unable to Perform	Initials and Date
Assessment				
1. Assess the client's knowledge of the therapy. *Comments:*	☐	☐	☐	
2. Check for an allergy to eggs. *Comments:*	☐	☐	☐	
3. Assess the client's veins. *Comments:*	☐	☐	☐	
4. Assess the client's IV site several times daily. *Comments:*	☐	☐	☐	
5. Assess for signs of sepsis. *Comments:*	☐	☐	☐	
6. Monitor blood sugars. *Comments:*	☐	☐	☐	
7. Check daily for changes in the written order. *Comments:*	☐	☐	☐	
8. Check the client's laboratory results daily. *Comments:*	☐	☐	☐	
9. Check that the peripheral parenteral nutrition (PPN) label exactly matches the PPN order. *Comments:*	☐	☐	☐	
10. Check identification band when hanging a new bottle of PPN. *Comments:*	☐	☐	☐	
11. Assess weight daily. *Comments:*	☐	☐	☐	

continued on the following page

continued from the previous page

Procedure 8-20	Able to Perform	Able to Perform with Assistance	Unable to Perform	Initials and Date
Planning/Expected Outcomes				
1. Client will receive adequate nutritional support via PPN. *Comments:*	☐	☐	☐	
2. Client will maintain weight. *Comments:*	☐	☐	☐	
3. There are no complications at peripheral site. *Comments:*	☐	☐	☐	
Implementation				
1. Check the label on the PPN bag against the written order. Check expiration date. *Comments:*	☐	☐	☐	
2. Inspect the PPN bag for precipitates, cloudiness, or leakage. *Comments:*	☐	☐	☐	
3. Inspect the lipid solution for separation, oiliness, or particles. *Comments:*	☐	☐	☐	
4. Check that the client does not have an allergy to eggs. *Comments:*	☐	☐	☐	
5. Gather IV controller tubing and a filter for the PPN. *Comments:*	☐	☐	☐	
6. Wash hands. *Comments:*	☐	☐	☐	
7. Attach the filter to the IV tubing and close the clamp. Spike the tubing into the bag. *Comments:*	☐	☐	☐	
8. Hang the PPN and prime the tubing. Date the tubing. *Comments:*	☐	☐	☐	
9. Remove the protective cap from the lipid container and cleanse the rubber stopper with alcohol. *Comments:*	☐	☐	☐	

Procedure 8-20	Able to Perform	Able to Perform with Assistance	Unable to Perform	Initials and Date
10. Close the clamp on the vented tubing and spike the tubing into the bottle using aseptic technique. *Comments:*	☐	☐	☐	
11. Hang the lipids and prime tubing. Date the tubing. *Comments:*	☐	☐	☐	
12. Attach the lipid tubing to the PPN tubing via the Y-connector. *Comments:*	☐	☐	☐	
13. Insert tubing for PPN and lipids into the IV pumps. *Comments:*	☐	☐	☐	
14. Check client's armband before beginning infusion. *Comments:*	☐	☐	☐	
15. Verify patency of IV site or perform venipuncture. *Comments:*	☐	☐	☐	
16. Wear gloves to connect the IV tubing to the IV catheter. Tape all connections. *Comments:*	☐	☐	☐	
17. Turn on IV pumps at the prescribed rate. Start at half the prescribed rate for the first 30–60 minutes. *Comments:*	☐	☐	☐	
18. Monitor client for allergic reactions during the initial lipid administration. *Comments:*	☐	☐	☐	
19. Record the PPN and lipid administration. *Comments:*	☐	☐	☐	

continued on the following page

continued from the previous page

Procedure 8-20	Able to Perform	Able to Perform with Assistance	Unable to Perform	Initials and Date
20. Check the IV site several times during the day for signs of infiltration or phlebitis. *Comments:*	☐	☐	☐	
21. Wash hands. *Comments:*	☐	☐	☐	

Checklist for Procedure 8-21 Hemodialysis Site Care

Name _____ Date _____

School _____

Instructor _____

Course _____

Procedure 8-21 Hemodialysis Site Care	Able to Perform	Able to Perform with Assistance	Unable to Perform	Initials and Date
Assessment				
1. Identify the client's renal failure and other chronic diseases. *Comments:*	☐	☐	☐	
2. Assess the venous access site. *Comments:*	☐	☐	☐	
3. Assess vital signs. *Comments:*	☐	☐	☐	
4. Check for pain or numbness in access site extremity. *Comments:*	☐	☐	☐	
5. Check for bruit and thrill in the fistula/graft. *Comments:*	☐	☐	☐	
6. Assess client's knowledge of site care and hemodialysis. *Comments:*	☐	☐	☐	
Planning/Expected Outcomes				
1. Access is patent for dialysis without evidence of complications. *Comments:*	☐	☐	☐	
2. Client is able to discuss access and self-care principles and practices. *Comments:*	☐	☐	☐	
Implementation				
Arteriovenous Fistula: Shunt or Graft 1. Wash hands. *Comments:*	☐	☐	☐	

continued on the following page

continued from the previous page

Procedure 8-21	Able to Perform	Able to Perform with Assistance	Unable to Perform	Initials and Date
2. Position extremity so that you can easily palpate the fistula. *Comments:*	☐	☐	☐	
3. Palpate over the area to feel for thrill (vibration). *Comments:*	☐	☐	☐	
4. Auscultate over the area to detect a bruit (swishing noise). *Comments:*	☐	☐	☐	
5. Palpate pulses and observe capillary refill distal to the fistula. *Comments:*	☐	☐	☐	
6. Assess for complications in the area around the fistula and the entire extremity. *Comments:*	☐	☐	☐	
7. Post signs noting to avoid venipuncture and blood pressure in the fistula extremity. *Comments:*	☐	☐	☐	
8. Inform client to avoid activities that will restrict blood flow or injure the affected extremity. *Comments:*	☐	☐	☐	
9. When the incision is healed, the skin over the fistula requires only routine care. *Comments:*	☐	☐	☐	
Double-Lumen Catheter 10. Wash hands. *Comments:*	☐	☐	☐	
11. Fill two syringes with heparin and saline. *Comments:*	☐	☐	☐	
12. If changing caps, prime with heparin and saline. *Comments:*	☐	☐	☐	

Procedure 8-21	Able to Perform	Able to Perform with Assistance	Unable to Perform	Initials and Date
13. Open care kit or assemble supplies and place on sterile field. *Comments:*	☐	☐	☐	
14. Put on mask and nonsterile gloves. *Comments:*	☐	☐	☐	
15. Remove old dressing and discard with gloves appropriately. *Comments:*	☐	☐	☐	
16. Put on sterile gloves. *Comments:*	☐	☐	☐	
17. Cleanse site with alcohol and assess site. *Comments:*	☐	☐	☐	
18. Cleanse surrounding area with povidone-iodine. *Comments:*	☐	☐	☐	
19. Let air dry and apply transparent dressing. *Comments:*	☐	☐	☐	
20. Close clamp to both lumens and remove and discard old caps. *Comments:*	☐	☐	☐	
21. Cleanse ends of catheter with alcohol and attach new, primed caps. *Comments:*	☐	☐	☐	
22. Unclamp lumens and flush with heparin and saline. *Comments:*	☐	☐	☐	
23. Some institutional policies will include aspirating the resident heparin solution before flushing. *Comments:*	☐	☐	☐	

Checklist for Procedure 8-22   Using an Implantable Venous Access Device

Name _____ Date _____

School _____

Instructor _____

Course _____

Procedure 8-22 Using an Implantable Venous Access Device	Able to Perform	Able to Perform with Assistance	Unable to Perform	Initials and Date
Assessment				
1. Assess for criteria favorable to port placement. *Comments:*	☐	☐	☐	
2. Determine the suitability of the treatment to be delivered via the port. *Comments:*	☐	☐	☐	
3. Assess the client's understanding of the procedure. *Comments:*	☐	☐	☐	
4. Assess the site condition and catheter patency. *Comments:*	☐	☐	☐	
Planning/Expected Outcomes				
1. The client describes the purpose, benefits, and risks of the implanted port. *Comments:*	☐	☐	☐	
2. The client reports minimal discomfort when the device is accessed. *Comments:*	☐	☐	☐	
3. The client completes therapy via the implanted device with minimal complications. *Comments:*	☐	☐	☐	
4. The client describes symptoms of complications and measures to manage these complications. *Comments:*	☐	☐	☐	
Implementation				
1. Review the written order. *Comments:*	☐	☐	☐	

continued on the following page

continued from the previous page

Procedure 8-22	Able to Perform	Able to Perform with Assistance	Unable to Perform	Initials and Date
2. Explain the procedure to the client. *Comments:*	☐	☐	☐	
3. Gather supplies. *Comments:*	☐	☐	☐	
4. Wash hands. *Comments:*	☐	☐	☐	
5. Expose skin and palpate port septum. *Comments:*	☐	☐	☐	
6. Administer local anesthetic if necessary. *Comments:*	☐	☐	☐	
7. Put on sterile gloves. *Comments:*	☐	☐	☐	
8. Clean area with alcohol and povidone-iodine. *Comments:*	☐	☐	☐	
9. Prime needle and extension set with saline solution. *Comments:*	☐	☐	☐	
10. Stabilize port and insert needle through the skin and septum. *Comments:*	☐	☐	☐	
11. Aspirate blood to verify needle placement and port function. *Comments:*	☐	☐	☐	
12. Obtain blood samples as prescribed. *Comments:*	☐	☐	☐	
13. Flush the line with saline solution to clear blood and establish patency of the line. *Comments:*	☐	☐	☐	

Procedure 8-22	Able to Perform	Able to Perform with Assistance	Unable to Perform	Initials and Date
14. Proceed with medication administration as indicated. *Comments:*	☐	☐	☐	
15. Secure needle with a sterile dressing. If left in place, change every 7 days. *Comments:*	☐	☐	☐	
16. When removing needle, flush with heparin solution, maintaining positive pressure at the end of the instillation. *Comments:*	☐	☐	☐	
17. Stabilize port and remove needle. *Comments:*	☐	☐	☐	
18. Apply pressure and dressing to needle insertion site. *Comments:*	☐	☐	☐	
19. Document interventions. *Comments:*	☐	☐	☐	

Checklist for Procedure 8-23   Caring for an Implanted Venous Access Device

Name _____ Date _____

School _____

Instructor _____

Course _____

Procedure 8-23 **Caring for an Implanted Venous Access Device**	Able to Perform	Able to Perform with Assistance	Unable to Perform	Initials and Date
Assessment				
1. Assess the type of venous access device (VAD) in place. *Comments:*	☐	☐	☐	
2. Assess the function and patency of the catheter. *Comments:*	☐	☐	☐	
3. Assess client's knowledge of the purpose of the catheter. *Comments:*	☐	☐	☐	
4. Check policies regarding maintaining patency of an implantable VAD. *Comments:*	☐	☐	☐	
Planning/Expected Outcomes				
1. The nurse will be able to aspirate blood through the catheter. *Comments:*	☐	☐	☐	
2. The nurse will be able to infuse fluid through the catheter. *Comments:*	☐	☐	☐	
3. The skin at the insertion site and the puncture site will remain intact. *Comments:*	☐	☐	☐	
4. The client will have no signs or symptoms of infection. *Comments:*	☐	☐	☐	
5. The catheter injection port will remain intact. *Comments:*	☐	☐	☐	
6. The client/caregiver will be able to explain the purpose and maintenance of the VAD. *Comments:*	☐	☐	☐	

continued on the following page

continued from the previous page

Procedure 8-23	Able to Perform	Able to Perform with Assistance	Unable to Perform	Initials and Date
7. The client/caregiver will be able to perform dressing changes and skin care. *Comments:*	☐	☐	☐	
8. The access site will be free of signs of infiltration. *Comments:*	☐	☐	☐	
Implementation				
1. Wash hands. Apply gown and mask, if required. *Comments:*	☐	☐	☐	
2. Prepare sterile field and lay out supplies. *Comments:*	☐	☐	☐	
3. Swab skin over port with alcohol and povidone-iodine. *Comments:*	☐	☐	☐	
4. Apply sterile gloves. *Comments:*	☐	☐	☐	
5. Prepare sterile syringe with 20 ml of normal saline. *Comments:*	☐	☐	☐	
6. Prepare Huber needle: • Attach extension tubing between saline syringe and Huber needle. • Fill tubing with saline solution. *Comments:*	☐	☐	☐	
7. Apply sterile drape to port site. *Comments:*	☐	☐	☐	
8. Access port: • Palpate port septum using aseptic technique. • Insert Huber needle through skin. • Push down until needle rests against needle stop. *Comments:*	☐	☐	☐	
9. Flush port with normal saline. *Comments:*	☐	☐	☐	

Procedure 8-23	Able to Perform	Able to Perform with Assistance	Unable to Perform	Initials and Date
10. Obtain blood sample if ordered: • Aspirate 5 ml of fluid and discard. • Aspirate blood with syringe size equal to desired amount. • Flush port with normal saline. • Flush port with heparin solution if no IV is started. *Comments:*	☐	☐	☐	
11. Set up IV infusion: • Secure Huber needle with sterile dressing. • Connect IV tubing to Huber needle. • Set flow rate of infusion as ordered. When the infusion is finished: • Flush port with normal saline. • Flush port with heparin solution if no further therapy is ordered. *Comments:*	☐	☐	☐	
12. Dispose of soiled equipment appropriately. Wash hands. *Comments:*	☐	☐	☐	

Checklist for Procedure 8-24   Obtaining an Arterial Blood Gas Specimen

Name _____ Date _____

School _____

Instructor _____

Course _____

Procedure 8-24 Obtaining an Arterial Blood Gas Specimen	Able to Perform	Able to Perform with Assistance	Unable to Perform	Initials and Date
Assessment				
1. Assess for symptoms that require an arterial blood gas sample. *Comments:*	☐	☐	☐	
2. Assess if the client has had a change in oxygenation less than 30 minutes ago. *Comments:*	☐	☐	☐	
3. Assess collateral blood flow by performing Allen's test. *Comments:*	☐	☐	☐	
4. Assess tissue surrounding artery. *Comments:*	☐	☐	☐	
5. Assess client's baseline or most recent ABG. *Comments:*	☐	☐	☐	
6. Assess client's knowledge about the procedure. *Comments:*	☐	☐	☐	
Planning/Expected Outcomes				
1. The client will have normal ABG results. *Comments:*	☐	☐	☐	
2. The extremity distal to the puncture will be unchanged. *Comments:*	☐	☐	☐	
3. The client will be calm and free of pain. *Comments:*	☐	☐	☐	
4. The client will have minimal bleeding from puncture site. *Comments:*	☐	☐	☐	

continued on the following page

continued from the previous page

Procedure 8-24	Able to Perform	Able to Perform with Assistance	Unable to Perform	Initials and Date
Implementation				
1. Explain procedure to client in calm tone of voice. *Comments:*	☐	☐	☐	

2. Prepare syringe with heparin:
  • Aspirate heparin into syringe from vial.
  • Withdraw plunger the entire length of syringe and eject all heparin.
Comments:
	☐	☐	☐	

3. Select safest and most accessible site for ABG sample.
  • Perform Allen's test. Select the radial artery if Allen's test is positive.
  • Brachial artery should be used if Allen's test is negative.
  • Femoral artery is used only by specially trained practitioners.
Comments:
	☐	☐	☐	

4. Wash hands and put on gloves. *Comments:*	☐	☐	☐	
5. Palpate radial site with fingertips and slightly hyperextend client's wrist. *Comments:*	☐	☐	☐	
6. Use alcohol to clean the area above the pulse. *Comments:*	☐	☐	☐	
7. Hold alcohol swab in one hand while keeping a fingertip from the other hand on the artery. *Comments:*	☐	☐	☐	
8. Insert needle with bevel up into artery at a 45° angle. *Comments:*	☐	☐	☐	
9. Hold the syringe still when blood appears in the syringe. *Comments:*	☐	☐	☐	
10. Allow arterial pulsing to pump blood into syringe. *Comments:*	☐	☐	☐	

Procedure 8-24	Able to Perform	Able to Perform with Assistance	Unable to Perform	Initials and Date
11. When finished, hold alcohol swab over the puncture site and withdraw needle. *Comments:*	☐	☐	☐	
12. Apply pressure with the alcohol swab over the puncture site. *Comments:*	☐	☐	☐	
13. Inspect site for signs of complications. *Comments:*	☐	☐	☐	
14. Remove gloves and wash hands. *Comments:*	☐	☐	☐	
15. Prepare sample for laboratory and send it: • Expel any air bubbles from syringe. • Label syringe with client identification. • Place syringe in cup of crushed ice. • Fill out requisition form. *Comments:*	☐	☐	☐	
16. Review ABG results and compare with normal values. *Comments:*	☐	☐	☐	
17. Report results and perform nursing measures accordingly. *Comments:*	☐	☐	☐	

Checklist for Procedure 8-25 Assisting with the Insertion and Maintenance of an Epidural Catheter

Name _____ Date _____

School _____

Instructor _____

Course _____

Procedure 8-25 Assisting with the Insertion and Maintenance of an Epidural Catheter	Able to Perform	Able to Perform with Assistance	Unable to Perform	Initials and Date
Assessment				
1. Perform a history and physical before epidural placement. *Comments:*	☐	☐	☐	
2. Assess baseline vital signs. *Comments:*	☐	☐	☐	
3. Assess client's ability to follow directions and communicate. *Comments:*	☐	☐	☐	
Planning/Expected Outcomes				
1. Client will experience sensation expected from the epidural. *Comments:*	☐	☐	☐	
2. Client will experience no untoward effects of epidural anesthesia. *Comments:*	☐	☐	☐	
3. Client will perform self-medication as appropriate. *Comments:*	☐	☐	☐	
4. Client will experience desired effect until it is appropriate to discontinue treatment. *Comments:*	☐	☐	☐	
Implementation				
1. Review preanesthesia orders. *Comments:*	☐	☐	☐	
2. Assemble equipment. *Comments:*	☐	☐	☐	

continued on the following page

continued from the previous page

Procedure 8-25	Able to Perform	Able to Perform with Assistance	Unable to Perform	Initials and Date
3. Apply client monitors in accordance with institutional policy. *Comments:*	☐	☐	☐	
4. Assist client to lying or sitting position. *Comments:*	☐	☐	☐	
5. Assess that the client is able to maintain a stable position. *Comments:*	☐	☐	☐	
6. Maintain calm milieu. *Comments:*	☐	☐	☐	
7. Monitor for: • Untoward effects of medication or anesthesia. • Untoward effects associated with a dural puncture. *Comments:*	☐	☐	☐	
8. Assist anesthesia practitioner to stabilize catheter. *Comments:*	☐	☐	☐	
9. Follow practitioner's direction for client positioning. *Comments:*	☐	☐	☐	
10. Initiate automatic drug delivery system. *Comments:*	☐	☐	☐	
11. Perform frequent blood pressure and neurologic exams. *Comments:*	☐	☐	☐	
12. Monitor client at frequent intervals for analgesic and/or anesthetic effects, and compliance with mobility limitations. *Comments:*	☐	☐	☐	

Checklist for Procedure 9-1   Bandaging

Name _____ Date _____

School _____

Instructor _____

Course _____

Procedure 9-1 Bandaging	Able to Perform	Able to Perform with Assistance	Unable to Perform	Initials and Date
Assessment				
1. Assess the wound to be covered if a wound is involved. *Comments:*	☐	☐	☐	
2. Assess the client's level of consciousness. *Comments:*	☐	☐	☐	
3. Assess the client's skin integrity. *Comments:*	☐	☐	☐	
4. Assess the neurovascular status. *Comments:*	☐	☐	☐	
5. Assess that client is not allergic to latex products. *Comments:*	☐	☐	☐	
Planning/Expected Outcomes				
1. The client does not become hypovolemic, and bleeding is controlled. *Comments:*	☐	☐	☐	
2. The wound is supported and in alignment. *Comments:*	☐	☐	☐	
3. The bandage is applied properly. *Comments:*	☐	☐	☐	
4. The client does not experience discomfort from the bandaging. *Comments:*	☐	☐	☐	
5. There is adequate circulation to the wound and distal body parts. *Comments:*	☐	☐	☐	

continued on the following page

continued from the previous page

Procedure 9-1	Able to Perform	Able to Perform with Assistance	Unable to Perform	Initials and Date
6. The client does not report any numbness or tingling. *Comments:*	☐	☐	☐	
7. The wound heals without skin breakdown or neurovascular damage. *Comments:*	☐	☐	☐	
Implementation				
1. Wash hands. *Comments:*	☐	☐	☐	
2. Determine the reason for the bandage. *Comments:*	☐	☐	☐	
3. Assess the neurovascular status. *Comments:*	☐	☐	☐	
4. Assess skin integrity. *Comments:*	☐	☐	☐	
5. Assess need for immobilization. *Comments:*	☐	☐	☐	
6. Assess client's comfort and level of consciousness. *Comments:*	☐	☐	☐	
7. Gather materials needed, based on assessment. *Comments:*	☐	☐	☐	
8. Apply the bandage. • Hold roll in dominant hand. Hold the loose end with the nondominant hand. • Unroll bandage proximally, applying slight tension. • Overlap the first two or three turns to secure the loose end. • The bandage can be transferred from hand to hand. Avoid bandaging too tightly. *Comments:*	☐	☐	☐	

Procedure 9-1	Able to Perform	Able to Perform with Assistance	Unable to Perform	Initials and Date
9. Common Bandaging Methods: • Figure eight: Ascend obliquely above and below joint, in a figure-eight fashion. • Spiral Wrap: Overlap upward/downward one-half to two-thirds width of the bandage with each turn. • Recurrent turns: Anchor bandage, then make a reverse turn taking roll of bandage over the distal end of the stump. Continue front to back with reverse turns until the wound is covered and then anchor. • Reverse spiral: Anchor bandage. Advance bandage proximally at about a 30° angle. Halfway through each turn, fold bandage toward the nurse and continue in a downward fashion. Secure the end. *Comments:*	☐	☐	☐	
10. Remove and appropriately dispose of gloves. Wash hands. *Comments:*	☐	☐	☐	

Checklist for Procedure 9-2   Applying a Dry Dressing

Name _____ Date _____

School _____

Instructor _____

Course _____

Procedure 9-2 Applying a Dry Dressing	Able to Perform	Able to Perform with Assistance	Unable to Perform	Initials and Date
Assessment				
1. Assess the client's comfort level. *Comments:*	☐	☐	☐	
2. Assess the external appearance of the initial and subsequent dressings. *Comments:*	☐	☐	☐	
3. Assess the appearance of the wound and drains once the dressing is removed. *Comments:*	☐	☐	☐	
4. Assess the client's understanding about the care of the surgical site. *Comments:*	☐	☐	☐	
5. If solutions are to be used on the wound, assess the client's allergy status and test a drop of solution on the skin. *Comments:*	☐	☐	☐	
Planning/Expected Outcomes				
1. The site will be inspected. *Comments:*	☐	☐	☐	
2. The initial dressing will be reinforced until changed by the qualified practitioner. *Comments:*	☐	☐	☐	
3. The site will have the appropriate dressing applied. *Comments:*	☐	☐	☐	
4. The client/family will demonstrate the ability to perform the wound care and dressing change. *Comments:*	☐	☐	☐	

continued on the following page

continued from the previous page

Procedure 9-2	Able to Perform	Able to Perform with Assistance	Unable to Perform	Initials and Date
Implementation				
1. Gather supplies. *Comments:*	☐	☐	☐	
2. Provide privacy. *Comments:*	☐	☐	☐	
3. Explain procedure to client. *Comments:*	☐	☐	☐	
4. Wash hands. *Comments:*	☐	☐	☐	
5. Apply clean exam gloves. *Comments:*	☐	☐	☐	
6. Remove dressing and place in appropriate receptacle. *Comments:*	☐	☐	☐	
7. Observe the undressed wound. *Comments:*	☐	☐	☐	
8. Cleanse around the incision with a warm, wet washcloth. • Cleanse the suture line with prescribed solution. • Used applicators should not be reintroduced into the sterile solution. *Comments:*	☐	☐	☐	
9. Remove used exam gloves. *Comments:*	☐	☐	☐	
10. Wash hands. *Comments:*	☐	☐	☐	
11. Set up supplies. *Comments:*	☐	☐	☐	
12. Apply a pair of clean exam gloves. *Comments:*	☐	☐	☐	

continued from the previous page

Procedure 9-2	Able to Perform	Able to Perform with Assistance	Unable to Perform	Initials and Date
13. Grasping just the edges, apply a new gauze dressing. Tape lightly or apply tubular mesh. *Comments:*	☐	☐	☐	
14. Remove gloves and wash hands. *Comments:*	☐	☐	☐	
15. Conduct client/family education about the dressing. *Comments:*	☐	☐	☐	

Checklist for Procedure 9-3 Applying a Wet to Damp Dressing (Wet to Dry to Moist Dressing)

Name _____ Date _____

School _____

Instructor _____

Course _____

Procedure 9-3 Applying a Wet to Damp Dressing (Wet to Dry to Moist Dressing)	Able to Perform	Able to Perform with Assistance	Unable to Perform	Initials and Date
Assessment				
1. Assess the client's comfort level. *Comments:*	☐	☐	☐	
2. Assess the external appearance of the dressing. *Comments:*	☐	☐	☐	
3. After the dressing is removed, assess the appearance of the wound and drains. *Comments:*	☐	☐	☐	
4. Assess the client's understanding of the dressing changes and wound care. *Comments:*	☐	☐	☐	
5. Assess the client's healing response to previous treatments. *Comments:*	☐	☐	☐	
Planning/Expected Outcomes				
1. The site will be inspected. *Comments:*	☐	☐	☐	
2. The site will have the appropriate dressing applied. *Comments:*	☐	☐	☐	
3. The client/family will demonstrate understanding and ability to perform the dressing change and wound care. *Comments:*	☐	☐	☐	
Implementation				
1. Gather supplies. *Comments:*	☐	☐	☐	
2. Provide privacy; draw curtains; close door. *Comments:*	☐	☐	☐	

continued on the following page

continued from the previous page

Procedure 9-3	Able to Perform	Able to Perform with Assistance	Unable to Perform	Initials and Date
3. Explain procedure to client. *Comments:*	☐	☐	☐	
4. Wash hands. *Comments:*	☐	☐	☐	
5. Apply clean gloves and other needed protective clothing. *Comments:*	☐	☐	☐	
6. Assess need for pain medication. *Comments:*	☐	☐	☐	
7. Inform client that the dressing is going to be removed. *Comments:*	☐	☐	☐	
8. Remove wet to damp dressing and dispose of appropriately. Note the makeup of the old dressing. *Comments:*	☐	☐	☐	
9. Observe the undressed wound. *Comments:*	☐	☐	☐	
10. Cleanse the skin around the incision, if necessary. *Comments:*	☐	☐	☐	
11. Remove used exam gloves. *Comments:*	☐	☐	☐	
12. Wash hands. *Comments:*	☐	☐	☐	
13. Set up supplies in a sterile field. *Comments:*	☐	☐	☐	
14. Apply sterile gloves. *Comments:*	☐	☐	☐	

Procedure 9-3	Able to Perform	Able to Perform with Assistance	Unable to Perform	Initials and Date
15. Place packing material in the bowl with the ordered solution. • Wring gauze or packing until damp. • Gently place wet gauze over the area. *Comments:*	☐	☐	☐	
16. Apply dry external dressing. • Secure dressing with tape, Montgomery straps, or tubular mesh. *Comments:*	☐	☐	☐	
17. Remove gloves and wash hands. *Comments:*	☐	☐	☐	
18. Mark the dressing with the date, time, and initials. *Comments:*	☐	☐	☐	
19. Conduct client/family education about the dressing. *Comments:*	☐	☐	☐	

Checklist for Procedure 9-4   Applying a Transparent Dressing

Name _____ Date _____

School _____

Instructor _____

Course _____

Procedure 9-4 Applying a Transparent Dressing	Able to Perform	Able to Perform with Assistance	Unable to Perform	Initials and Date
Assessment				
1. Question the client about any reactions to adhesive products. *Comments:*	☐	☐	☐	
2. Assess the client's skin and wound site. *Comments:*	☐	☐	☐	
3. Assess the client for skin reaction to transparent dressing products. *Comments:*	☐	☐	☐	
Planning/Expected Outcomes				
1. The client will have promotion of healing process. *Comments:*	☐	☐	☐	
2. The client will have no adverse reaction to adhesive material. *Comments:*	☐	☐	☐	
Implementation				
1. Check the client's medical record for previous reactions to adhesives and date of last dressing change. *Comments:*	☐	☐	☐	
2. Wash hands. *Comments:*	☐	☐	☐	
3. Expose the area and put on gloves. *Comments:*	☐	☐	☐	
4. Remove any clothes or coverings from area of dressing change and put on examination gloves. *Comments:*	☐	☐	☐	

continued on the following page

continued from the previous page

Procedure 9-4	Able to Perform	Able to Perform with Assistance	Unable to Perform	Initials and Date
5. Remove old dressing. Hold the client's skin taut and pull off the dressing in the direction of hair growth. *Comments:*	☐	☐	☐	
6. Discard the used dressing in disposable bag. *Comments:*	☐	☐	☐	
7. Assess the wound. *Comments:*	☐	☐	☐	
8. Remove and discard the gloves. *Comments:*	☐	☐	☐	
9. Reglove in clean or sterile gloves. *Comments:*	☐	☐	☐	
10. Open the package with transparent dressing. *Comments:*	☐	☐	☐	
11. Grasp the tab on the back of the dressing and separate about 1 inch of the backing from the dressing. *Comments:*	☐	☐	☐	
12. Place the adhesive side on the skin. Hold the dressing in place and peel the backing off the dressing, smoothing it over the site. *Comments:*	☐	☐	☐	
13. Press gently and smooth out any wrinkles. *Comments:*	☐	☐	☐	
14. Reinforce edges with tape as needed. *Comments:*	☐	☐	☐	
15. Date and initial the dressing. *Comments:*	☐	☐	☐	

Checklist for Procedure 9-5   Applying a Pressure Bandage

Name _____   Date _____

School _____

Instructor _____

Course _____

Procedure 9-5 Applying a Pressure Bandage	Able to Perform	Able to Perform with Assistance	Unable to Perform	Initials and Date
Assessment				
1. Observation, rapid assessment of bleeding site, and immediate action are required. *Comments:*	☐	☐	☐	
2. Identify the origin of bleeding. *Comments:*	☐	☐	☐	
3. Assess vital signs and general client condition. *Comments:*	☐	☐	☐	
Planning/Expected Outcomes				
1. Bleeding is stopped. *Comments:*	☐	☐	☐	
2. Circulating blood volume is maintained and the client has no adverse consequences. *Comments:*	☐	☐	☐	
3. Underlying causes are identified and treated. *Comments:*	☐	☐	☐	
4. If there is debridement, sterile technique is used and infection is prevented. *Comments:*	☐	☐	☐	
5. If suicide was attempted, the client is referred appropriately. *Comments:*	☐	☐	☐	
Implementation				
1. Wash hands and apply protective gear as time permits. *Comments:*	☐	☐	☐	

continued on the following page

continued from the previous page

Procedure 9-5	Able to Perform	Able to Perform with Assistance	Unable to Perform	Initials and Date
2. Rapidly assess the wound and determine origin of bleeding. *Comments:*	☐	☐	☐	
3. Call for assistance as needed. *Comments:*	☐	☐	☐	
4. Apply firm pressure with sterile gauze. *Comments:*	☐	☐	☐	
5. Cover the wound and apply pressure. Do not remove blood-soaked gauze; add additional layers and maintain pressure. Elevate the extremity. *Comments:*	☐	☐	☐	
6. Apply tape firmly over site, maintaining pressure. *Comments:*	☐	☐	☐	
7. Apply an Ace bandage or elastic wrap over the sterile dressings. *Comments:*	☐	☐	☐	
8. Remove gloves and wash hands. *Comments:*	☐	☐	☐	
9. Check the client's pulses distal to the wound. *Comments:*	☐	☐	☐	
10. Assess the client and obtain a complete set of vital signs. *Comments:*	☐	☐	☐	
11. If hemorrhage was large or unexpected, initiate intravenous fluids. *Comments:*	☐	☐	☐	
12. Monitor vital signs every 15 minutes or more often if necessary. *Comments:*	☐	☐	☐	
13. Wash hands. *Comments:*	☐	☐	☐	

Checklist for Procedure 9-6 Changing Dressings around Therapeutic Puncture Sites

Name _____ Date _____

School _____

Instructor _____

Course _____

Procedure 9-6 **Changing Dressings around Therapeutic Puncture Sites**	Able to Perform	Able to Perform with Assistance	Unable to Perform	Initials and Date
Assessment				
1. Assess the client's comfort level. *Comments:*	☐	☐	☐	
2. Assess the appearance of the therapeutic puncture site. *Comments:*	☐	☐	☐	
3. Assess the position and condition of any therapeutic devices. *Comments:*	☐	☐	☐	
4. Assess the client's understanding about the care of the puncture site. *Comments:*	☐	☐	☐	
Planning/Expected Outcomes				
1. The puncture site will be free from complications. *Comments:*	☐	☐	☐	
2. The puncture site will be cleaned and dressed appropriately. *Comments:*	☐	☐	☐	
3. The client will verbalize and/or demonstrate understanding about the therapeutic puncture site. *Comments:*	☐	☐	☐	
Implementation				
Dressing Removal and Site Inspection (All Therapeutic Puncture Sites)				
1. Gather supplies. *Comments:*	☐	☐	☐	
2. Provide privacy; draw curtains; close door. *Comments:*	☐	☐	☐	

continued on the following page

continued from the previous page

Procedure 9-6	Able to Perform	Able to Perform with Assistance	Unable to Perform	Initials and Date
3. Explain procedure to client. *Comments:*	☐	☐	☐	
4. Wash hands and set up supplies. *Comments:*	☐	☐	☐	
5. Apply clean gloves. Nurse and client mask for central line dressing changes. *Comments:*	☐	☐	☐	
6. Remove dressing and place in appropriate receptacle. *Comments:*	☐	☐	☐	
Dressing Applications for Peripheral IV Cannulas Newly Inserted 7. Place a transparent semipermeable (TSM) dressing over the newly placed cannula. *Comments:*	☐	☐	☐	
8. Tape the cannula and tubing over the TSM dressing. *Comments:*	☐	☐	☐	
9. Document the time and date of the dressing change. *Comments:*	☐	☐	☐	
Dressing Applications for PICC Line, Triple Lumen Catheter (TLC), or Single Subclavian Line, and Central Venous Access Devices Needing Redressing 10. Review agency policy for dressing change procedure. *Comments:*	☐	☐	☐	
11. Repeat Actions 1–6. *Comments:*	☐	☐	☐	
12. Observe site. • Check for unusual findings at the site. • Note the position of therapeutic devices. *Comments:*	☐	☐	☐	
13. Apply sterile gloves. *Comments:*	☐	☐	☐	

Procedure 9-6	Able to Perform	Able to Perform with Assistance	Unable to Perform	Initials and Date
14. Cleanse around line with sterile saline and sterile cotton-tip applicators. Dry with dry applicator. *Comments:*	☐	☐	☐	
15. Cleanse around line with povidone-iodine. Let it dry. *Comments:*	☐	☐	☐	
16. Remove dried povidone-iodine with alcohol swabs. Allow alcohol to dry. *Comments:*	☐	☐	☐	
17. Apply dressing to site. PICC Line: • Apply new stabilizing Steri-strips if (necessary). • Apply a TSM dressing. Triple Lumen Catheter: • Apply a TSM dressing. External Long-Term Venous Access Device, Tunneled with Cuff: • Apply one folded 2 × 2 under the line and one flat 2 × 2 on top; tape in place. *Comments:*	☐	☐	☐	
18. Apply necessary tape to indwelling line or tubing. *Comments:*	☐	☐	☐	
19. Conduct client/family education about the dressing. *Comments:*	☐	☐	☐	
Dressing Applications for Peripherally Inserted Drainage Tubes 20. Repeat Actions 10–17. *Comments:*	☐	☐	☐	
21. Apply folded gauze under tube. Apply flat gauze pads on top of tube. Tape securely. *Comments:*	☐	☐	☐	
22. Apply necessary tape to tube. *Comments:*	☐	☐	☐	
23. Empty or change the drainage collection container and record the amount. *Comments:*	☐	☐	☐	

continued on the following page

continued from the previous page

Procedure 9-6	Able to Perform	Able to Perform with Assistance	Unable to Perform	Initials and Date
24. Conduct client/family education about the dressing. *Comments:*	☐	☐	☐	
Dressing Applications for Puncture Sites Following Diagnostic Procedures 25. Review agency policy for dressing change procedure. *Comments:*	☐	☐	☐	
26. Repeat Actions 1–5. *Comments:*	☐	☐	☐	
27. Apply clean gloves unless sterile gloves are indicated. *Comments:*	☐	☐	☐	
28. Observe site. *Comments:*	☐	☐	☐	
29. Apply dressing to site. Lumbar Puncture: • Band-Aid is applied following brief pressure to the site. Thoracentesis: • Sterile petrolatum gauze, 4 × 4 and 2-inch tape. Paracentesis: • Apply several thicknesses of 4 × 4 gauze and tape to secure. Angiography: • A Band-Aid or 4 × 4 gauze pad is placed following pressure being applied to the site. Needle Biopsy Sites: • Tape a Band-Aid or 2 × 2 gauze pad in place. *Comments:*	☐	☐	☐	
30. Conduct client/family education about the dressing and any limitations. *Comments:*	☐	☐	☐	

Checklist for Procedure 9-7 Irrigating a Wound

Name _____ Date _____

School _____

Instructor _____

Course _____

Procedure 9-7 Irrigating a Wound	Able to Perform	Able to Perform with Assistance	Unable to Perform	Initials and Date
Assessment				
1. Assess the current dressing. *Comments:*	☐	☐	☐	
2. Assess the client. *Comments:*	☐	☐	☐	
3. Assess client concerns regarding this wound and the irrigation. *Comments:*	☐	☐	☐	
4. Assess the client's environment. *Comments:*	☐	☐	☐	
Planning/Expected Outcomes				
1. The wound will be free of exudate, drainage, and debris. *Comments:*	☐	☐	☐	
2. The wound will be free of signs and symptoms of infection. *Comments:*	☐	☐	☐	
3. The procedure will be performed with a minimum of trauma to the client. *Comments:*	☐	☐	☐	
Implementation				
1. Confirm the written order for wound irrigation. *Comments:*	☐	☐	☐	
2. Assess the client's pain level and medicate if needed. *Comments:*	☐	☐	☐	
3. Explain the procedure to the client. *Comments:*	☐	☐	☐	

continued on the following page

continued from the previous page

Procedure 9-7	Able to Perform	Able to Perform with Assistance	Unable to Perform	Initials and Date
4. Assist the client onto a waterproof pad in a position that will allow the irrigant to flow from the clean to dirty areas of the wound. *Comments:*	☐	☐	☐	
5. Wash hands and apply gloves; remove and discard the old dressing. *Comments:*	☐	☐	☐	
6. Assess the wound's appearance. *Comments:*	☐	☐	☐	
7. Remove and discard the gloves, and wash hands. *Comments:*	☐	☐	☐	
8. Prepare the sterile irrigation tray and dressing supplies. *Comments:*	☐	☐	☐	
9. Apply sterile gloves (and goggles if needed). *Comments:*	☐	☐	☐	
10. Position the sterile basin so the irrigant will flow into the basin. *Comments:*	☐	☐	☐	
11. Fill the syringe with irrigant and gently flush the wound. Repeat until clear or the ordered amount of fluid has been used. *Comments:*	☐	☐	☐	
12. Dry the edges of the wound with sterile gauze. *Comments:*	☐	☐	☐	
13. Assess the wound's appearance and drainage. *Comments:*	☐	☐	☐	
14. Apply a sterile dressing. Remove gloves and dispose of properly. Wash hands. *Comments:*	☐	☐	☐	
15. Document all assessment findings and actions taken. *Comments:*	☐	☐	☐	

Checklist for Procedure 9-8 Packing a Wound

Name _____ Date _____

School _____

Instructor _____

Course _____

Procedure 9-8 Packing a Wound	Able to Perform	Able to Perform with Assistance	Unable to Perform	Initials and Date
Assessment				
1. Assess the dressing currently in place. *Comments:*	☐	☐	☐	
2. Assess the client's comfort level. *Comments:*	☐	☐	☐	
3. Assess the client's understanding of the healing process and the procedure. *Comments:*	☐	☐	☐	
4. Assess the wound for healing. *Comments:*	☐	☐	☐	
5. Assess the wound size and depth. *Comments:*	☐	☐	☐	
Planning/Expected Outcomes				
1. The wound will not exhibit signs or symptoms of infection. *Comments:*	☐	☐	☐	
2. The client will experience a minimum of trauma related to the procedure. *Comments:*	☐	☐	☐	
3. The client will understand the reason for the wound care regimen. *Comments:*	☐	☐	☐	
4. The client/caregiver will be able to demonstrate appropriate wound care. *Comments:*	☐	☐	☐	

continued on the following page

continued from the previous page

Procedure 9-8	Able to Perform	Able to Perform with Assistance	Unable to Perform	Initials and Date
5. The wound will measurably heal. *Comments:*	☐	☐	☐	
6. Wound drainage will be adequately absorbed. *Comments:*	☐	☐	☐	
Implementation				
1. Wash hands. *Comments:*	☐	☐	☐	
2. Provide for client privacy. *Comments:*	☐	☐	☐	
3. Assemble dressing change material at bedside. *Comments:*	☐	☐	☐	
4. Apply gloves. *Comments:*	☐	☐	☐	
5. Remove the old dressing, noting the way it was applied. *Comments:*	☐	☐	☐	
6. Dispose of the old dressing appropriately. *Comments:*	☐	☐	☐	
7. Remove gloves and dispose of them appropriately. *Comments:*	☐	☐	☐	
8. Open and prepare the dressing materials. *Comments:*	☐	☐	☐	
9. Apply sterile gloves or a clean set of disposable gloves. *Comments:*	☐	☐	☐	
10. Inspect and measure the wound. *Comments:*	☐	☐	☐	
11. Treat the wound according to the prescribed wound regimen. *Comments:*	☐	☐	☐	

Procedure 9-8	Able to Perform	Able to Perform with Assistance	Unable to Perform	Initials and Date
12. Using the old dressing as a template, place the prescribed packing material into the wound. *Comments:*	☐	☐	☐	
13. If there is debridement, be sure the packing material contacts all the surfaces to be debrided. *Comments:*	☐	☐	☐	
14. If absorbing drainage, fluff the gauze prior to packing. *Comments:*	☐	☐	☐	
15. Pack all tunneled areas loosely. *Comments:*	☐	☐	☐	
16. Apply any secondary dressing. *Comments:*	☐	☐	☐	
17. Secure the dressing in place. *Comments:*	☐	☐	☐	
18. Dispose of any waste appropriately. *Comments:*	☐	☐	☐	
19. Remove gloves and dispose of properly. *Comments:*	☐	☐	☐	
20. Remove any soiled bedding or foul-smelling waste. Freshen the air if necessary. *Comments:*	☐	☐	☐	
21. Wash hands. *Comments:*	☐	☐	☐	

Checklist for Procedure 9-9   Cleaning and Dressing a Wound with an Open Drain

Name _____ Date _____

School _____

Instructor _____

Course _____

Procedure 9-9 **Cleaning and Dressing a Wound with an Open Drain**	Able to Perform	Able to Perform with Assistance	Unable to Perform	Initials and Date
Assessment				
1. Assess the client's comfort level. *Comments:*	☐	☐	☐	
2. Assess the appearance of the dressing. *Comments:*	☐	☐	☐	
3. Assess the appearance of the wound. *Comments:*	☐	☐	☐	
4. Assess the client's understanding about the post-operative care of the surgical wound site. *Comments:*	☐	☐	☐	
Planning/Expected Outcomes				
1. The site and drains will be inspected. *Comments:*	☐	☐	☐	
2. The site will have the appropriate dressing applied. *Comments:*	☐	☐	☐	
3. The drains will be monitored for proper function. *Comments:*	☐	☐	☐	
4. The client/family will demonstrate understanding of the purpose of the drains and care of the wound site. *Comments:*	☐	☐	☐	
Implementation				
1. Gather supplies. *Comments:*	☐	☐	☐	
2. Provide privacy; draw curtains; close door. *Comments:*	☐	☐	☐	

continued on the following page

continued from the previous page

Procedure 9-9	Able to Perform	Able to Perform with Assistance	Unable to Perform	Initials and Date
3. Explain procedure to client. *Comments:*	☐	☐	☐	
4. Wash hands. *Comments:*	☐	☐	☐	
5. Apply clean gloves and any other needed protection. *Comments:*	☐	☐	☐	
6. Remove dressing and place in appropriate receptacle. *Comments:*	☐	☐	☐	
7. Observe the drain and undressed wound. *Comments:*	☐	☐	☐	
8. Cleanse the skin around the incision if necessary. *Comments:*	☐	☐	☐	
9. Remove used exam gloves. *Comments:*	☐	☐	☐	
10. Wash hands. *Comments:*	☐	☐	☐	
11. Set up supplies. *Comments:*	☐	☐	☐	
12. Set up a sterile field and apply sterile gloves. *Comments:*	☐	☐	☐	
13. • Cleanse the suture line using sterile saline and sterile cotton-tip applicators. • Use one applicator then discard. • Dry with dry cotton-tip applicators. Perform wound care. *Comments:*	☐	☐	☐	
14. Cleanse the area under the drain. *Comments:*	☐	☐	☐	

Procedure 9-9	Able to Perform	Able to Perform with Assistance	Unable to Perform	Initials and Date
15. Apply precut drain sponges around the drain. Top with 1–2 layers of uncut drain sponges. *Comments:*	☐	☐	☐	
16. If necessary, apply a new pair of sterile gloves. *Comments:*	☐	☐	☐	
17. • Apply dry external dressing. • Secure dressing in place. *Comments:*	☐	☐	☐	
18. Conduct client/family education about the dressing. *Comments:*	☐	☐	☐	

Checklist for Procedure 9-10   Dressing a Wound with Retention Sutures

Name _____ Date _____

School _____

Instructor _____

Course _____

Procedure 9-10 Dressing a Wound with Retention Sutures	Able to Perform	Able to Perform with Assistance	Unable to Perform	Initials and Date
Assessment				
1. Assess the client's comfort level postoperatively. *Comments:*	☐	☐	☐	
2. Assess the appearance of the initial postoperative dressing. *Comments:*	☐	☐	☐	
3. Assess the appearance of the wound and drains once the dressing is removed. *Comments:*	☐	☐	☐	
4. Assess the client's understanding about the care of the wound site. *Comments:*	☐	☐	☐	
Planning/Expected Outcomes				
1. The site will be inspected. *Comments:*	☐	☐	☐	
2. The site will have the appropriate dressing applied. *Comments:*	☐	☐	☐	
3. Drains will be monitored for proper functioning. *Comments:*	☐	☐	☐	
4. The client/family will demonstrate understanding of the dressing change and wound care. *Comments:*	☐	☐	☐	
Implementation				
Dressing Application for Closed Surgical Wounds with Wire Retention Sutures				
1. Gather supplies. *Comments:*	☐	☐	☐	

continued on the following page

continued from the previous page

Procedure 9-10	Able to Perform	Able to Perform with Assistance	Unable to Perform	Initials and Date
2. Provide privacy; draw curtains; close door. *Comments:*	☐	☐	☐	
3. Explain procedure to client. *Comments:*	☐	☐	☐	
4. Wash hands. *Comments:*	☐	☐	☐	
5. Apply clean exam gloves. *Comments:*	☐	☐	☐	
6. Remove dressing and place in an appropriate receptacle. *Comments:*	☐	☐	☐	
7. Observe the undressed wound. *Comments:*	☐	☐	☐	
8. Cleanse the skin around the incision (if necessary). *Comments:*	☐	☐	☐	
9. Remove used exam gloves. *Comments:*	☐	☐	☐	
10. Wash hands. *Comments:*	☐	☐	☐	
11. Set up supplies. *Comments:*	☐	☐	☐	
12. Set up a sterile field and apply sterile gloves. *Comments:*	☐	☐	☐	
13. Gently cleanse the suture line, the retention sutures, and plastic guard devices using sterile saline and sterile cotton-tip applicators. Dry with dry cotton-tip applicators. *Comments:*	☐	☐	☐	

Procedure 9-10	Able to Perform	Able to Perform with Assistance	Unable to Perform	Initials and Date
14. Optional: Apply a hydrocolloid self-adhesive pad under each plastic guard. *Comments:*	☐	☐	☐	
15. Apply a new dressing to incision line. Tuck dressings under the retention sutures. If necessary, apply a new pair of sterile gloves. *Comments:*	☐	☐	☐	
16. Apply external dry dressing. Secure dressing in place. *Comments:*	☐	☐	☐	
17. Educate client/family about dressing care. *Comments:*	☐	☐	☐	

Checklist for Procedure 9-11   Obtaining a Wound Drainage Specimen for Culturing

Name _____ Date _____

School _____

Instructor _____

Course _____

Procedure 9-11 Obtaining a Wound Drainage Specimen for Culturing	Able to Perform	Able to Perform with Assistance	Unable to Perform	Initials and Date
Assessment				
1. Assess the wound and the surrounding tissues. *Comments:*	☐	☐	☐	
2. Assess the client's overall status. *Comments:*	☐	☐	☐	
Planning/Expected Outcomes				
1. The culture will be collected with a minimum of trauma to the client. *Comments:*	☐	☐	☐	
2. The culture will be representative of the wound flora. *Comments:*	☐	☐	☐	
Implementation				
1. • Wash hands and apply gloves. • Remove old dressing. • Dispose of dressing and gloves appropriately. • Wash hands again. *Comments:*	☐	☐	☐	
2. Open the dressing supplies aseptically and apply gloves. *Comments:*	☐	☐	☐	
3. Assess the wound's appearance. *Comments:*	☐	☐	☐	
4. Irrigate the wound with normal saline prior to collecting the culture. *Comments:*	☐	☐	☐	
5. Blot the excess saline with a sterile gauze pad. *Comments:*	☐	☐	☐	

continued on the following page

continued from the previous page

Procedure 9-11	Able to Perform	Able to Perform with Assistance	Unable to Perform	Initials and Date
6. Remove the culture swab from the tube and roll the swab over the granulation tissue. *Comments:*	☐	☐	☐	
7. • Replace the swab into the culture tube. • Recap the tube. • Crush the medium located in the bottom or cap of the tube. *Comments:*	☐	☐	☐	
8. Remove gloves, wash hands, and apply sterile gloves. Dress the wound. *Comments:*	☐	☐	☐	
9. Label and transport the specimen to the laboratory. *Comments:*	☐	☐	☐	
10. Remove gloves and wash hands. *Comments:*	☐	☐	☐	
11. Document all assessment findings and actions taken. *Comments:*	☐	☐	☐	

Checklist for Procedure 9-12   Maintaining a Closed Wound Drainage System

Name _____ Date _____

School _____

Instructor _____

Course _____

Procedure 9-12 **Maintaining a Closed Wound Drainage System**	Able to Perform	Able to Perform with Assistance	Unable to Perform	Initials and Date
Assessment				
1. Identify the type and amount of drainage from the wound. *Comments:*	☐	☐	☐	
2. Inspect the condition of the skin surrounding the wound. *Comments:*	☐	☐	☐	
3. Measure the dimensions of the wound or determine the type of drainage system previously used. *Comments:*	☐	☐	☐	
Planning/Expected Outcomes				
1. The skin around the wound will be protected from drainage. *Comments:*	☐	☐	☐	
2. Wound drainage will be contained in the drainage system. *Comments:*	☐	☐	☐	
3. Odor from the wound will be controlled. *Comments:*	☐	☐	☐	
4. The drainage system will not decrease the client's comfort. *Comments:*	☐	☐	☐	
5. Drainage will be accurately measured and documented. *Comments:*	☐	☐	☐	
6. The drainage system will not decrease the client's mobility. *Comments:*	☐	☐	☐	
7. The drainage system will cost less than dressing changes. *Comments:*	☐	☐	☐	

continued on the following page

continued from the previous page

Procedure 9-12	Able to Perform	Able to Perform with Assistance	Unable to Perform	Initials and Date
Implementation				
1. Assess client's comfort level prior to beginning procedure. *Comments:*	☐	☐	☐	
2. Medicate client for pain, if needed. *Comments:*	☐	☐	☐	
3. Wash hands. *Comments:*	☐	☐	☐	
4. Assemble equipment. *Comments:*	☐	☐	☐	
5. Open sterile packages. *Comments:*	☐	☐	☐	
6. Apply clean gloves and remove old dressing. *Comments:*	☐	☐	☐	
7. Change to a new pair of clean or sterile gloves. *Comments:*	☐	☐	☐	
8. Moisten several packages of gauze with normal saline. *Comments:*	☐	☐	☐	
9. Cleanse wound bed with moistened gauze pads. *Comments:*	☐	☐	☐	
10. Lay drain/catheter over the fistula site in wound bed. *Comments:*	☐	☐	☐	
11. Lay fresh moistened gauze pads in the wound bed over the drain. *Comments:*	☐	☐	☐	
12. Cover the entire wound with occlusive dressing. *Comments:*	☐	☐	☐	
13. Attach drain/catheter to intermittent low wall suction. *Comments:*	☐	☐	☐	

Procedure 9-12	Able to Perform	Able to Perform with Assistance	Unable to Perform	Initials and Date
14. Empty and record drainage at least every 8 hours. *Comments:*	☐	☐	☐	
15. Change dressing system as needed. *Comments:*	☐	☐	☐	

Checklist for Procedure 9-13 Care of the Jackson-Pratt (JP) Drain Site and Emptying the Drain Bulb

Name _____ Date _____

School _____

Instructor _____

Course _____

Procedure 9-13 Care of the Jackson-Pratt (JP) Drain Site and Emptying the Drain Bulb	Able to Perform	Able to Perform with Assistance	Unable to Perform	Initials and Date
Assessment				
1. Assess the client's understanding about the procedure. *Comments:*	☐	☐	☐	
2. Assess the external appearance of the dressed drain exit site. *Comments:*	☐	☐	☐	
3. Assess the drain exit site once the dressing is removed. *Comments:*	☐	☐	☐	
4. Assess the client/family response to the drain care procedure. *Comments:*	☐	☐	☐	
Planning/Expected Outcomes				
1. The JP drain exit site will be inspected. *Comments:*	☐	☐	☐	
2. The JP drain site will be cleansed and redressed. *Comments:*	☐	☐	☐	
3. The external JP will be inspected for proper functioning. *Comments:*	☐	☐	☐	
4. The JP drainage bulb will be emptied. *Comments:*	☐	☐	☐	
5. The client/family will demonstrate understanding about the procedure. *Comments:*	☐	☐	☐	
6. The drain site will remain free of infection. *Comments:*	☐	☐	☐	

continued on the following page

continued from the previous page

Procedure 9-13	Able to Perform	Able to Perform with Assistance	Unable to Perform	Initials and Date
7. The client will not experience discomfort due to site inspection or care. *Comments:*	☐	☐	☐	
Implementation				
1. Review written orders. *Comments:*	☐	☐	☐	
2. Gather supplies. *Comments:*	☐	☐	☐	
3. Provide privacy; draw curtains; close door. *Comments:*	☐	☐	☐	
4. Explain procedure to client/family. *Comments:*	☐	☐	☐	
5. Wash hands and set up supplies. *Comments:*	☐	☐	☐	
6. Apply clean exam gloves. *Comments:*	☐	☐	☐	
7. Unpin drain tube from gown. Remove old dressing and dispose of appropriately. *Comments:*	☐	☐	☐	
8. Assess site. *Comments:*	☐	☐	☐	
9. • Cleanse around drain with sterile cotton-tip applicator. • Dry with dry applicators. *Comments:*	☐	☐	☐	
10. Avoid contamination of the swabs and solutions. *Comments:*	☐	☐	☐	
11. Cleanse around drain with an iodine swab and let it dry. *Comments:*	☐	☐	☐	

Procedure 9-13	Able to Perform	Able to Perform with Assistance	Unable to Perform	Initials and Date
12. If necessary, apply new, clean exam gloves. *Comments:*	☐	☐	☐	
13. Apply folded 4 × 4s under and over the drain and tape in place. *Comments:*	☐	☐	☐	
14. Secure drain tube to dressing. Then secure to gown/clothing. *Comments:*	☐	☐	☐	
15. Assess the bulb for contents and compression. *Comments:*	☐	☐	☐	
16. To empty the bulb, wash hands, set up supplies, and apply gloves. *Comments:*	☐	☐	☐	
17. Wipe the drainage spout with iodine or alcohol. *Comments:*	☐	☐	☐	
18. Remove the cap to the spout. *Comments:*	☐	☐	☐	
19. Pour the collected drainage into the measuring container. *Comments:*	☐	☐	☐	
20. While the cap is still off, squeeze the bulb and, while compressed, reapply the cap to the spout. *Comments:*	☐	☐	☐	
21. Use an iodine swab or alcohol to wipe around the spout. *Comments:*	☐	☐	☐	
22. Record the drainage and dispose of the drainage. *Comments:*	☐	☐	☐	
23. Remove and properly dispose of gloves. Wash hands. *Comments:*	☐	☐	☐	

Checklist for Procedure 9-14   Removing Skin Sutures and Staples

Name _____ Date _____

School _____

Instructor _____

Course _____

Procedure 9-14 Removing Skin Sutures and Staples	Able to Perform	Able to Perform with Assistance	Unable to Perform	Initials and Date
Assessment				
1. Assess the wound. *Comments:*	☐	☐	☐	
2. Assess for any signs of infection. *Comments:*	☐	☐	☐	
3. Assess for any conditions that impede the healing process. *Comments:*	☐	☐	☐	
Planning/Expected Outcomes				
1. The wound is healing, with the edges well approximated. *Comments:*	☐	☐	☐	
2. There is no redness or signs of infection. *Comments:*	☐	☐	☐	
3. There is an absence of pain. *Comments:*	☐	☐	☐	
Implementation				
1. Wash hands. *Comments:*	☐	☐	☐	
2. Assess the wound to determine whether healing has occurred. *Comments:*	☐	☐	☐	
3. Explain the procedure. *Comments:*	☐	☐	☐	
4. Close the door and curtains around the client's bed. *Comments:*	☐	☐	☐	

continued on the following page

continued from the previous page

Procedure 9-14	Able to Perform	Able to Perform with Assistance	Unable to Perform	Initials and Date
5. Raise the bed to a comfortable level. *Comments:*	☐	☐	☐	
6. Position the client for easy access to the suture line. *Comments:*	☐	☐	☐	
7. Drape the client so that only the suture area is exposed. *Comments:*	☐	☐	☐	
8. Open the suture removal kit, and assemble supplies. *Comments:*	☐	☐	☐	
9. Apply clean gloves; remove old dressing and dispose of appropriately. *Comments:*	☐	☐	☐	
10. Remove gloves and rewash hands. *Comments:*	☐	☐	☐	
11. If dressings are to be used, assemble equipment and supplies. *Comments:*	☐	☐	☐	
12. • Apply sterile gloves. • Clean the incision. *Comments:*	☐	☐	☐	
13. Removing an interrupted suture: • Use forceps to grasp the suture near the knot. *Comments:*	☐	☐	☐	
14. Place the curved edge of the scissors under the suture or near the knot. *Comments:*	☐	☐	☐	
15. Cut the suture close to the skin. Pull the long end and remove in one piece. *Comments:*	☐	☐	☐	
16. Removing a continuous suture: • Cut both the first and second suture before removing them. *Comments:*	☐	☐	☐	

continued from the previous page

Procedure 9-14	Able to Perform	Able to Perform with Assistance	Unable to Perform	Initials and Date
17. Some policies require removal of every other suture, with the remaining sutures removed later. *Comments:*	☐	☐	☐	
18. Discard removed sutures onto the gauze squares. Dispose of gauze squares appropriately. *Comments:*	☐	☐	☐	
19. Assess the suture line to ensure that the edges remain approximated and that all sutures have been removed. *Comments:*	☐	☐	☐	
20. Apply adhesive strips or butterfly strips across the suture line to secure the edges. *Comments:*	☐	☐	☐	
21. Dispose of the soiled equipment. *Comments:*	☐	☐	☐	
22. Remove gloves and wash hands. *Comments:*	☐	☐	☐	
23. If removing staples: • Repeat Actions 2–12. • Use a staple extractor to remove every other staple. Place the lower tip of staple remover under the staple and squeeze the handles together. • Repeat Actions 20–22. *Comments:*	☐	☐	☐	

Checklist for Procedure 9-15   Preventing and Managing the Pressure Ulcer

Name _____ Date _____

School _____

Instructor _____

Course _____

Procedure 9-15 **Preventing and Managing the Pressure Ulcer**	Able to Perform	Able to Perform with Assistance	Unable to Perform	Initials and Date
Assessment				
1. Assess client's level of mobility. *Comments:*	☐	☐	☐	
2. Assess client's control over bowel and bladder. *Comments:*	☐	☐	☐	
3. Assess client's sensation. *Comments:*	☐	☐	☐	
4. Assess client's nutritional status. *Comments:*	☐	☐	☐	
5. Assess client's hemoglobin and hematocrit levels. *Comments:*	☐	☐	☐	
6. Assess client's temperature. *Comments:*	☐	☐	☐	
7. Assess client's weight. *Comments:*	☐	☐	☐	
8. Assess client's hydration level. *Comments:*	☐	☐	☐	
9. Assess client for edema. *Comments:*	☐	☐	☐	
10. Assess whether the client has equipment that is in prolonged contact with skin. *Comments:*	☐	☐	☐	

continued on the following page

continued from the previous page

Procedure 9-15	Able to Perform	Able to Perform with Assistance	Unable to Perform	Initials and Date
11. Assess client's skin for early signs of breakdown or progression of healing. *Comments:*	☐	☐	☐	
Planning/Expected Outcomes				
1. The client will not experience a disruption of skin integrity. *Comments:*	☐	☐	☐	
2. The client will benefit from wound care and supportive measures to begin tissue healing. *Comments:*	☐	☐	☐	
3. The client will experience regular turning and passive range of motion. *Comments:*	☐	☐	☐	
4. The client will increase nutrition to meet metabolic demands. *Comments:*	☐	☐	☐	
5. The client will not experience signs or symptoms of infection. *Comments:*	☐	☐	☐	
6. The client will be pain free. *Comments:*	☐	☐	☐	
7. The client will cope with the pressure ulcer positively. *Comments:*	☐	☐	☐	
8. The client will verbalize and demonstrate techniques to prevent pressure ulcers. *Comments:*	☐	☐	☐	
Implementation				
1. Check the written order for positioning and dressing change instructions. *Comments:*	☐	☐	☐	
2. Gather equipment. *Comments:*	☐	☐	☐	

Procedure 9-15	Able to Perform	Able to Perform with Assistance	Unable to Perform	Initials and Date
3. Identify the client and explain the procedure. *Comments:*	☐	☐	☐	
4. Wash your hands. *Comments:*	☐	☐	☐	
5. Provide for client privacy and apply gloves. *Comments:*	☐	☐	☐	
6. Adjust the bed to your level and lower the side rail nearest you. *Comments:*	☐	☐	☐	
7. Assess client's risk for developing pressure ulcers by using a risk chart. *Comments:*	☐	☐	☐	
8. Assess client's skin for pressure points. *Comments:*	☐	☐	☐	
9. Assess for potential areas of pressure points. *Comments:* .	☐	☐	☐	
10. Change client's position. *Comments:*	☐	☐	☐	
11. Keep client's position at 30° or less. *Comments:*	☐	☐	☐	
12. Provide skin care; don't massage pressure points. *Comments:*	☐	☐	☐	
13. Use support devices to protect and support the body. *Comments:*	☐	☐	☐	
14. Perform dressing change to a pressure ulcer as ordered. *Comments:*	☐	☐	☐	
15. Return side rail to the upright position and lower the bed. *Comments:*	☐	☐	☐	

continued on the following page

continued from the previous page

Procedure 9-15	Able to Perform	Able to Perform with Assistance	Unable to Perform	Initials and Date
16. Remove gloves and wash hands. *Comments:*	☐	☐	☐	
17. Document pressure points and/or ulcers, skin and wound care provided, and position changes. *Comments:*	☐	☐	☐	
18. Create an every-2-hours turning schedule. *Comments:*	☐	☐	☐	

Checklist for Procedure 9-16   Managing Irritated Peristomal Skin

Name _____ Date _____

School _____

Instructor _____

Course _____

Procedure 9-16 **Managing Irritated Peristomal Skin**	Able to Perform	Able to Perform with Assistance	Unable to Perform	Initials and Date
Assessment				
1. Inspect the stoma for color and appearance. *Comments:*	☐	☐	☐	
2. Inspect the condition of the skin surrounding the stoma. *Comments:*	☐	☐	☐	
3. Measure the dimensions of the stoma prior to ordering an appliance. *Comments:*	☐	☐	☐	
Planning/Expected Outcomes				
1. Client exhibits improved or healed areas of peristomal skin. *Comments:*	☐	☐	☐	
2. Client reports increased comfort. *Comments:*	☐	☐	☐	
3. Client is able to identify factors that lead to breakdown and interventions to prevent breakdown. *Comments:*	☐	☐	☐	
4. Client is able to demonstrate skin care regimen. *Comments:*	☐	☐	☐	
5. Client voices feelings about change in body image. *Comments:*	☐	☐	☐	
Implementation				
1. Wash hands. *Comments:*	☐	☐	☐	

continued on the following page

continued from the previous page

Procedure 9-16	Able to Perform	Able to Perform with Assistance	Unable to Perform	Initials and Date
2. Assemble appropriate supplies. *Comments:*	☐	☐	☐	
3. Apply clean gloves. *Comments:*	☐	☐	☐	
4. Empty pouch. Remove current ostomy appliance. *Comments:*	☐	☐	☐	
5. Dispose of appliance appropriately. *Comments:*	☐	☐	☐	
6. Wash hands. *Comments:*	☐	☐	☐	
7. Apply clean gloves. *Comments:*	☐	☐	☐	
8. Cleanse stoma and skin with warm tap water. Pat dry. *Comments:*	☐	☐	☐	
9. Measure stoma at base. *Comments:*	☐	☐	☐	
10. Place gauze pad over orifice of stoma. *Comments:*	☐	☐	☐	
11. Trace pattern onto paper backing of wafer. *Comments:*	☐	☐	☐	
12. Cut wafer as traced. *Comments:*	☐	☐	☐	
13. Attach clean pouch to wafer. Make sure port is closed. Set aside. *Comments:*	☐	☐	☐	
14. Sprinkle pectin powder onto the irritated peristomal skin. *Comments:*	☐	☐	☐	

Procedure 9-16	Able to Perform	Able to Perform with Assistance	Unable to Perform	Initials and Date
15. Brush off any excess pectin powder using a gauze pad. *Comments:*	☐	☐	☐	
16. Dab the skin sealant over the pectin powder. Allow to dry. *Comments:*	☐	☐	☐	
17. Remove gauze pad from orifice of stoma. *Comments:*	☐	☐	☐	
18. Remove paper backing from wafer and place with stoma centered in opening of wafer. *Comments:*	☐	☐	☐	
19. Apply a ring of pectin paste onto the wafer at the edge of the stoma opening. *Comments:*	☐	☐	☐	
20. Cover edges of wafer with hypoallergenic tape. *Comments:*	☐	☐	☐	
21. Wash hands. *Comments:*	☐	☐	☐	

Checklist for Procedure 9-17   Pouching a Draining Wound

Name _____ Date _____

School _____

Instructor _____

Course _____

Procedure 9-17 Pouching a Draining Wound	Able to Perform	Able to Perform with Assistance	Unable to Perform	Initials and Date
Assessment				
1. Identify the type and amount of wound drainage. *Comments:*	☐	☐	☐	
2. Inspect the condition of the skin surrounding the wound. *Comments:*	☐	☐	☐	
3. Measure the wound prior to obtaining a drainage system. *Comments:*	☐	☐	☐	
Planning/Expected Outcomes				
1. The skin around the wound will be protected. *Comments:*	☐	☐	☐	
2. The drainage from the wound will be contained in the pouch. *Comments:*	☐	☐	☐	
3. Odor from the wound will be minimized. *Comments:*	☐	☐	☐	
4. The pouch will not increase the client's discomfort. *Comments:*	☐	☐	☐	
5. The pouch will facilitate measurement of wound drainage. *Comments:*	☐	☐	☐	
6. The pouch will not impair the client's mobility. *Comments:*	☐	☐	☐	

continued on the following page

continued from the previous page

Procedure 9-17	Able to Perform	Able to Perform with Assistance	Unable to Perform	Initials and Date
Implementation				
1. Wash hands. *Comments:*	☐	☐	☐	
2. Assemble appropriate pouch and wafer. *Comments:*	☐	☐	☐	
3. Apply clean gloves. *Comments:*	☐	☐	☐	
4. After emptying pouch remove current appliance. *Comments:*	☐	☐	☐	
5. Dispose of appliance appropriately. *Comments:*	☐	☐	☐	
6. Wash hands. *Comments:*	☐	☐	☐	
7. Apply clean gloves. *Comments:*	☐	☐	☐	
8. Cleanse periwound area with normal saline. Pat dry. *Comments:*	☐	☐	☐	
9. Measure fistula/wound opening, adding a one-eighth-inch clearance from edge of fistula. *Comments:*	☐	☐	☐	
10. Place gauze pad over orifice of fistula. *Comments:*	☐	☐	☐	
11. Trace pattern onto paper backing of wafer. *Comments:*	☐	☐	☐	
12. Cut wafer as traced. *Comments:*	☐	☐	☐	
13. Remove gauze pad from orifice of fistula. *Comments:*	☐	☐	☐	

Procedure 9-17	Able to Perform	Able to Perform with Assistance	Unable to Perform	Initials and Date
14. Attach clean pouch to wafer, then wafer to skin. *Comments:*	☐	☐	☐	
15. To attach wafer to skin, remove paper backing and place the cutout hole over the fistula. *Comments:*	☐	☐	☐	
16. To attach pouch to wafer, close port of pouch, remove adhesive backing and place on wafer. *Comments:*	☐	☐	☐	
17. Cover exposed areas of the wafer with hypoallergenic tape. *Comments:*	☐	☐	☐	
18. Wash hands. *Comments:*	☐	☐	☐	

Checklist for Procedure 10-1 Applying an Elastic Bandage

Name _____ Date _____

School _____

Instructor _____

Course _____

Procedure 10-1 Applying an Elastic Bandage	Able to Perform	Able to Perform with Assistance	Unable to Perform	Initials and Date
Assessment				
1. Check the client's skin integrity. *Comments:*	☐	☐	☐	
2. Assess circulation and neurovascular status. *Comments:*	☐	☐	☐	
3. Assess for the presence of a wound. *Comments:*	☐	☐	☐	
Planning/Expected Outcomes				
1. The client will have decreased edema. *Comments:*	☐	☐	☐	
2. The client will have decreased pain. *Comments:*	☐	☐	☐	
3. The client's body will be supported and in good alignment. *Comments:*	☐	☐	☐	
4. The client will not have tingling and numbness distal to the bandage. *Comments:*	☐	☐	☐	
5. The client will have good perfusion distal to the bandage. *Comments:*	☐	☐	☐	
6. The bandage will be properly anchored. *Comments:*	☐	☐	☐	
7. The client will not experience skin irritation or decreased skin integrity related to the bandage. *Comments:*	☐	☐	☐	

continued on the following page

continued from the previous page

Procedure 10-1	Able to Perform	Able to Perform with Assistance	Unable to Perform	Initials and Date
Implementation				
1. Assess size of material needed and gather materials. *Comments:*	☐	☐	☐	
2. Wash hands. *Comments:*	☐	☐	☐	
3. Explain purpose and need for bandages to client. *Comments:*	☐	☐	☐	
4. Assess the skin to be covered. Assess that the client is in a correct position. *Comments:*	☐	☐	☐	
5. Apply the bandage. *Comments:*	☐	☐	☐	
6. Secure in place. *Comments:*	☐	☐	☐	
7. Check for wrinkles and areas of constriction. Check warmth, color, and CMS (circulation, movement, sensation) distal to wrap. *Comments:*	☐	☐	☐	
8. Wash hands. *Comments:*	☐	☐	☐	

Checklist for Procedure 10-2   Applying a Splint

Name _____ Date _____

School _____

Instructor _____

Course _____

Procedure 10-2 Applying a Splint	Able to Perform	Able to Perform with Assistance	Unable to Perform	Initials and Date
Assessment				
1. Assess the area where the splint is to be applied. *Comments:*	☐	☐	☐	
2. Assess the client's skin integrity. *Comments:*	☐	☐	☐	
3. Assess the neurovascular status. *Comments:*	☐	☐	☐	
4. Assess the client's level of pain and how he or she is dealing with it. *Comments:*	☐	☐	☐	
Planning/Expected Outcomes				
1. The client will not experience unnecessary pain. *Comments:*	☐	☐	☐	
2. The client will not sustain further injury. *Comments:*	☐	☐	☐	
3. The injury will be well supported and immobilized. *Comments:*	☐	☐	☐	
4. There will be adequate circulation to the wound and distal body part. *Comments:*	☐	☐	☐	
5. The client will not experience any skin breakdown. *Comments:*	☐	☐	☐	
6. The client will verbalize an understanding regarding the procedure. *Comments:*	☐	☐	☐	

continued on the following page

continued from the previous page

Procedure 10-2	Able to Perform	Able to Perform with Assistance	Unable to Perform	Initials and Date
Implementation				
1. Wash hands. *Comments:*	☐	☐	☐	
2. Assess the need for a dressing. *Comments:*	☐	☐	☐	
3. Check the written orders. *Comments:*	☐	☐	☐	
4. Measure the area to be splinted. Check for left- or right-sided splints. *Comments:*	☐	☐	☐	
5. Apply the splint by sliding it over the area to be immobilized and securing it. *Comments:*	☐	☐	☐	
6. Check the neurovascular status of the area distal to the splint. *Comments:*	☐	☐	☐	
7. If the client will be removing and applying the splint, instruct him or her regarding the procedure. *Comments:*	☐	☐	☐	
8. Check the neurovascular status of the area distal to the splint prior to discharge. *Comments:*	☐	☐	☐	
9. Wash hands. *Comments:*	☐	☐	☐	

Checklist for Procedure 10-3   Applying an Arm Sling

Name _____ Date _____

School _____

Instructor _____

Course _____

Procedure 10-3 Applying an Arm Sling	Able to Perform	Able to Perform with Assistance	Unable to Perform	Initials and Date
Assessment				
1. Assess the area that is to have the sling applied. *Comments:*	☐	☐	☐	
2. Assess the client's skin integrity on the upper extremity and neck. *Comments:*	☐	☐	☐	
3. Assess the client's level of consciousness. *Comments:*	☐	☐	☐	
4. Assess the client's level of pain. *Comments:*	☐	☐	☐	
Planning/Expected Outcomes				
1. The client will not experience any unnecessary pain. *Comments:*	☐	☐	☐	
2. The procedure will be performed with a minimum of trauma. *Comments:*	☐	☐	☐	
3. The injured area is adequately supported. *Comments:*	☐	☐	☐	
4. The client will not experience any skin breakdown or neurovascular damage. *Comments:*	☐	☐	☐	
Implementation				
1. Wash hands. *Comments:*	☐	☐	☐	

continued on the following page

continued from the previous page

Procedure 10-3	Able to Perform	Able to Perform with Assistance	Unable to Perform	Initials and Date
Applying the Triangular Sling				
2. Place the affected arm across the client's chest. Flex the elbow to 90°. *Comments:*	☐	☐	☐	
3. Place the base of the triangle under the client's wrist with the apex of the triangle under the client's elbow. *Comments:*	☐	☐	☐	
4. Pull the lower point up over the affected arm to meet with the upper point. Tie the two points together with a square knot. *Comments:*	☐	☐	☐	
5. Fold the apex of the triangle around the elbow and secure. *Comments:*	☐	☐	☐	
6. Pad any areas where the sling presses against soft tissues. *Comments:*	☐	☐	☐	
7. Have the client sit or stand and check the alignment of the arm. *Comments:*	☐	☐	☐	
Applying a Manufactured Sling				
8. Position the sling next to the arm. *Comments:*	☐	☐	☐	
9. Support the arm as you guide it into the sleeve. *Comments:*	☐	☐	☐	
10. Adjust the shoulder strap. *Comments:*	☐	☐	☐	
11. Adjust the waist strap. *Comments:*	☐	☐	☐	
12. If appropriate, teach the client/caregiver how to apply and remove the sling. *Comments:*	☐	☐	☐	
13. Wash hands. *Comments:*	☐	☐	☐	

Checklist for Procedure 10-4   Applying Antiembolic Stockings

Name _____ Date _____

School _____

Instructor _____

Course _____

Procedure 10-4 Applying Antiembolic Stockings	Able to Perform	Able to Perform with Assistance	Unable to Perform	Initials and Date
Assessment				
1. Assess the condition of the client's lower extremities. *Comments:*	☐	☐	☐	
2. Assess the quality and equality of peripheral pulses. *Comments:*	☐	☐	☐	
3. Assess the client's understanding of the procedure. *Comments:*	☐	☐	☐	
4. Assess for signs and symptoms of deep vein thrombosis. *Comments:*	☐	☐	☐	
Planning/Expected Outcomes				
1. The client will not experience deep venous thrombosis. *Comments:*	☐	☐	☐	
2. The client's venous return will be improved. *Comments:*	☐	☐	☐	
3. The client's peripheral pulses will remain intact while stockings are in place. *Comments:*	☐	☐	☐	
4. The client will have good circulation while stockings are in place. *Comments:*	☐	☐	☐	
Implementation				
1. Wash hands. *Comments:*	☐	☐	☐	
2. Review the orders with the client. *Comments:*	☐	☐	☐	

continued on the following page

continued from the previous page

Procedure 10-4	Able to Perform	Able to Perform with Assistance	Unable to Perform	Initials and Date
3. Explain the purpose of stockings and the procedure to the client. *Comments:*	☐	☐	☐	
4. With the client supine, measure the leg for the correct size. *Comments:*	☐	☐	☐	
5. Compare the obtained measurements with the package to ascertain proper size. *Comments:*	☐	☐	☐	
6. Evenly apply talc or cornstarch on the client's legs and feet. *Comments:*	☐	☐	☐	
7. Apply stockings. *Comments:*	☐	☐	☐	
8. Turn stockings inside out. Place hand inside stocking and grasp the stocking toe. *Comments:*	☐	☐	☐	
9. Hold the client's toe with the stockinged hand. Pull the stocking over the hand and the client's toes. Release toes. *Comments:*	☐	☐	☐	
10. Hold each side of the stocking and pull it over the toes to the heel. *Comments:*	☐	☐	☐	
11. Holding each side of the stocking, pull up, using the thumbs to guide the stocking upward. *Comments:*	☐	☐	☐	
12. Repeat with the other leg, if necessary. *Comments:*	☐	☐	☐	
13. Smooth and remove any wrinkles in the stockings. *Comments:*	☐	☐	☐	
14. Wash hands. *Comments:*	☐	☐	☐	

Checklist for Procedure 10-5   Applying a Pneumatic Compression Device

Name _____ Date _____

School _____

Instructor _____

Course _____

Procedure 10-5 Applying a Pneumatic Compression Device	Able to Perform	Able to Perform with Assistance	Unable to Perform	Initials and Date
Assessment				
1. Assess the condition of the client's lower extremities. *Comments:*	☐	☐	☐	
2. Assess the quality and equality of peripheral pulses. *Comments:*	☐	☐	☐	
3. Assess the client's understanding of the procedure. *Comments:*	☐	☐	☐	
4. Assess the client for symptoms of deep vein thrombosis. *Comments:*	☐	☐	☐	
Planning/Expected Outcomes				
1. The client's venous circulation will be improved. *Comments:*	☐	☐	☐	
2. The client will not develop deep venous thrombosis. *Comments:*	☐	☐	☐	
3. The client's skin will remain intact. *Comments:*	☐	☐	☐	
Implementation				
1. Wash hands. *Comments:*	☐	☐	☐	
2. Explain procedure to client. *Comments:*	☐	☐	☐	
3. Measure the leg according to recommendations. *Comments:*	☐	☐	☐	

continued on the following page

continued from the previous page

Procedure 10-5	Able to Perform	Able to Perform with Assistance	Unable to Perform	Initials and Date
4. Check that pneumatic cuffs match the mechanical unit. *Comments:*	☐	☐	☐	
5. Check client's elastic stockings for wrinkles and folds. *Comments:*	☐	☐	☐	
6. Palpate peripheral pulses for presence and equality. • Perform baseline neurovascular assessment. • Note evidence of skin breakdown, infection, or arterial insufficiency. *Comments:*	☐	☐	☐	
7. Position the cuff flat on the bed next to the client's leg. *Comments:*	☐	☐	☐	
8. Center the client's leg in the cuff. Align the knee with the cuff opening. *Comments:*	☐	☐	☐	
9. Wrap the cuff around the leg with the front opening over the knee. *Comments:*	☐	☐	☐	
10. Secure the cuff, making sure two fingers fit between the leg and the cuff. *Comments:*	☐	☐	☐	
11. Attach the cuff to the mechanical unit. *Comments:*	☐	☐	☐	
12. Turn the unit on and watch the movement for one cycle. *Comments:*	☐	☐	☐	
13. At least every 4 hours, unplug the unit and remove the cuff. • Inspect the skin and provide skin care. • Perform a neurovascular assessment. • Compare both extremities and baseline assessment. *Comments:*	☐	☐	☐	
14. Wash hands. *Comments:*	☐	☐	☐	

Checklist for Procedure 10-6   Applying Abdominal, T-, or Breast Binders

Name _____ Date _____

School _____

Instructor _____

Course _____

Procedure 10-6 Applying Abdominal, T-, or Breast Binders	Able to Perform	Able to Perform with Assistance	Unable to Perform	Initials and Date
Assessment				
1. Assess the reason the binder is needed. Comments:	☐	☐	☐	
2. Assess the client's skin condition. Comments:	☐	☐	☐	
3. Assess and measure the client. Comments:	☐	☐	☐	
4. Assess for any special placement circumstances. Comments:	☐	☐	☐	
5. Assess the client's understanding of the procedure. Comments:	☐	☐	☐	
Planning/Expected Outcomes				
1. For breast binder, lactation will be suppressed. Comments:	☐	☐	☐	
2. Binder will provide support for dressings or soft tissue. Comments:	☐	☐	☐	
3. Binder will not be too tight, or compress the skin. Comments:	☐	☐	☐	
4. T-binder in a male client will not compress the testicles. Comments:	☐	☐	☐	
5. Client will assist in the placement of the binder. Comments:	☐	☐	☐	
Implementation				
Bra Binder 1. Wash hands. Comments:	☐	☐	☐	

continued on the following page

continued from the previous page

Procedure 10-6	Able to Perform	Able to Perform with Assistance	Unable to Perform	Initials and Date
2. Assist the client to a sitting position. *Comments:*	☐	☐	☐	
3. Apply bra, adjusting for a snug fit. *Comments:*	☐	☐	☐	
4. Adjust if necessary. *Comments:*	☐	☐	☐	
5. Add use of adjunctive treatments, if needed. *Comments:*	☐	☐	☐	
6. Wash hands. *Comments:*	☐	☐	☐	
Other Binders 7. Wash hands. *Comments:*	☐	☐	☐	
8. Choose correct binder. *Comments:*	☐	☐	☐	
9. Help the client into the proper position to place the binder. *Comments:*	☐	☐	☐	
10. Wrap the abdominal binder snugly around client's waist. • Bring the tail(s) of the T-binder up between the client's legs. *Comments:*	☐	☐	☐	
11. Secure binders with fasteners. *Comments:*	☐	☐	☐	
12. Adjust if necessary. *Comments:*	☐	☐	☐	
13. Wash hands. *Comments:*	☐	☐	☐	

Checklist for Procedure 10-7   Applying Skin Traction—Adhesive and Nonadhesive

Name _____ Date _____

School _____

Instructor _____

Course _____

Procedure 10-7 Applying Skin Traction—Adhesive and Nonadhesive	Able to Perform	Able to Perform with Assistance	Unable to Perform	Initials and Date
Assessment				
1. Assess skin integrity. *Comments:*	☐	☐	☐	
2. Assess neurovascular status in the affected area. *Comments:*	☐	☐	☐	
3. Assess the client's understanding of and need for the treatment. *Comments:*	☐	☐	☐	
4. Assess for complications of traction and immobility. *Comments:*	☐	☐	☐	
Planning/Expected Outcomes				
1. The affected part will have adequate neurovascular perfusion. *Comments:*	☐	☐	☐	
2. The client will understand the reason for and cooperate with the treatment. *Comments:*	☐	☐	☐	
3. The client will experience a minimum of discomfort. *Comments:*	☐	☐	☐	
Implementation				
Applying Skin Traction 1. Wash hands. *Comments:*	☐	☐	☐	
2. Assemble the overhead traction bars, if needed. *Comments:*	☐	☐	☐	

continued on the following page

continued from the previous page

Procedure 10-7	Able to Perform	Able to Perform with Assistance	Unable to Perform	Initials and Date
3. Clean and assess the area of traction application. *Comments:*	☐	☐	☐	
4. Know the type of traction being applied. *Comments:*	☐	☐	☐	
Adhesive Traction 5. Shave the area if there is a large amount of hair. *Comments:*	☐	☐	☐	
6. Apply tincture of benzoin to the area to be taped. *Comments:*	☐	☐	☐	
7. Place the adhesive traction tape on the body part. Add any spreader bars or hooks needed. *Comments:*	☐	☐	☐	
8. Wrap the body part with an elastic bandage. *Comments:*	☐	☐	☐	
Nonadhesive Traction 9. Apply the traction appliance to the appropriate body part. *Comments:*	☐	☐	☐	
10. Secure it with the fasteners provided. *Comments:*	☐	☐	☐	
11. If needed, attach the appropriate hardware. *Comments:*	☐	☐	☐	
12. Apply the amount of traction ordered for the correct amount of time. *Comments:*	☐	☐	☐	
Traction with Weights 13. Attach pulleys in the appropriate places. *Comments:*	☐	☐	☐	
14. Tie the traction rope in a knot that will hold without slipping. *Comments:*	☐	☐	☐	

Procedure 10-7	Able to Perform	Able to Perform with Assistance	Unable to Perform	Initials and Date
15. Apply the ordered weight to the traction rope. *Comments:*	☐	☐	☐	
16. Monitor the client while in traction. *Comments:*	☐	☐	☐	
17. Wash hands. *Comments:*	☐	☐	☐	

Checklist for Procedure 10-8   Maintaining and Monitoring Skeletal Traction

Name _____ Date _____

School _____

Instructor _____

Course _____

Procedure 10-8 Maintaining and Monitoring Skeletal Traction	Able to Perform	Able to Perform with Assistance	Unable to Perform	Initials and Date
Assessment				
1. Assess the client for position, alignment, skin condition, CSM, and movement of the extremity. *Comments:*	☐	☐	☐	
2. Assess pain location, intensity, and duration. *Comments:*	☐	☐	☐	
3. Determine from the chart what type of traction and how much weight is ordered for the client. *Comments:*	☐	☐	☐	
4. Assess general skin condition and pressure points. It is important to record any changes and care for emerging pressure sores. *Comments:*	☐	☐	☐	
Planning/Expected Outcomes				
1. Traction will be maintained as ordered. *Comments:*	☐	☐	☐	
2. Client will maintain body alignment while in traction. *Comments:*	☐	☐	☐	
3. Client will maintain good skin condition. *Comments:*	☐	☐	☐	
Implementation				
1. Assess CSM after placement, hourly for at least 4 hours, then every 4 hours, and then every shift. *Comments:*	☐	☐	☐	
2. Acquire the necessary number of people to accomplish the task. *Comments:*	☐	☐	☐	

continued on the following page

continued from the previous page

Procedure 10-8	Able to Perform	Able to Perform with Assistance	Unable to Perform	Initials and Date
3. Explain the procedure to the client. *Comments:*	☐	☐	☐	
4. The traction setup. Be sure the lines and weights hang freely and the structural frame is secure. *Comments:*	☐	☐	☐	
5. Wash hands. *Comments:*	☐	☐	☐	
6. One person will monitor the traction and fractured extremity. *Comments:*	☐	☐	☐	
7. Turn the client. • For a client who is unable to assist, two people are on the side that will lift the client's body, and one person is on the opposite side to stuff pillows. • For a client who is able to assist, leave the bed rail up so the client can use it to pull the upper body across. • For a client with a fractured hip, be careful where pillows are placed beneath the fracture. There should be enough support without misaligning the bones. *Comments:*	☐	☐	☐	
8. Reassess CMS, body alignment, and pain. *Comments:*	☐	☐	☐	
Transferring from Bed to Gurney 9. See Actions 1–5. *Comments:*	☐	☐	☐	
10. Assess the gurney or bed to be sure the correct traction setup and equipment are available. *Comments:*	☐	☐	☐	
11. One person applies manual traction to the arch—the metal piece that joins the sides of the pin where the rope attaches—while another removes the weights and rope. *Comments:*	☐	☐	☐	
12. Use a slide board to transfer client from bed to bed. Be certain one person is monitoring the broken extremity, moving it with the rest of the body. *Comments:*	☐	☐	☐	

Procedure 10-8	Able to Perform	Able to Perform with Assistance	Unable to Perform	Initials and Date
13. Once the client is straight in the new bed, reapply traction slowly. The person holding manual traction should not let go until the weights are freely hanging. *Comments:*	☐	☐	☐	
14. Once the client is settled, reassess CMS, body alignment, and pain. *Comments:*	☐	☐	☐	
15. Wash hands. *Comments:*	☐	☐	☐	

Checklist for Procedure 10-9   External Fixation or Skeletal Pin Care

Name _____ Date _____

School _____

Instructor _____

Course _____

Procedure 10-9 External Fixation or Skeletal Pin Care	Able to Perform	Able to Perform with Assistance	Unable to Perform	Initials and Date
Assessment				
1. Assess the client's knowledge or previous experience with the procedure. *Comments:*	☐	☐	☐	
2. Assess client for pain, proper alignment, positioning, skin condition, and overall health. Also assess for circulation, movement, and sensation (CMS). *Comments:*	☐	☐	☐	
3. Assess client's chart for anticipated length of treatment via traction. *Comments:*	☐	☐	☐	
4. Document the neuromuscular status and any skin problems. *Comments:*	☐	☐	☐	
5. Assess the client's current level of mobility. *Comments:*	☐	☐	☐	
Planning/Expected Outcomes				
1. Traction will be maintained throughout care. *Comments:*	☐	☐	☐	
2. Client will maintain proper body alignment. *Comments:*	☐	☐	☐	
3. Client will maintain good skin condition and CMS in the affected extremity. *Comments:*	☐	☐	☐	
4. Client will show no signs or symptoms of infection. *Comments:*	☐	☐	☐	

continued on the following page

continued from the previous page

Procedure 10-9	Able to Perform	Able to Perform with Assistance	Unable to Perform	Initials and Date
5. Client will not experience excessive pain. *Comments:*	☐	☐	☐	
Implementation				
1. Wash hands. *Comments:*	☐	☐	☐	
2. Premedicate with analgesics (if necessary). *Comments:*	☐	☐	☐	
3. Assess CMS and skin condition. *Comments:*	☐	☐	☐	
4. Assess for proper alignment and positioning. Check that traction lines are free from the bed and linens. *Comments:*	☐	☐	☐	
5. Prepare materials and mix solution in a sterile manner. *Comments:*	☐	☐	☐	
6. Put gloves on and replace as needed if soiled. *Comments:*	☐	☐	☐	
7. Remove current dressing around each pin site. *Comments:*	☐	☐	☐	
8. Soak cotton tip applicator with clean solution. Swipe around each pin site once per swab. *Comments:*	☐	☐	☐	
9. Remove gloves and wash hands. *Comments:*	☐	☐	☐	

Checklist for Procedure 10-10   Assisting with Casting—Plaster and Fiberglass

Name _____ Date _____

School _____

Instructor _____

Course _____

Procedure 10-10 Assisting with Casting—Plaster and Fiberglass	Able to Perform	Able to Perform with Assistance	Unable to Perform	Initials and Date
Assessment				
1. Assess the client for acute pain or anxiety. *Comments:*	☐	☐	☐	
2. Assess the neurovascular status of the area before and after casting. *Comments:*	☐	☐	☐	
3. Understand the kind of injury and the type of cast being applied. *Comments:*	☐	☐	☐	
4. Assess the skin. *Comments:*	☐	☐	☐	
5. Assess the client's understanding of the procedure. *Comments:*	☐	☐	☐	
Planning/Expected Outcomes				
1. The cast will maintain good bone alignment. *Comments:*	☐	☐	☐	
2. A cast will be applied with minimal trauma to the client. *Comments:*	☐	☐	☐	
3. There will be no vascular compromise during or after the procedure. *Comments:*	☐	☐	☐	
Implementation				
1. Introduce yourself. Assess current vascular status. *Comments:*	☐	☐	☐	
2. Assess client's ability to communicate. *Comments:*	☐	☐	☐	

continued on the following page

continued from the previous page

Procedure 10-10	Able to Perform	Able to Perform with Assistance	Unable to Perform	Initials and Date
3. Prepare all equipment. *Comments:*	☐	☐	☐	
4. If necessary, protect the bed and client from water and casting residue. *Comments:*	☐	☐	☐	
5. Have the client in the proper position for reduction and casting. *Comments:*	☐	☐	☐	
6. Wash hands. Wear gloves and protective clothing as needed. Assess neurovascular status (CMS). *Comments:*	☐	☐	☐	
7. Plaster cast: • Place the roll into warm water on its end until the bubbles stop rising. • Remove it from the water and squeeze gently. • Hand the roll to the person applying the cast. *Comments:*	☐	☐	☐	
8. Fiberglass cast: • Open the sealed fiberglass rolls as needed. • Hold the package for the person applying the cast. *Comments:*	☐	☐	☐	
9. Assist the person applying the cast. *Comments:*	☐	☐	☐	
10. Swelling may occur after casting. If the cast is bivalved, wrap the cast in Ace wraps to hold it in place. *Comments:*	☐	☐	☐	
11. A window may be cut in the cast to relieve pressure. *Comments:*	☐	☐	☐	
12. Elevate cast site when complete. *Comments:*	☐	☐	☐	

Procedure 10-10	Able to Perform	Able to Perform with Assistance	Unable to Perform	Initials and Date
13. For plaster casts, leave the cast uncovered while it is drying. *Comments:*	☐	☐	☐	
14. Reassess vascular status. *Comments:*	☐	☐	☐	
15. Clean the bed and remove casting materials, if needed. *Comments:*	☐	☐	☐	
16. Prepare client for post reduction x-ray as necessary. *Comments:*	☐	☐	☐	
17. Wash hands. *Comments:*	☐	☐	☐	

Checklist for Procedure 10-11   Cast Care and Comfort

Name _____ Date _____

School _____

Instructor _____

Course _____

Procedure 10-11 Cast Care and Comfort	Able to Perform	Able to Perform with Assistance	Unable to Perform	Initials and Date
Assessment				
1. Assess the CSM every 8 hours. *Comments:*	☐	☐	☐	
2. Assess for color, temperature, edema, pain, skin irritation, capillary refill, and drainage. *Comments:*	☐	☐	☐	
3. Assess for severe pain over bony prominences. *Comments:*	☐	☐	☐	
4. Assess the condition of the cast. *Comments:*	☐	☐	☐	
5. Assess the client's understanding of the cast and its care. *Comments:*	☐	☐	☐	
Planning/Expected Outcomes				
1. There will be no vascular compromise while the cast is in place. *Comments:*	☐	☐	☐	
2. The cast will remain intact. *Comments:*	☐	☐	☐	
3. The client will be comfortable while the cast is in place. *Comments:*	☐	☐	☐	
Implementation				
1. Wash hands. *Comments:*	☐	☐	☐	
2. Check circulation, movement, and sensation. *Comments:*	☐	☐	☐	

continued on the following page

continued from the previous page

Procedure 10-11	Able to Perform	Able to Perform with Assistance	Unable to Perform	Initials and Date
3. Assess skin. *Comments:*	☐	☐	☐	
4. Assess pain or soreness. • Reposition the extremity q2h. • Elevate the extremity and apply ice. *Comments:*	☐	☐	☐	
5. Assess cast for intact cotton padding. *Comments:*	☐	☐	☐	
6. Assess cast for intact edges. • Use tape to petal the edges. • Do not allow the cast to get wet. *Comments:*	☐	☐	☐	
7. Assess safety. *Comments:*	☐	☐	☐	
8. Instruct client/caregiver about symptoms to report. *Comments:*	☐	☐	☐	
9. Support the cast. *Comments:*	☐	☐	☐	
10. Assess for infection. Mark drainage and date on cast. *Comments:*	☐	☐	☐	
11. Synthetic casts should be kept dry. *Comments:*	☐	☐	☐	
12. Wash hands. *Comments:*	☐	☐	☐	

Checklist for Procedure 10-12   Cast Bivalving and Windowing

Name _____ Date _____

School _____

Instructor _____

Course _____

Procedure 10-12 Cast Bivalving and Windowing	Able to Perform	Able to Perform with Assistance	Unable to Perform	Initials and Date
Assessment				
1. Assess CSM q1 hour × 4, q2 hours × 4, q4 hours × 4 then q8 hours × 24. *Comments:*	☐	☐	☐	
2. Pain that is severe and unrelieved by medication or by repositioning, and is not proportional to the severity of the injury, requires immediate investigation by the health care provider. *Comments:*	☐	☐	☐	
3. Assess for pain over bony prominences, odor, or drainage on the cast. *Comments:*	☐	☐	☐	
Planning/Expected Outcomes				
1. Complaints and signs of pressure will diminish. *Comments:*	☐	☐	☐	
2. The correct area will be exposed. *Comments:*	☐	☐	☐	
Implementation				
1. Wash hands. *Comments:*	☐	☐	☐	
2. Assess for intact cotton padding underneath the cast. *Comments:*	☐	☐	☐	
3. Remind the client that the blade will not cut. *Comments:*	☐	☐	☐	
4. Medicate the client for pain, if needed. *Comments:*	☐	☐	☐	

continued on the following page

continued from the previous page

Procedure 10-12	Able to Perform	Able to Perform with Assistance	Unable to Perform	Initials and Date
5. Assist the client to place the extremity. *Comments:*	☐	☐	☐	
6. Assist in cutting the cast as requested. *Comments:*	☐	☐	☐	
7. To window a cast, cut lightly over the appropriate area. *Comments:*	☐	☐	☐	
8. Remove the window. *Comments:*	☐	☐	☐	
9. Cut the padding away to inspect the skin. *Comments:*	☐	☐	☐	
10. When bivalving a cast: • The technician will cut the cast on each side of the limb. • Assist in using cast spreaders. • Cut the padding underneath. *Comments:*	☐	☐	☐	
11. Petal the edges of the new window or bivalve. *Comments:*	☐	☐	☐	
12. Secure the cast together with Velcro, Ace wrap, or tape. *Comments:*	☐	☐	☐	
13. Wash hands. *Comments:*	☐	☐	☐	

Checklist for Procedure 10-13   Cast Removal

Name _____ Date _____

School _____

Instructor _____

Course _____

Procedure 10-13 Cast Removal	Able to Perform	Able to Perform with Assistance	Unable to Perform	Initials and Date
Assessment				
1. Determine if this is a cast change or permanent removal. *Comments:*	☐	☐	☐	
2. Determine if there is any suspected disruption in skin integrity. *Comments:*	☐	☐	☐	
3. Determine how many weeks the fracture has been healing. *Comments:*	☐	☐	☐	
4. Determine the condition of the cast. *Comments:*	☐	☐	☐	
5. If this is a final removal, assess ROM and muscle strength. *Comments:*	☐	☐	☐	
Planning/Expected Outcomes				
1. Cast will be removed successfully from the client. *Comments:*	☐	☐	☐	
2. Client will remain safe after the removal of the cast. *Comments:*	☐	☐	☐	
3. Proper equipment will be given to the client on discharge. *Comments:*	☐	☐	☐	
Implementation				
1. Wash hands. *Comments:*	☐	☐	☐	
2. Introduce yourself to client. *Comments:*	☐	☐	☐	
3. Assess vascular status. *Comments:*	☐	☐	☐	

continued on the following page

continued from the previous page

Procedure 10-13	Able to Perform	Able to Perform with Assistance	Unable to Perform	Initials and Date
4. Assess client's ability to communicate. *Comments:*	☐	☐	☐	
5. Prepare equipment and have it at bedside. *Comments:*	☐	☐	☐	
6. Prepare environment and client. *Comments:*	☐	☐	☐	
7. Wash hands and wear protective clothing as needed. *Comments:*	☐	☐	☐	
8. Prepare client for how extremity will look after removal. *Comments:*	☐	☐	☐	
9. Client may continue to need supportive aids. *Comments:*	☐	☐	☐	
10. The technician will cut the cast with the saw. Support the limb as requested. *Comments:*	☐	☐	☐	
11. The technician will split the cast and cut the padding. *Comments:*	☐	☐	☐	
12. The technician will then remove the cast, support the limb, and reassure the client. *Comments:*	☐	☐	☐	
13. Assess the skin underneath the cast. Gently clean the skin. *Comments:*	☐	☐	☐	
14. May need to apply Ace wrap after cast removal. *Comments:*	☐	☐	☐	
15. Assess the extremity where the cast was removed and document how the extremity looks. *Comments:*	☐	☐	☐	
16. Wash hands. *Comments:*	☐	☐	☐	

continued from the previous page

Checklist for Procedure 10-14   Assisting with a Continuous Passive Motion Device

Name _____ Date _____

School _____

Instructor _____

Course _____

Procedure 10-14 **Assisting with a Continuous Passive Motion Device**	Able to Perform	Able to Perform with Assistance	Unable to Perform	Initials and Date
Assessment				
1. Assess the written orders for continuous passive motion (CPM) usage. *Comments:*	☐	☐	☐	
2. Assess the neurovascular status of the involved extremity. *Comments:*	☐	☐	☐	
3. Assess movement of the involved extremity. *Comments:*	☐	☐	☐	
4. Pay attention to client's report of pain and discomfort. *Comments:*	☐	☐	☐	
Planning/Expected Outcomes				
1. Will facilitate joint range of motion. *Comments:*	☐	☐	☐	
2. Will promote wound healing. *Comments:*	☐	☐	☐	
3. Will prevent formation of adhesions. *Comments:*	☐	☐	☐	
4. Edema, both peripheral and central, will be decreased. *Comments:*	☐	☐	☐	
5. Effects of immobility will be decreased. *Comments:*	☐	☐	☐	
Implementation				
1. Wash hands. *Comments:*	☐	☐	☐	

continued on the following page

continued from the previous page

Procedure 10-14	Able to Perform	Able to Perform with Assistance	Unable to Perform	Initials and Date
2. Explain procedure to client. *Comments:*	☐	☐	☐	
3. Raise bed to comfortable working height and lower side rails. *Comments:*	☐	☐	☐	
4. Position CPM device upon the bed and install client softgoods kit to unit. *Comments:*	☐	☐	☐	
5. Set CPM controls according to the written orders. *Comments:*	☐	☐	☐	
6. Adjust length of CPM device to correspond to extremity measurements. *Comments:*	☐	☐	☐	
7. Affirm that CPM device is adjusted to accept appropriate extremity. *Comments:*	☐	☐	☐	
8. Position client in the middle of the bed with involved extremity slightly abducted. *Comments:*	☐	☐	☐	
9. Place client's extremity in unit, maintaining proper anatomical placement of extremity in relation to CPM device. *Comments:*	☐	☐	☐	
10. Adjust the footpad. *Comments:*	☐	☐	☐	
11. Apply CPM restraining straps. *Comments:*	☐	☐	☐	
12. Start the CPM unit. The unit should be monitored for several cycles. *Comments:*	☐	☐	☐	

Procedure 10-14	Able to Perform	Able to Perform with Assistance	Unable to Perform	Initials and Date
13. Give the client the CPM stop and go switch. *Comments:*	☐	☐	☐	
14. Replace side rails to upright position and lower the bed. *Comments:*	☐	☐	☐	
15. Place the call light within reach. Place items of frequent use within reach of the client. *Comments:*	☐	☐	☐	
16. Wash hands. *Comments:*	☐	☐	☐	
17. Chart the treatment and the response of the client. *Comments:*	☐	☐	☐	

Checklist for Procedure 10-15   Assisting with Crutches, Cane, or Walker

Name _____ Date _____

School _____

Instructor _____

Course _____

Procedure 10-15 Assisting with Crutches, Cane, or Walker	Able to Perform	Able to Perform with Assistance	Unable to Perform	Initials and Date
Assessment				
1. Assess the reason the client requires an assistive device. *Comments:*	☐	☐	☐	
2. Assess the client's physical limitations. *Comments:*	☐	☐	☐	
3. Assess the client's physical environment. *Comments:*	☐	☐	☐	
4. Assess the client's ability to understand and follow directions. *Comments:*	☐	☐	☐	
Planning/Expected Outcomes				
1. The client will ambulate safely with an assistive device. *Comments:*	☐	☐	☐	
2. The client will feel confident while using the assistive device. *Comments:*	☐	☐	☐	
Implementation				
Crutch Walking				
1. Inform client you will be teaching crutch ambulation. *Comments:*	☐	☐	☐	
2. Assess client for strength, mobility, range of motion, visual acuity, perceptual difficulties, and balance. *Comments:*	☐	☐	☐	
3. Adjust crutches to fit the client. The crutch pad should fit 1.5–2 inches below the axilla. The hand grip should keep the elbows bent at 30° flexion. *Comments:*	☐	☐	☐	

continued on the following page

continued from the previous page

Procedure 10-15	Able to Perform	Able to Perform with Assistance	Unable to Perform	Initials and Date
4. Provide a robe or other covering as well as nonslip foot coverings or shoes. *Comments:*	☐	☐	☐	
5. Lower the height of the bed. *Comments:*	☐	☐	☐	
6. Dangle the client. Assess for vertigo. *Comments:*	☐	☐	☐	
7. Apply the gait belt around the client's waist, if needed. *Comments:*	☐	☐	☐	
8. Instruct client on method of holding crutches while he or she remains seated. This should be with elbows bent 30° while hands are on the hand grips and pads are 1.5 to 2 inches below the axilla. *Comments:*	☐	☐	☐	
9. Assist the client to a standing position by placing both crutches in the non-dominant hand. *Comments:*	☐	☐	☐	
10. Instruct the client to remain still for a few seconds while assessing for vertigo or nausea. *Comments:*	☐	☐	☐	
Four-Point Gait 11. • Position crutches to the side and in front of each foot. • Move the right crutch forward 4–6 inches. • Move the left foot forward, even with the left crutch. • Move the left crutch forward 4–6 inches. • Move the right foot forward, even with the right crutch. • Repeat the four-point gait. *Comments:*	☐	☐	☐	
Three-Point Gait 12. • Advance both crutches and the weaker leg forward together. • Move the stronger leg forward, even with the crutches. • Repeat the three-point gait. *Comments:*	☐	☐	☐	

Procedure 10-15	Able to Perform	Able to Perform with Assistance	Unable to Perform	Initials and Date
Two-Point Gait 13. • Move the left crutch and right leg forward 4–6 inches. • Move the right crutch and left leg forward 4–6 inches. • Repeat the two-point gait. *Comments:*	☐	☐	☐	
Swing-Through Gait 14. • Move both crutches forward together 4–6 inches. • Move both legs forward, even with the crutches. • Repeat the swing-through gait. *Comments:*	☐	☐	☐	
Walking Up Stairs 15. • Instruct client to position the crutches as if walking. • Place the strong leg on the first step. • Pull the weak leg up and move the crutches up to the first step. • Repeat for all steps. *Comments:*	☐	☐	☐	
Walking Down Stairs 16. • Position the crutches as if walking. • Place weight on the strong leg. • Move the crutches down to the next lower step. • Place partial weight on hands and crutches. • Move the weak leg down to the step with the crutches. • Put total weight on arms and crutches. • Move strong leg to same step as weak leg and crutches. • Repeat for all steps. *Comments:*	☐	☐	☐	
17. Set realistic goals. *Comments:*	☐	☐	☐	
18. Consult with a physical therapist. *Comments:*	☐	☐	☐	
19. Wash hands. *Comments:*	☐	☐	☐	
Sitting with Crutches 20. Instruct client to back up to chair until it is felt with the back of the legs. *Comments:*	☐	☐	☐	

continued on the following page

continued from the previous page

Procedure 10-15	Able to Perform	Able to Perform with Assistance	Unable to Perform	Initials and Date
21. Place both crutches in the non-dominant hand and use the dominant hand to reach back to the chair. *Comments:*	☐	☐	☐	
22. Instruct client to lower slowly into the chair. *Comments:*	☐	☐	☐	
Walking with a Cane 23. Repeat Actions 1–7. *Comments:*	☐	☐	☐	
24. Have the client hold the cane in the hand opposite the affected leg. *Comments:*	☐	☐	☐	
25. Have the client push up from sitting while pushing down on the bed with his or her arms. *Comments:*	☐	☐	☐	
26. Have the client stand at the bedside for a few moments. *Comments:*	☐	☐	☐	
27. Assess the height of the cane. *Comments:*	☐	☐	☐	
28. Walk to the side and slightly behind the client. *Comments:*	☐	☐	☐	
The Cane Gait 29. • Move the cane and the weaker leg forward at the same time for the same distance. • Place weight on the weaker leg and the cane. • Move the strong leg forward. • Place weight on the strong leg. *Comments:*	☐	☐	☐	
Sitting with a Cane 30. • Have client turn around and back up to the chair. • Client grasps the arm of the chair with the free hand and lowers him- or herself into the chair. • Place the cane out of the way but within reach. *Comments:*	☐	☐	☐	

Procedure 10-15	Able to Perform	Able to Perform with Assistance	Unable to Perform	Initials and Date
31. Set realistic goals. *Comments:*	☐	☐	☐	
32. Consult with a physical therapist. *Comments:*	☐	☐	☐	
33. Wash hands. *Comments:*	☐	☐	☐	
Walking with a Walker 34. Repeat Actions 1–7. *Comments:*	☐	☐	☐	
35. Place the walker in front of the client. *Comments:*	☐	☐	☐	
36. Have the client put the nondominant hand on the front bar of the walker or on the hand grip for that hand, whichever is more comfortable. Then, using the dominant hand to push off from the bed and the nondominant hand for stabilization, help the client to an upright position. *Comments:*	☐	☐	☐	
37. Have the client transfer his hands to the walker, one at a time. *Comments:*	☐	☐	☐	
38. The handgrips should be just below waist level. *Comments:*	☐	☐	☐	
39. Walk to the side and slightly behind the client. *Comments:*	☐	☐	☐	
The Walker Gait 40. • Move the walker and weaker leg forward at the same time. • Place as much weight as allowed on the weaker leg. • Move the strong leg forward. • Shift the weight to the strong leg. *Comments:*	☐	☐	☐	

continued on the following page

continued from the previous page

Procedure 10-15	Able to Perform	Able to Perform with Assistance	Unable to Perform	Initials and Date
Sitting with a Walker 41. • Have client turn around and back up to the chair. • Have him or her place hands on the chair armrests, one hand at a time. • Using the armrests for support, client will lower body slowly into the chair. *Comments:*	☐	☐	☐	
42. Set realistic goals. *Comments:*	☐	☐	☐	
43. Consult with a physical therapist. *Comments:*	☐	☐	☐	
44. Wash hands. *Comments:*	☐	☐	☐	

Checklist for Procedure 11-1   Administering an Electrocardiogram

Name _____ Date _____

School _____

Instructor _____

Course _____

Procedure 11-1 Administering an Electrocardiogram	Able to Perform	Able to Perform with Assistance	Unable to Perform	Initials and Date
Assessment				
1. Assess age, gender, and current medication history. Comments:	☐	☐	☐	
2. Assess the availability of electrode placement sites and client's ability to lie supine. Comments:	☐	☐	☐	
3. Determine presence of pain with possible cardiac origin. Comments:	☐	☐	☐	
4. Assess client need for information about the procedure. Comments:	☐	☐	☐	
Planning/Expected Outcomes				
1. The client will be able to cooperate with procedure. Comments:	☐	☐	☐	
2. The client will not be anxious. Comments:	☐	☐	☐	
3. The client will be able to describe the reason for the electrocardiogram (ECG). Comments:	☐	☐	☐	
Implementation				
1. Wash hands. Comments:	☐	☐	☐	
2. Close door and curtains. Comments:	☐	☐	☐	
3. Explain the procedure and rationale for ECG. Comments:	☐	☐	☐	

continued on the following page

continued from the previous page

Procedure 11-1	Able to Perform	Able to Perform with Assistance	Unable to Perform	Initials and Date
4. Bring ECG machine to the bedside and open electrode packages. *Comments:*	☐	☐	☐	
5. Enter all demographic data into the machine. *Comments:*	☐	☐	☐	
6. Position the client in a supine position. *Comments:*	☐	☐	☐	
7. Remove moisture, oil, and excess hair from electrode sites. *Comments:*	☐	☐	☐	
8. Apply electrode paste and attach electrodes to the chest and extremities. *Comments:*	☐	☐	☐	
9. Attach lead wires to electrodes. *Comments:*	☐	☐	☐	
10. Obtain a tracing as ordered. *Comments:*	☐	☐	☐	
11. Inspect tracing for adequate quality. *Comments:*	☐	☐	☐	
12. Remove leads and electrodes. Wipe paste from skin. *Comments:*	☐	☐	☐	
13. Notify physician or qualified practitioner of abnormalities. *Comments:*	☐	☐	☐	
14. Wash hands. *Comments:*	☐	☐	☐	
15. Return machine and replace supplies. *Comments:*	☐	☐	☐	

continued from the previous page

Checklist for Procedure 11-2   Magnetic Resonance Imaging (MRI)

Name _____ Date _____

School _____

Instructor _____

Course _____

Procedure 11-2 Magnetic Resonance Imaging (MRI)	Able to Perform	Able to Perform with Assistance	Unable to Perform	Initials and Date
Assessment				
1. Assess the client's knowledge of the procedure. *Comments:*	☐	☐	☐	
2. Review the client's signature on the informed consent form. *Comments:*	☐	☐	☐	
3. Assess client's weight. *Comments:*	☐	☐	☐	
4. Assess the client for metal objects in the body. *Comments:*	☐	☐	☐	
5. Assess client for claustrophobia. *Comments:*	☐	☐	☐	
6. Assess client for pregnancy. *Comments:*	☐	☐	☐	
7. Assess client's ability to remain still for 30–90 minutes. *Comments:*	☐	☐	☐	
8. Assess client for allergies to dye or contrast medium. *Comments:*	☐	☐	☐	
9. Assess the client's veins for adequate venous access. *Comments:*	☐	☐	☐	
Planning/Expected Outcomes				
1. The client will tolerate the procedure without anxiety. *Comments:*	☐	☐	☐	

continued on the following page

continued from the previous page

Procedure 11-2	Able to Perform	Able to Perform with Assistance	Unable to Perform	Initials and Date
2. The client will remain still during the procedure. *Comments:*	☐	☐	☐	
3. Successful images will be obtained for diagnosis. *Comments:*	☐	☐	☐	
4. The client will not experience a reaction to contrast medium. *Comments:*	☐	☐	☐	
Implementation				
1. Provide teaching regarding the MRI machine. *Comments:*	☐	☐	☐	
2. Have client remove all metallic objects. *Comments:*	☐	☐	☐	
3. Instruct client to void. *Comments:*	☐	☐	☐	
4. Assist client onto padded table. • Secure client on table with Velcro straps. • Provide client with hearing protection. • Place any special equipment. *Comments:*	☐	☐	☐	
5. Observe client for claustrophobia or inability to remain still. *Comments:*	☐	☐	☐	
6. Assess for an allergic reaction to contrast medium. *Comments:*	☐	☐	☐	
7. Technologist performs MRI. *Comments:*	☐	☐	☐	
8. After study, assist client to sitting and standing position. *Comments:*	☐	☐	☐	
9. Wash hands. *Comments:*	☐	☐	☐	

Checklist for Procedure 11-3   Assisting with Computed Tomography (CT) Scanning

Name _____ Date _____

School _____

Instructor _____

Course _____

Procedure 11-3 Assisting with Computed Tomography (CT) Scanning	Able to Perform	Able to Perform with Assistance	Unable to Perform	Initials and Date
Assessment				
1. Confirm client's identity and knowledge level concerning the procedure. *Comments:*	☐	☐	☐	
2. Determine the need for and presence of informed consent. *Comments:*	☐	☐	☐	
3. Determine the client's ability to lie still and supine for up to 1 hour. *Comments:*	☐	☐	☐	
4. Assess the client for feelings of claustrophobia. *Comments:*	☐	☐	☐	
5. Assess the client for an allergy to contrast agents. *Comments:*	☐	☐	☐	
6. Determine if the client has a history of compromised renal function. *Comments:*	☐	☐	☐	
7. Assess the client's need for sedation during procedure. *Comments:*	☐	☐	☐	
Planning/Expected Outcomes				
1. The client will cooperate and be free from anxiety. *Comments:*	☐	☐	☐	
2. The client will be comfortable during and after the procedure. *Comments:*	☐	☐	☐	
3. Satisfactory images will be obtained for diagnosis. *Comments:*	☐	☐	☐	

continued on the following page

continued from the previous page

Procedure 11-3	Able to Perform	Able to Perform with Assistance	Unable to Perform	Initials and Date
4. The client will understand what results are being sought and when he or she will be informed of the results. Comments:	☐	☐	☐	
Implementation				
1. Wash hands. Comments:	☐	☐	☐	
2. Confirm identity of client. Comments:	☐	☐	☐	
3. Explain procedure and rationale to client. Comments:	☐	☐	☐	
4. Confirm that client has signed informed consent. Comments:	☐	☐	☐	
5. Start IV if contrast dye is to be given. Comments:	☐	☐	☐	
6. Give sedation to client if ordered. Comments:	☐	☐	☐	
7. Instruct client on position during scan: • Lie still. • Do not be afraid of whirring and clicking noises. • Breathe deeply and relax. Comments:	☐	☐	☐	

Checklist for Procedure 11-4   Assisting with a Liver Biopsy

Name _____ Date _____

School _____

Instructor _____

Course _____

Procedure 11-4 Assisting with a Liver Biopsy	Able to Perform	Able to Perform with Assistance	Unable to Perform	Initials and Date
Assessment				
1. Assess the client's knowledge of the procedure. *Comments:*	☐	☐	☐	
2. Review the client's signature on the informed consent form. *Comments:*	☐	☐	☐	
3. Assess the client's ability to remain still in the supine position and the right lateral position. *Comments:*	☐	☐	☐	
4. Assess the client for ability to cooperate and hold breath for 15 seconds. *Comments:*	☐	☐	☐	
5. Assess vital signs as baseline data. *Comments:*	☐	☐	☐	
6. Review the medical record for the client's risk of bleeding. *Comments:*	☐	☐	☐	
7. Assess for a history of allergic reactions to antiseptic or anesthetic solutions. *Comments:*	☐	☐	☐	
8. Assess the client for ascites. *Comments:*	☐	☐	☐	
9. Assess the client for pneumonia. *Comments:*	☐	☐	☐	
10. Assess client's understanding of risk and ability to sign consent form. *Comments:*	☐	☐	☐	

continued on the following page

continued from the previous page

Procedure 11-4	Able to Perform	Able to Perform with Assistance	Unable to Perform	Initials and Date
Planning/Expected Outcomes				
1. The client will understand the procedure and tolerate it without anxiety. *Comments:*	☐	☐	☐	
2. The client will remain still in the required position during and after the procedure. *Comments:*	☐	☐	☐	
3. The client will experience minimal pain. *Comments:*	☐	☐	☐	
4. There will be no bleeding or infectious complications. *Comments:*	☐	☐	☐	
5. The biopsy will be sufficient for diagnostic testing. *Comments:*	☐	☐	☐	
Implementation				
1. Have client void. *Comments:*	☐	☐	☐	
2. Wash hands. *Comments:*	☐	☐	☐	
3. Administer medication for sedation or pain. *Comments:*	☐	☐	☐	
4. Take vital signs and record. *Comments:*	☐	☐	☐	
5. Set up sterile tray. *Comments:*	☐	☐	☐	
6. Assist client in maintaining correct position: • Have client lay supine on bed with right arm under head. • Have client place left arm at side or under head. *Comments:*	☐	☐	☐	

Procedure 11-4	Able to Perform	Able to Perform with Assistance	Unable to Perform	Initials and Date
7. Instruct the client that the physician or qualified practitioner will ask him or her to hold breath during the procedure. *Comments:*	☐	☐	☐	
8. Nurse supports the client and assists during the procedure: • Reassure client while explaining each step of procedure. • Assess client's condition during the procedure. • Coach client on breathing and holding the breath. *Comments:*	☐	☐	☐	
9. Physician or qualified practitioner performs the aspiration; the nurse assists as needed. *Comments:*	☐	☐	☐	
10. After the procedure, apply pressure to biopsy site: • Instruct client to roll onto the right side and remain in that position for 2 hours. *Comments:*	☐	☐	☐	
11. Label the specimen with client's name and send to laboratory. *Comments:*	☐	☐	☐	
12. Assess vital signs every 15 minutes for an hour, every 30 minutes for 2 hours, then every hour for 4 hours. *Comments:*	☐	☐	☐	
13. Put on gloves and discard used supplies appropriately. *Comments:*	☐	☐	☐	
14. Wash hands. *Comments:*	☐	☐	☐	

Checklist for Procedure 11-5   Assisting with a Thoracentesis

Name _____ Date _____

School _____

Instructor _____

Course _____

Procedure 11-5 **Assisting with a Thoracentesis**	Able to Perform	Able to Perform with Assistance	Unable to Perform	Initials and Date
Assessment				
1. Assess the necessary pretests and their purpose. *Comments:*	☐	☐	☐	
2. Obtain client consent per institutional policy. *Comments:*	☐	☐	☐	
3. Obtain baseline vital signs and medical history. *Comments:*	☐	☐	☐	
4. Determine client's knowledge of and prior experience with thoracentesis. *Comments:*	☐	☐	☐	
5. Assess the need for sedation, premedications, or restraints. *Comments:*	☐	☐	☐	
6. Assess ability to sign consent form. *Comments:*	☐	☐	☐	
Planning/Expected Outcomes				
1. The client's pain will decrease or cease. *Comments:*	☐	☐	☐	
2. Respirations will show no evidence of distress. *Comments:*	☐	☐	☐	
3. Diagnostic tests will improve. *Comments:*	☐	☐	☐	
4. The client will experience a minimal amount of discomfort during the procedure. *Comments:*	☐	☐	☐	

continued on the following page

continued from the previous page

Procedure 11-5	Able to Perform	Able to Perform with Assistance	Unable to Perform	Initials and Date
5. The client will not experience any injury or infection related to the procedure. *Comments:*	☐	☐	☐	
Implementation				
1. Wash hands as necessary throughout the procedure. *Comments:*	☐	☐	☐	
2. Identify client, and obtain baseline assessment and medical history. *Comments:*	☐	☐	☐	
3. Be sure a signed consent has been completed. *Comments:*	☐	☐	☐	
4. Review necessary pretests and have information available. *Comments:*	☐	☐	☐	
5. Prepare necessary laboratory/cytology labels and requisitions. *Comments:*	☐	☐	☐	
6. Review client teaching and assess anxiety. *Comments:*	☐	☐	☐	
7. Reidentify client, assess allergy history, and premedicate as ordered. *Comments:*	☐	☐	☐	
8. Prepare the necessary equipment and sterile field. *Comments:*	☐	☐	☐	
9. Assist in client positioning: • Sitting at edge of bed with arms on bedside table • Sitting straddled on chair • Lying on unaffected side *Comments:*	☐	☐	☐	
10. Assist throughout procedure. *Comments:*	☐	☐	☐	

Procedure 11-5	Able to Perform	Able to Perform with Assistance	Unable to Perform	Initials and Date
11. Upon completion of procedure: • Apply occlusive dressing to site. • Position client on unaffected side. • Appropriately dispose of contaminated equipment. • Label and send out specimens for testing. *Comments:*	☐	☐	☐	
12. Assess client for complications. *Comments:*	☐	☐	☐	
13. Wash hands. *Comments:*	☐	☐	☐	

Checklist for Procedure 11-6   Assisting with an Abdominal Paracentesis

Name _____ Date _____

School _____

Instructor _____

Course _____

Procedure 11-6 Assisting with an Abdominal Paracentesis	Able to Perform	Able to Perform with Assistance	Unable to Perform	Initials and Date
Assessment				
1. Identify the purpose for the abdominal paracentesis. *Comments:*	☐	☐	☐	
2. Check allergies, bleeding problems, current medications, or if the client might be pregnant. *Comments:*	☐	☐	☐	
3. Assess client's knowledge regarding the procedure. *Comments:*	☐	☐	☐	
4. Assess the client for bleeding tendencies. *Comments:*	☐	☐	☐	
5. Assess client's ability to sign consent form. *Comments:*	☐	☐	☐	
Planning/Expected Outcomes				
1. Client will experience minimal discomfort during the procedure. *Comments:*	☐	☐	☐	
2. Client will not suffer any adverse effects following the procedure. *Comments:*	☐	☐	☐	
3. Client will experience relief of symptoms. *Comments:*	☐	☐	☐	
Implementation				
1. Wash hands. *Comments:*	☐	☐	☐	
2. Instruct the client regarding the procedure. *Comments:*	☐	☐	☐	

continued on the following page

continued from the previous page

Procedure 11-6	Able to Perform	Able to Perform with Assistance	Unable to Perform	Initials and Date
3. Check the written order. *Comments:*	☐	☐	☐	
4. Verify that the client has signed a consent form. *Comments:*	☐	☐	☐	
5. Assess for allergies to local anesthetics or antiseptic solutions. *Comments:*	☐	☐	☐	
6. Ask the client to void as completely as possible. *Comments:*	☐	☐	☐	
7. Measure the client's abdominal girth and weight. *Comments:*	☐	☐	☐	
8. Help the client to assume a fully supported upright position. *Comments:*	☐	☐	☐	
9. Wash your hands again. *Comments:*	☐	☐	☐	
10. Assemble equipment. Open the sterile tray if requested by practitioner. *Comments:*	☐	☐	☐	
11. Place a blood pressure cuff on one of the client's arms. *Comments:*	☐	☐	☐	
12. Help the client maintain position during the procedure. Assist as needed. *Comments:*	☐	☐	☐	
13. Reassure the client during the procedure. *Comments:*	☐	☐	☐	
14. Record the client's blood pressure readings and pulse and observe the client. *Comments:*	☐	☐	☐	

Procedure 11-6	Able to Perform	Able to Perform with Assistance	Unable to Perform	Initials and Date
15. When the procedure is completed, assist the client to a comfortable position. *Comments:*	☐	☐	☐	
16. Measure the client's abdominal girth and weight. *Comments:*	☐	☐	☐	
17. Monitor the client's vital signs, urine output, and drainage every 15 minutes for 1 hour. *Comments:*	☐	☐	☐	
18. Label the specimen, place in biohazard bag, and send to the laboratory. *Comments:*	☐	☐	☐	
19. Record and describe the amount of fluid drained. *Comments:*	☐	☐	☐	
20. Dispose of equipment appropriately. *Comments:*	☐	☐	☐	
21. Wash hands. *Comments:*	☐	☐	☐	
22. Assess the laboratory results. *Comments:*	☐	☐	☐	

Checklist for Procedure 11-7   Assisting with a Bone Marrow Biopsy/Aspiration

Name _____ Date _____

School _____

Instructor _____

Course _____

Procedure 11-7 Assisting with a Bone Marrow Biopsy/Aspiration	Able to Perform	Able to Perform with Assistance	Unable to Perform	Initials and Date
Assessment				
1. Assess the client's knowledge of the procedure. *Comments:*	☐	☐	☐	
2. Review the client's signature on the informed consent form. *Comments:*	☐	☐	☐	
3. Assess the client's ability to remain still and in the proper position during the procedure. *Comments:*	☐	☐	☐	
4. Assess vital signs as baseline data. *Comments:*	☐	☐	☐	
5. Review the medical record for the client's risk of bleeding. *Comments:*	☐	☐	☐	
6. Assess for a history of allergies to antiseptic or anesthetic solutions. *Comments:*	☐	☐	☐	
7. Assess client's ability to sign consent form. *Comments:*	☐	☐	☐	
Planning/Expected Outcomes				
1. The client will understand the procedure and tolerate it without anxiety. *Comments:*	☐	☐	☐	
2. The client will remain still and in the required position during the procedure. *Comments:*	☐	☐	☐	
3. The client will experience minimal pain. *Comments:*	☐	☐	☐	

continued on the following page

continued from the previous page

Procedure 11-7	Able to Perform	Able to Perform with Assistance	Unable to Perform	Initials and Date
4. There will be no bleeding or infectious complications. *Comments:*	☐	☐	☐	
5. The specimen will be sufficient for diagnostic testing. *Comments:*	☐	☐	☐	
Implementation				
1. Have the client void. *Comments:*	☐	☐	☐	
2. Administer medication for sedation or pain. *Comments:*	☐	☐	☐	
3. Wash hands. *Comments:*	☐	☐	☐	
4. Set up sterile tray. *Comments:*	☐	☐	☐	
5. Assist client in maintaining correct position. *Comments:*	☐	☐	☐	
6. Reassure client while explaining each step of procedure. *Comments:*	☐	☐	☐	
7. Assess client's condition during the procedure. *Comments:*	☐	☐	☐	
8. The qualified practitioner performs the aspiration or biopsy. The nurse assists as needed. *Comments:*	☐	☐	☐	
9. Nurse may assist with applying pressure and dressing to the site. Prepare, label, and send the slides or test tubes with the specimen. *Comments:*	☐	☐	☐	
10. Assist client into a comfortable position. *Comments:*	☐	☐	☐	
11. Put on gloves and discard supplies appropriately. *Comments:*	☐	☐	☐	
12. Wash hands. *Comments:*	☐	☐	☐	

Checklist for Procedure 11-8   Assisting with a Lumbar Puncture

Name _____   Date _____

School _____

Instructor _____

Course _____

Procedure 11-8 Assisting with a Lumbar Puncture	Able to Perform	Able to Perform with Assistance	Unable to Perform	Initials and Date
Assessment				
1. Assess the client's ability to understand and follow instructions. *Comments:*	☐	☐	☐	
2. Assess the client's ability to assume the necessary position. *Comments:*	☐	☐	☐	
3. Assess the ability of the client to maintain the fetal position. *Comments:*	☐	☐	☐	
4. Review the medical record for indications that contraindicate the procedure. *Comments:*	☐	☐	☐	
5. Assess the client for allergies to local anesthetic agents. *Comments:*	☐	☐	☐	
6. Check the client's signature on the informed consent form. *Comments:*	☐	☐	☐	
7. Assess the client's knowledge about the procedure. *Comments:*	☐	☐	☐	
8. Assess vital signs and neurologic reactions of legs. *Comments:*	☐	☐	☐	
9. Assess client's ability to sign consent form. *Comments:*	☐	☐	☐	
Planning/Expected Outcomes				
1. Client will understand the procedure and its rationale. *Comments:*	☐	☐	☐	

continued on the following page

continued from the previous page

Procedure 11-8	Able to Perform	Able to Perform with Assistance	Unable to Perform	Initials and Date
2. Client will be comfortable and not anxious. *Comments:*	☐	☐	☐	
3. There will be minimal bleeding or leakage of cerebrospinal fluid (CSF). *Comments:*	☐	☐	☐	
4. The client will not experience a postprocedure headache. *Comments:*	☐	☐	☐	
5. The test results of the CSF will be normal. *Comments:*	☐	☐	☐	
Implementation				
1. Explain the procedure to client. *Comments:*	☐	☐	☐	
2. Have the client void before the procedure. *Comments:*	☐	☐	☐	
3. Prepare labels and requisitions for specimens. *Comments:*	☐	☐	☐	
4. Position client in the fetal position. Turn on the side with back facing you. *Comments:*	☐	☐	☐	
5. Expose the spine. *Comments:*	☐	☐	☐	
6. The qualified practitioner performs the procedure. *Comments:*	☐	☐	☐	
7. Observe client during and after procedure for neurologic changes. *Comments:*	☐	☐	☐	
8. Assist client in maintaining position while talking to client throughout the procedure. *Comments:*	☐	☐	☐	

Procedure 11-8	Able to Perform	Able to Perform with Assistance	Unable to Perform	Initials and Date
9. Put on gloves. *Comments:*	☐	☐	☐	
10. Assist with direct pressure and application of antibiotic ointment and dressing as needed. *Comments:*	☐	☐	☐	
11. Label specimens with name, date, and time, as well as the order in which specimens were taken. *Comments:*	☐	☐	☐	
12. Assist client to a comfortable position flat in the bed. *Comments:*	☐	☐	☐	
13. Encourage fluid intake. Assess and manage pain as needed. *Comments:*				
14. Wash hands. *Comments:*	☐	☐	☐	

Checklist for Procedure 11-9   Assisting with Amniocentesis

Name _____ Date _____

School _____

Instructor _____

Course _____

Procedure 11-9 Assisting with Amniocentesis	Able to Perform	Able to Perform with Assistance	Unable to Perform	Initials and Date
Assessment				
1. Assess gestational age of the baby. *Comments:*	☐	☐	☐	
2. Ascertain family's understanding of the procedure. *Comments:*	☐	☐	☐	
3. Assess client's emotional status. *Comments:*	☐	☐	☐	
4. Assess fetal heart rate and long-term variability before procedure. *Comments:*	☐	☐	☐	
5. Assess maternal vital signs. *Comments:*	☐	☐	☐	
6. Assess client's ability to sign a consent form. *Comments:*	☐	☐	☐	
Planning/Expected Outcomes				
1. The client will experience no episode of vena caval syndrome. *Comments:*	☐	☐	☐	
2. Postprocedural contractions will subside within 1 hour. *Comments:*	☐	☐	☐	
3. The fetal heart rate, variability, and periodic changes will remain stable. *Comments:*	☐	☐	☐	
4. The family will be told when to expect a report of findings. *Comments:*	☐	☐	☐	

continued on the following page

continued from the previous page

Procedure 11-9	Able to Perform	Able to Perform with Assistance	Unable to Perform	Initials and Date
5. The family will discuss implications of findings. *Comments:*	☐	☐	☐	
6. Follow-up care will be arranged in a timely manner. *Comments:*	☐	☐	☐	
Implementation				
1. Wash hands. *Comments:*	☐	☐	☐	
2. Arrange amniocentesis equipment and specimen containers. *Comments:*	☐	☐	☐	
3. Position client in left lateral tilt (if greater than 20 weeks gestation). *Comments:*	☐	☐	☐	
4. Provide ultrasound technologist with warm ultrasound gel. *Comments:*	☐	☐	☐	
5. The practitioner will perform the procedure. • Encourage the client to relax. • Explain the procedure as it is being performed. *Comments:*	☐	☐	☐	
6. After the procedure, clean gel from client's abdomen. Apply a Band-Aid to site. *Comments:*	☐	☐	☐	
7. Label and transport specimens to laboratory. *Comments:*	☐	☐	☐	
8. Monitor fetal heart rate, if ordered. *Comments:*	☐	☐	☐	
9. Ascertain that client understands signs and symptoms to report after discharge. *Comments:*	☐	☐	☐	
10. Arrange for follow-up to obtain test results. *Comments:*	☐	☐	☐	
11. Wash hands. *Comments:*	☐	☐	☐	

Checklist for Procedure 11-10   Assisting with Bronchoscopy

Name _____ Date _____ ,

School _____

Instructor _____

Course _____

Procedure 11-10 Assisting with Bronchoscopy	Able to Perform	Able to Perform with Assistance	Unable to Perform	Initials and Date
Assessment				
1. Determine whether the client has been NPO (had anything to eat or drink) for 4–8 hours. Comments:	☐	☐	☐	
2. Determine the presence of a current chest x-ray and blood work. Comments:	☐	☐	☐	
3. Assess where the procedure will be done. Comments:	☐	☐	☐	
4. Identify the drugs ordered. Comments:	☐	☐	☐	
5. Assess the client's vital signs, lung sounds, and blood oxygen levels. Comments:	☐	☐	☐	
6. Assess the client's chart for a signed consent form. Comments:	☐	☐	☐	
7. Assess the client's understanding regarding the procedure. Comments:	☐	☐	☐	
8. Assess client's ability to understand risks and sign a consent form. Comments:	☐	☐	☐	
Planning/Expected Outcomes				
1. The client will express understanding of the procedure. Comments:	☐	☐	☐	
2. The client will tolerate the procedure with a minimum of discomfort. Comments:	☐	☐	☐	

continued on the following page

continued from the previous page

Procedure 11-10	Able to Perform	Able to Perform with Assistance	Unable to Perform	Initials and Date
3. The purpose of the bronchoscopy will be achieved. *Comments:*	☐	☐	☐	
4. Usable samples will be obtained, labeled, and processed. *Comments:*	☐	☐	☐	
5. The client will not suffer any adverse effects. *Comments:*	☐	☐	☐	
Implementation				
1. Wash hands. *Comments:*	☐	☐	☐	
2. Set up for the bronchoscopy. *Comments:*	☐	☐	☐	
3. Draw up medication per the written orders and label each syringe. *Comments:*	☐	☐	☐	
4. Ready syringes of saline for the lavage and saline washes. *Comments:*	☐	☐	☐	
5. Lay out equipment needed. *Comments:*	☐	☐	☐	
6. Make sure all paperwork is filled out and ready. *Comments:*	☐	☐	☐	
7. Check that emergency medications and supplies are available. *Comments:*	☐	☐	☐	
8. Verify client's identity. *Comments:*	☐	☐	☐	
9. Have client put on a gown if he or she is an outpatient. *Comments:*	☐	☐	☐	

Procedure 11-10	Able to Perform	Able to Perform with Assistance	Unable to Perform	Initials and Date
10. Place vital signs monitors. Record vital signs and continue to monitor every 5–15 minutes. *Comments:*	☐	☐	☐	
11. Confirm safe transport following the procedure. *Comments:*	☐	☐	☐	
12. Obtain informed consent. *Comments:*	☐	☐	☐	
13. Start supplemental oxygen. *Comments:*	☐	☐	☐	
14. Have client remove false teeth. *Comments:*	☐	☐	☐	
15. Give the anticholinergic agent, if ordered. *Comments:*	☐	☐	☐	
16. Give a nebulizer with a bronchodilator and lidocaine, if ordered. *Comments:*	☐	☐	☐	
17. Anesthetize the nares and throat with topical lidocaine and cocaine. *Comments:*	☐	☐	☐	
18. Give first dose of intravenous sedation. *Comments:*	☐	☐	☐	
19. Lubricate the distal end of the scope with water-soluble lubricant. *Comments:*	☐	☐	☐	
20. Place a mouth guard in client's mouth for oral route. *Comments:*	☐	☐	☐	
21. As the practitioner passes the scope, the assistant will inject lidocaine into the scope, numbing the airways. *Comments:*	☐	☐	☐	

continued on the following page

continued from the previous page

Procedure 11-10	Able to Perform	Able to Perform with Assistance	Unable to Perform	Initials and Date
22. Instruct the client not to talk. *Comments:*	☐	☐	☐	
23. Assist the physician or qualified practitioner in obtaining samples: *Bronchoalveolar lavage* • Place a large suction trap on the suction port of the scope. Reconnect the suction. • Introduce sterile saline through the biopsy port. • Monitor the return suctioned back into the trap. • Repeat until an adequate sample is obtained. • Remove the suction trap from the scope carefully. *Cytology brush* • Open the package. Make sure the brush is inside the protective sheath. • Carefully push the brush down through the biopsy port. • Slowly advance it until the practitioner tells you to stop. • Push the brush out and move it back and forth 3 or 4 times. • Pull the brush back into the sheath. • Pull the brush and sheath out of the scope. • Prepare the sample according to hospital policy. *Protective brush* • Remove from packaging and carefully uncoil. • Push the brush through the biopsy port on the scope. • Advance until the practitioner tells you to stop. • Pull the two sheaths together and push out the wax plug. • Move the brush back and forth inside the airway. • Pull the brush back into the protective sheath. • Pull the brush and sheath out of the scope. • Use sterile wire cutters to cut the brush off into a sterile specimen cup. *Biopsies* • Remove the biopsy forceps from the package and test them. • The practitioner may want to instill epinephrine at this time. • Push the biopsy forceps through the biopsy port. • Advance until the practitioner tells you to stop. • Open the forceps and push forward. • Close and hold when told to and give a tug, pulling the forceps out of the scope. • Place biopsy in a container of formalin. • Rinse the formalin off in alcohol. • Repeat actions for another biopsy. *Comments:*	☐	☐	☐	

Procedure 11-10	Able to Perform	Able to Perform with Assistance	Unable to Perform	Initials and Date
24. Label the samples immediately. *Comments:*	☐	☐	☐	
25. Rinse the scope after the procedure. *Comments:*	☐	☐	☐	
26. During recovery, wean the client off the oxygen. *Comments:*	☐	☐	☐	
27. Watch the oxygen saturation and vital signs. *Comments:*	☐	☐	☐	
28. When client is awake and vital signs have returned to baseline, take out the IV. Instruct the client not to eat or drink for 2 hours. *Comments:*	☐	☐	☐	
29. Instruct the client/caregiver about possible side effects. • Do not drive for at least 6 hours after the bronchoscopy. • For inpatients, call a report to the floor. *Comments:*	☐	☐	☐	
30. Deliver samples to the laboratory. *Comments:*	☐	☐	☐	
31. Check the scope for any leaks or damage. *Comments:*	☐	☐	☐	
32. Clean the scope inside and out. Rinse well and sterilize. *Comments:*	☐	☐	☐	
33. Follow-up monitoring is advisable. Outpatients should be instructed regarding symptoms requiring them to contact the practitioner. *Comments:*	☐	☐	☐	
34. Wash hands. *Comments:*	☐	☐	☐	

Checklist for Procedure 11-11   Assisting with Gastrointestinal Endoscopy

Name _____ Date _____

School _____

Instructor _____

Course _____

Procedure 11-11 **Assisting with Gastrointestinal Endoscopy**	Able to Perform	Able to Perform with Assistance	Unable to Perform	Initials and Date
Assessment				
1. Assess the client's knowledge of and preparation for the procedure. *Comments:*	☐	☐	☐	
2. Perform a brief health assessment. *Comments:*	☐	☐	☐	
3. Assess for substance abuse or chemical dependencies. *Comments:*	☐	☐	☐	
4. Check for allergies to drugs. *Comments:*	☐	☐	☐	
5. Ask about current medications. *Comments:*	☐	☐	☐	
6. Check for dentures or loose teeth for esophagogastroduodenoscopy (EGD) and endoscopic retrograde cholangiopancreatography (ERCP). *Comments:*	☐	☐	☐	
7. Verify plans for transportation home if client is an outpatient. *Comments:*	☐	☐	☐	
8. Assess client's ability to sign a consent form. *Comments:*	☐	☐	☐	
Planning/Expected Outcomes				
1. Client will have no signs of bleeding or perforation. *Comments:*	☐	☐	☐	
2. Client will have a stable airway and respiratory status. *Comments:*	☐	☐	☐	

continued on the following page

continued from the previous page

Procedure 11-11	Able to Perform	Able to Perform with Assistance	Unable to Perform	Initials and Date
3. Client will have stable cardiovascular status. *Comments:*	☐	☐	☐	
4. Client will be easily aroused and able to talk. *Comments:*	☐	☐	☐	
5. Gag reflex will be intact. *Comments:*	☐	☐	☐	
6. Client will be able to move with minimal assistance. *Comments:*	☐	☐	☐	
7. Client will be transferred back to the unit or discharged home. *Comments:*	☐	☐	☐	
Implementation				
1. Wash hands. *Comments:*	☐	☐	☐	
2. Check equipment to be sure it is functioning. *Comments:*	☐	☐	☐	
3. Prepare for possible biopsies, polyp removal, or photos. *Comments:*	☐	☐	☐	
4. Check that emergency equipment is available. *Comments:*	☐	☐	☐	
5. Verify client identification. *Comments:*	☐	☐	☐	
6. Perform brief nursing assessment. *Comments:*	☐	☐	☐	
7. Check for drug allergies or unusual reactions to medications. *Comments:*	☐	☐	☐	
8. Verify NPO status and procedure prep. *Comments:*	☐	☐	☐	

Procedure 11-11	Able to Perform	Able to Perform with Assistance	Unable to Perform	Initials and Date
9. Verify that the consent for procedure is signed. *Comments:*	☐	☐	☐	
10. Verify client has a ride home if using conscious sedation. *Comments:*	☐	☐	☐	
11. Answer any questions. *Comments:*	☐	☐	☐	
12. Start IV and IV fluids, if indicated. *Comments:*	☐	☐	☐	
13. Connect to vital sign monitors. *Comments:*	☐	☐	☐	
14. Check baseline vital signs. *Comments:*	☐	☐	☐	
15. Start oxygen. *Comments:*	☐	☐	☐	
16. Wear appropriate protective garb. *Comments:*	☐	☐	☐	
17. Position client on left side with head of bed flat. *Comments:*	☐	☐	☐	
18. Ensure client privacy and dignity during the exam. *Comments:*	☐	☐	☐	
19. For an oral procedure, instruct client that the throat will be numbed and a mouthpiece inserted. *Comments:*	☐	☐	☐	
20. Administer IV medications for sedation per written orders. *Comments:*	☐	☐	☐	

continued on the following page

continued from the previous page

Procedure 11-11	Able to Perform	Able to Perform with Assistance	Unable to Perform	Initials and Date
21. While giving sedation, monitor vital signs and level of consciousness. *Comments:*	☐	☐	☐	
22. Document vital signs and level of consciousness after medications and at least every 15 minutes. *Comments:*	☐	☐	☐	
23. Notify practitioner of vital signs that deviate more than 20% from the baseline. *Comments:*	☐	☐	☐	
24. If cautery is used, apply a grounding pad to the thigh or hip. *Comments:*	☐	☐	☐	
25. Assist with biopsies or other specimens as needed. *Comments:*	☐	☐	☐	
26. Keep side rails up until sedation has worn off, monitor airway, and assess gag reflex. *Comments:*	☐	☐	☐	
27. Document all medications given. *Comments:*	☐	☐	☐	
28. Assess for signs of bleeding and perforation. *Comments:*	☐	☐	☐	
29. Monitor vital signs and level of consciousness every 15 minutes for at least 1 hour. *Comments:*	☐	☐	☐	
30. Provide written discharge instructions. *Comments:*	☐	☐	☐	
31. Discontinue outpatient IV access, observe site, and apply dressing. *Comments:*	☐	☐	☐	

Checklist for Procedure 11-12   Assisting with Proctosigmoidoscopy

Name _____ Date _____

School _____

Instructor _____

Course _____

Procedure 11-12 **Assisting with Proctosigmoidoscopy**	Able to Perform	Able to Perform with Assistance	Unable to Perform	Initials and Date
Assessment				
1. Auscultate the abdomen for bowel sounds. *Comments:*	☐	☐	☐	
2. Assess client's understanding of the procedure. *Comments:*	☐	☐	☐	
3. Assess client's compliance with bowel preparation. *Comments:*	☐	☐	☐	
4. Inspect the perianal skin. *Comments:*	☐	☐	☐	
5. Assess client's ability to sign a consent form. *Comments:*	☐	☐	☐	
Planning/Expected Outcomes				
1. Client will tolerate the procedure without undue anxiety. *Comments:*	☐	☐	☐	
2. The client will not experience pain related to the procedure. *Comments:*	☐	☐	☐	
3. The client will not experience injury related to the procedure. *Comments:*	☐	☐	☐	
4. The procedure will visualize the client's distal colon, rectum and anal canal. *Comments:*	☐	☐	☐	
Implementation				
1. Obtain informed consent. *Comments:*	☐	☐	☐	

continued on the following page

continued from the previous page

Procedure 11-12	Able to Perform	Able to Perform with Assistance	Unable to Perform	Initials and Date
2. Wash hands. *Comments:*	☐	☐	☐	
3. Assemble equipment. *Comments:*	☐	☐	☐	
4. Explain procedure to client. *Comments:*	☐	☐	☐	
5. Instruct client to apply hospital gown. Protect privacy. *Comments:*	☐	☐	☐	
6. Apply monitoring equipment. *Comments:*	☐	☐	☐	
7. Position client in the knee-chest or left lateral Sim's position. *Comments:*	☐	☐	☐	
8. Help the client maintain position. *Comments:*	☐	☐	☐	
9. Apply gloves. *Comments:*	☐	☐	☐	
10. Continue to explain the procedure as it progresses. *Comments:*	☐	☐	☐	
11. Apply lubricant to a gloved finger. *Comments:*	☐	☐	☐	
12. Use lubricated finger to check for possible rectal obstructions. *Comments:*	☐	☐	☐	
13. Lubricate end of endoscope. *Comments:*	☐	☐	☐	
14. Insert endoscope into anal canal and colon. *Comments:*	☐	☐	☐	

Procedure 11-12	Able to Perform	Able to Perform with Assistance	Unable to Perform	Initials and Date
15. Examine the distal sigmoid colon, rectum, and anal canal. *Comments:*	☐	☐	☐	
16. Slowly remove endoscope at completion of exam. *Comments:*	☐	☐	☐	
17. Place endoscope in appropriate container. *Comments:*	☐	☐	☐	
18. Remove soiled gloves and place in appropriate receptacle. *Comments:*	☐	☐	☐	
19. Wash hands. *Comments:*	☐	☐	☐	

Checklist for Procedure 11-13   Assisting with Arteriography

Name _____ Date _____

School _____

Instructor _____

Course _____

Procedure 11-13 Assisting with Arteriography	Able to Perform	Able to Perform with Assistance	Unable to Perform	Initials and Date
Assessment				
1. Confirm the client's identity and understanding of the procedure. *Comments:*	☐	☐	☐	
2. Determine the presence of informed consent and signatures of client and witness. *Comments:*	☐	☐	☐	
3. Determine allergy or reaction to iodine or contrast agents. *Comments:*	☐	☐	☐	
4. Determine baseline vital signs. *Comments:*	☐	☐	☐	
5. Determine the presence and character of peripheral pulses. *Comments:*	☐	☐	☐	
6. Determine need for baseline renal function tests. *Comments:*	☐	☐	☐	
7. Determine last oral intake of client. *Comments:*	☐	☐	☐	
8. Assess the client's ability to sign a consent form. *Comments:*	☐	☐	☐	
Planning/Expected Outcomes				
1. Client will identify general purpose and nature of procedure. *Comments:*	☐	☐	☐	
2. Client will verbalize anxiety. *Comments:*	☐	☐	☐	
3. Client will verbalize pain and obtain relief. *Comments:*	☐	☐	☐	

continued on the following page

continued from the previous page

Procedure 11-13	Able to Perform	Able to Perform with Assistance	Unable to Perform	Initials and Date
Implementation				
1. Confirm identity. *Comments:*	☐	☐	☐	
2. Explain procedure and rationale for procedure. *Comments:*	☐	☐	☐	
3. Confirm the presence of a signed consent. *Comments:*	☐	☐	☐	
4. Confirm presence of any allergies. *Comments:*	☐	☐	☐	
5. Wash hands. *Comments:*	☐	☐	☐	
6. Clip and shave arterial access site. *Comments:*	☐	☐	☐	
7. Obtain baseline vital signs. *Comments:*	☐	☐	☐	
8. Obtain baseline pulses and pulse characteristics. Mark sites. *Comments:*	☐	☐	☐	
9. Arrange for transport to radiology department. *Comments:*	☐	☐	☐	
10. A physician will perform the procedure. • A small incision is made in the groin or the arm for catheter insertion. • Following the procedure, the catheter is removed and pressure is applied to the insertion site. *Comments:*	☐	☐	☐	
11. Gather postprocedure equipment. *Comments:*	☐	☐	☐	
12. Wash hands and apply gloves, as needed. *Comments:*	☐	☐	☐	
13. Assess vital signs, level of consciousness, and pain. Assess the access site and downstream circulation. *Comments:*	☐	☐	☐	

Checklist for Procedure 11-14 Positron-Emission Tomography Scanning

Name _____ Date _____

School _____

Instructor _____

Course _____

Procedure 11-14 Positron-Emission Tomography Scanning	Able to Perform	Able to Perform with Assistance	Unable to Perform	Initials and Date
Assessment				
1. Assess the client's knowledge of the procedure. *Comments:*	☐	☐	☐	
2. Review the client's signature on the informed consent form. *Comments:*	☐	☐	☐	
3. Assess the client's use of alcohol, caffeine, sedatives, tranquilizers, or tobacco within 24 hours of the test. *Comments:*	☐	☐	☐	
4. Assess the client's veins. *Comments:*	☐	☐	☐	
5. Assess for the possibility of pregnancy. *Comments:*	☐	☐	☐	
6. Assess recent glucose intake. *Comments:*	☐	☐	☐	
Planning/Expected Outcomes				
1. The client will tolerate the procedure without anxiety. *Comments:*	☐	☐	☐	
2. The client will maintain the required procedural positions. *Comments:*	☐	☐	☐	
3. Successful images will be obtained for diagnosis. *Comments:*	☐	☐	☐	
4. The client will not experience any adverse effects secondary to being NPO. *Comments:*	☐	☐	☐	

continued on the following page

continued from the previous page

Procedure 11-14	Able to Perform	Able to Perform with Assistance	Unable to Perform	Initials and Date
Implementation				
1. Wash hands. Comments:	☐	☐	☐	
2. Cover the scanner bed with a clean sheet and a pillow. Comments:	☐	☐	☐	
3. Provide teaching regarding the positron-emission tomography (PET) scan and the scanner. Comments:	☐	☐	☐	
4. Ask client about alcohol, caffeine, sedatives, tranquilizers, or tobacco use in the last 24 hours. Determine NPO status. Comments:	☐	☐	☐	
5. Instruct client to void. Comments:	☐	☐	☐	
6. Start a saline IV for administration of radioactive material. A blood sample is collected from the other arm. Comments:	☐	☐	☐	
7. Assist client into the scanning bed. Comments:	☐	☐	☐	
8. Secure the client and place stabilizing devices as needed. Comments:	☐	☐	☐	
9. Administer additional radioactive material as ordered. Comments:	☐	☐	☐	
10. The client must lie quietly for 1–2 hours. Comments:	☐	☐	☐	
11. For brain scans, the client may be asked to perform mental exercises or undergo reduced sensory input. Comments:	☐	☐	☐	
12. After the test, remove the IVs and apply a dressing. Comments:	☐	☐	☐	

Procedure 11-14	Able to Perform	Able to Perform with Assistance	Unable to Perform	Initials and Date
13. Assist the client to a sitting and then standing position. *Comments:*	☐	☐	☐	
14. Encourage client to drink fluids. *Comments:*	☐	☐	☐	
15. Dispose of all equipment in appropriate radioactive waste containers. *Comments:*	☐	☐	☐	
16. Wash hands. *Comments:*	☐	☐	☐	

NOTES

NOTES

NOTES

NOTES

NOTES

NOTES

NOTES

NOTES

NOTES